Y0-BZD-562

EXTENSILE EXPOSURE

CHURCHILL LIVINGSTONE

Medical Division of Longman Group Limited

Distributed in the United States of America by
Churchill Livingstone Inc., 1560 Broadway, New York,
N.Y. 10036 and by associated companies, branches and
representatives throughout the world.

© Longman Group Limited, 1970

*All rights reserved. No part of this publication may
be reproduced, stored in a retrieval system, or transmitted in any form or by any means, electronic,
mechanical, photocopying, recording or otherwise,
without the prior permission of the publishers (Churchill
Livingstone, Robert Stevenson House, 1–3 Baxter's Place,
Leith Walk, Edinburgh, EH1 3AF).*

First Edition	1945
Reprinted	1946
Reprinted	1948
Reprinted	1950
Reprinted	1952
Second Edition	1957
Reprinted	1960
Reprinted	1962
Reprinted	1966
Reprinted	1970
Reprinted	1973
Reprinted	1977
Reprinted	1979
Reprinted	1982

Translated into Spanish	1953

ISBN 0 443 00226 6

.

*Printed and bound in Great Britain by
William Clowes (Beccles) Limited, Beccles and London*

EXTENSILE EXPOSURE

by

ARNOLD K. HENRY

M.B., Dublin ; M.Ch.(Hon.), Trinity College, Dublin, and Cairo ;
F.R.C.S.I. ; Chevalier de la Légion d'Honneur

Emeritus Professor of Clinical Surgery in the
University of Egypt ; Professor of Anatomy
in the Royal College of Surgeons, Ireland

" 'tis not so deep as a well, nor so wide as a church door ;
but . . . 'twill serve."

SECOND EDITION

CHURCHILL LIVINGSTONE

EDINBURGH LONDON AND NEW YORK

1973

TO MY WIFE

PREFACE TO SECOND EDITION

IF, as one keeps on hearing, the sort of anatomy untastefully called 'gross' were really finished, this re-edition would count only as a further impertinence. But while its predecessor was received with unexpected kindliness, the not-intolerant climate held just the echo of a salutary feline note : " It's all very interesting," said the Miller's Cat to the Mill-race, " but if you could manage to do your work—whose value I don't in the least dispute—a little more soberly, I for one should be grateful." Meanwhile, however, Time, which finds ways of settling sobriety's worse disorders, has not been idle.

The former edition was written firstly for my friends, and it is by the wish of some of them that I include (or, if you will, thrust in) old and more recent work for convenient access. And since several of these adjuncts go beyond the scope of limbs, the re-edition's title, though still ' Extensile,' is shorter by a tail. Otherwise I have left the text much as it was so that parts of it will ' date '—perhaps respectably like things men excavate which keep about them " glories of their fallen day " ; for instance, bipp—in Richard Stoney's hands. But bipp, some find, has strong survival value ; and lately, like the coelacanth, it has turned up again.

The present progress in surgery is so rapid that one year now is like a former hundred, and ten can leave us not outstripped but at the post. Even simple straight incisions have been altered, and I am most grateful for the chance of taking my impressions of their modern trends from a variety of patients, with scars long-healed and admirable, put at my disposal by the courtesy of Mr J. C. Sugars of the Adelaide Hospital, Dublin.

Approaching recent art one has at times to wrench oneself towards acceptance. Yet, after all, I should not grumble ; these new cuts suit my thesis : their turnings keep incisions long.

Let me revert to the gross anatomy which I have tried to teach
for almost ten years in the uniquely happy circumstance of this
old College. Some while back a distinguished exponent of my
subject told me that his first answer to new students asking what
they should read was, " A dictionary." That sound advice gains,
I find, with experience. " Light dies before the uncreating word."

Our own terms are Greek or Latin—' Greek ' sometimes to
ourselves. Yet when an Oriental candidate writes " the pulmonary
of the sacrum " or " aleolar tis," we suffer shock. How fortunate
for us that Sanscrit or Arabic did not preponderate directly in
forming current medical nomenclature !

For good or ill there will always be division between the arts
and the bleakness of science. It need not be absolute : like
earth and sky they are apart but they communicate at times by
flashes. A rare example must serve in lieu of portrait of a friend
and colleague whose name and work recurs through the text.
Once, after a class on the larynx at which I had to confess that
I did not know the meaning of the word ' arytenoid,' I met T. P.
Garry on my way out and enquired. " Arytenoid . . .? " he
said ; " shaped like a vase : Ruth at the well with her pitcher
balanced uneasily on her shoulder like the arytenoid on the
shoulder of the cricoid."

The reader who would wish to match that satisfying gleam with
competence in practice may note—if he have patience to arrive
so far—the explanation of how a finger working blindly deep in
the pelvis can with quasi-certainty (the only sort anatomy will
grant) find and pick up a hip-joint twig and part it from the
main sciatic stem. Yet the talk is that gross anatomy has died.
One might imagine it instead decrassified and taking wing.

In a former preface I tried to specify my gratitude to those
who helped me with the first edition. Some of them through
the past ten years have never ceased in helping me to re-edit—
Miss Zita Stead, my artist ; Mr Charles Macmillan, Managing
Director of Messrs E. & S. Livingstone, my publishers ; more
recently my indispensable secretary, Miss D. MacDaniel. Repeated

thanks are apt to seem like hollow resonance, so I will only say that patience—tried as theirs—is rare indeed.

My friend, Col. G. M. Irvine, till recently my colleague, has warded off, and even assumed, many distracting burdens on my behalf.

I have attempted to acknowledge other debts in relevant parts of the text: to my former Surgical Demonstrator, Mr W. A. L. Macgowan, and to Mr M. Stranc. Thanks are due in a special degree to my present Lecturer, Dr M. Levine, and to Dr O. Singer for their sketches; also to my Demonstrator, Mr M. S. Matharu, for his clear photography.

Not least am I grateful for the loyal collaboration of my technical staff in and out of the Dissecting Room: Robert Syms, William White, and that wise and kindly person Harry McCabe, who died recently and whom I knew during most of the forty years of his honourable service to these famous Dublin "Schools of Surgery," thus curiously named since 1789, but in fact the modern school of medicine of this Royal College and a lively source of world-wide education. It is a School unique, I think, in several respects, notably perhaps for quiet friendliness, of which I know its students carry much that matters to their patients.

ARNOLD K. HENRY

THE ROYAL COLLEGE OF SURGEONS,
DUBLIN.

May, 1957.

PREFACE TO FIRST EDITION

EXPOSURE that will vie effectively with the " great arsenal of chance " must be a match for every shift, and therefore have a range, *extensile*, like the tongue of the chameleon, to reach where it requires. This book, accordingly, seeks to enlarge the scope of certain set and parcelled methods of approach. It deals with means in which my confidence has grown from using them myself and watching others try them. And while a smooth success with first attempts pleased all concerned, mistakes (made as they were by persons of intelligence) proved real auxiliaries : they marked exactly what was ill-conceived or insufficiently described, and gave the chance for second thoughts—a chance these pages strive to seize.

Bone carries our anatomy and forms its central fact, and bone wherever possible is made the core of each exposure. Even the few confined to nerves and vessels bring in a glimpse of skeleton ; and some of these (though well rehearsed in other books and easily accessible) are borrowed here again. They form the roots from which exposures spread, and serve—like roots—to bind irrelative surroundings. The presence, too, of things so instantly attractive has let me note where charm may breed a moth-and-lamp effect that makes us " strut to our confusion."

The page who sings in *As You Like It* is correct : " hawking, or spitting, or saying we are hoarse " are only prologues to a bad voice ; and books, like songs, should be their own interpreters. But it is rare that one unaided person can write, print, illustrate and publish them. So debts alone may justify a preface ; and mine are large. My secretary, Mrs A. Wenham Brown—as quietly concerned for " a mistake in the dust of a butterfly's wing as in the disk of the sun "—has given deft, invaluable help at every stage, and latterly with indexing. Miss Zita Stead, the artist, adds to her gift the knowledge gained from actual dissection— a rare concurrence, used by her with scrupulous regard. Then, too, I have been fortunate to meet with a collaborator at once so expert, sterling and considerate as Mr Charles Macmillan, of Messrs E. & S. Livingstone Ltd., my publishers ; he puts a Scottish heart into his work.

To Professor J. H. Dible and the staff of his department I venture to express my gratitude for opportunities of contact with a welcome, stimulating climate—the evidence and birthright of a university. Dr J. Pritchard, too, at the Department of Anatomy, St. Mary's Hospital, has given me much friendly help.

That excellent technician, Mr J. Robson (now in the R.A.F.), has earned my special thanks, together with his friend, Mr V. Willmott, a very skilled photographer : their cheerful courtesy, and that of Section Commander C. Ward, was aid indeed.

The text in a superlative degree owes weeding and correction to my wife.

Lastly, a debt is due throughout to surgeons from every quarter of the Commonwealth. In friendly groups they formed (unwittingly) a panel whose jurors brought me verdicts ; and so these pages print what seemed to win, if not their full, unqualified approval, at least an *imprimatur*. Should I be wrong in that belief, the process of acquiring illusion for once sits smiling to the memory.

ARNOLD K. HENRY.

July, 1945.

CONTENTS

SECTION IV

THE LOWER LIMB

INTRODUCTION

NOMENCLATURE

. . . d'abord la clarté, puis encore la clarté et enfin la clarté.
—ANATOLE FRANCE.

Throughout the world in general—and, notably, in that of those who think and write—I find it only in the ratio of the diamond to the mass of the planet.
—PAUL VALÉRY.

A NEW nomenclature has recently appeared amongst anatomists—the third in thirty years; and so, for men of different age, a class to-day in operative surgery is something like a class in Babel: one does not speak to it collectively.[1]

I hold no brief for any terminology; the new, the old, the Basle have each their points. The new, for instance, turns from the vague " axillary " nerve of Basle back to the old and graphic circumflex. But change which darkens what was clear is less commendable. The trunk, for instance, that we knew (and still know well) as musculospiral, ended by forking into branches named respectively the " radial " and " posterior interosseous." This trunk then fell in line with continental usage and became the radial of Basle nomenclature; its terminal divisions, too, were well described as " deep " and " superficial." The third and new nomenclature confounds the trunk and superficial branch, and *both* are now called " radial." With that peculiar precedent of lost distinction the internal popliteal nerve (*alias* the tibial, *alias* the medial popliteal) might easily—in mounds of new editions—be called " sciatic."

An opportunity is ripening; like us, America and the Dominions have now had time to sift the question of nomenclature in English. Is it too much to hope that any joint, definitive agreement will bear convincing signatures which prove

---

[1] This flux is not peculiar to anatomy. Dons have it too; Hilaire Belloc records the fact : " They have turned the pronunciation of Latin (whereof we might have made a common tongue for general intercourse) quite upside down, consonants and vowels and diphthongs, so that my contemporaries can remember at least three quite different ways of pronouncing the simplest Latin phrase, three different fashions in the short space of a human life. Perhaps a fourth is coming." For Dons, he adds, are capable of anything.

it acceptable to those who work in *live* anatomy? Till then let criticisms rain, but may there be a truce to efforts at establishing parochial adjustments!

And meanwhile with Herodotus, who cared for clarity and was (like us) unsettled by kaleidoscopic terms, " I shall continue to employ the names which custom sanctions,"—names which I know our surgeons understand. So without fear of puzzling anyone I say " the upper end " of humerus, or, if I wish, its " proximal extremity." Nor shall I waive the right to use " inner " and " outer "; " internal to," " external to "; " inwards " or " outwards." " Medial " and " lateral " are useful words; I shall employ them too, but not *ad nauseam*; the English tongue resents a curb, and answers best when reined discreetly. Perhaps for reasons similar the French (who then had much to lose) refused to bow the knee to ' Basle.'

We recognise [1] at once the inner aspect of the thigh (or arm or leg), so why not speak of it? And though the present fiat of anatomists restricts the term of " inner surface " to linings of the hollow organs, yet, if I write that certain nerves lie to the inner side of arteries, will someone really think they lie within the lumen?

Such things, of course, are trifles weighed against the fact that every terminology has pockets of resistance to surgical approach. And these (within the boundary of my text) I am resolved to liquidate.

ON CERTAIN AIDS DERIVED FROM STRUCTURAL ARRANGEMENT

The operations of our intellect tend to geometry.
—HENRI BERGSON.

Que ferions nous sans le secours de ce qui n'existe pas ? . . . Les mythes sont les âmes de nos actions.—PAUL VALÉRY.

Some general considerations.—Few that invade the structure of anatomy are artists; the great majority take care, for the convenience of their memories, to force its details into shapes of Euclid—triangles, quadrilaterals, circles of peculiar form. The few (and they are very few) need no such framework; like painters who from scribbled notes of " green " or " yellow " produce a replica with tone and shade in exquisite gradation,

---

[1] *Recognise, recognize; mobilise, mobilize,* etc. The *Oxford English Dictionary* is strong for " z." But Pater who was ' Oxford ' allows the " s "—like Quiller-Couch of Oxford *and* of Cambridge. I shall abide by *Kent's* uncompromising verdict (*King Lear*, Act II, Sc. 2).

these few as easily recall the un-Euclidean visage of anatomy and deal with it as though by instinct.

The many (like myself) who fail to share the artist's gift are glad of aids—despised by those who do not need them. And here the targets for their scorn are plentiful : these pages nowhere scruple to include whatever crutch or simile or dodge has proved its worth repeatedly to groups or individuals. I am, indeed, convinced (like Tristram Shandy's father) that there exists " a North-west passage to the intellectual world, and that the soul of man has shorter ways of going to work, in furnishing itself with knowledge and instruction." Things, therefore, such as satellites, loop-holes, half-sleeves, shoulder-straps, cloaks, seams, leashes, bucket-handles, lids, sandwiches, V's, and manual mnemonics—these myths are rife throughout. Let us examine one or two more closely.

The half-sleeve.—By this I do not mean a sleeve cut short across but one divided lengthwise, covering subjacent structures somewhat in the way a cradle covers patients suffering from shock. We come upon such half-sleeve muscular investments behind the shaft of humerus ; in front of the femur ; at the back of the calf. In each half-sleeve there is a seam to find and rip —giving the latter word precise, housewifely meaning, remote from crime or even butchery.

Loop-holes.—A muscle in the space between attachments must have a portion of its belly 'free,' that is to say continuous with everything surrounding it in such a way as to allow of normal action and harmless instrumental separation. These parts when short and when we separate them out will form the boundary of a loop-hole which may give initial access to a deep and perilous position. A useful fingerbreadth of biceps, for example, close to the distal end of femur, lies free behind the intermuscular septum ; a touch will make the belly bound a loop-hole which can then be widened safely.

Satellites.—This term of satellite denotes a state of linked companionship, like that of median nerve with the sublimis belly, or of its ulnar neighbour with profundus ; for, coming from behind into the forearm, the latter trunk is fastened to the deeper muscle. A satellite relation thus implies reciprocal divorce from other structures. Specific application of this knowledge— of union as distinct from mere proximity—prevents much futile groping (pp. 100 and 221).

Other aids.—We should contrive to wring the utmost benefit from details of anatomy ; examples of this kind of exploitation are scattered through the text. Contributors in this respect are planes of cleavage, and I try to show how best to find them. Other aids abound. A bursa, for example, may help to make our surgical approach as smooth and easy as the gliding of its own

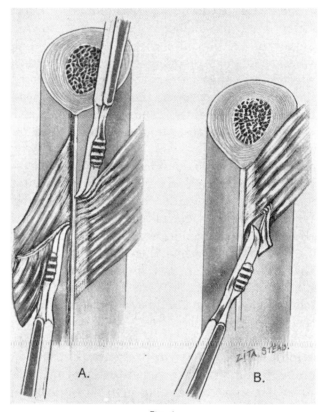

Fig. 1

The stripping angle

Work the rugine into the acute angle which fibres of muscle or interosseous membrane make with bone. (B shows how the rugine tears into a muscle when used in the reverse direction —against the obtuse angle.)

tendon (p. 101). Or fibres from another source may cross and bind the grain, say of the popliteus—a muscle that when split gives only meagre access. The crossing fibres then will mark a line for sectioning the muscle and also stop the creep of sutures through the grain (p. 261). A structure tethered on a single border will move more readily towards its tether, uncovering objectives deep to it ; so, to reach them easily, divide the skin along the border *opposite* the tether (p. 268). Angles of attachment help or impede the separation of fibres from bone. And muscles grasped and moved across their fixed companions provide the surgeon with a kind of tangible mnemonic which helps him for incising skin and separating structures (*The Lancet*, 1940, **1**, 125). Allusion to these angles and mobilities are frequent in the text and need some further explanation.

THE ACUTE OR STRIPPING ANGLE.—A shaft is stripped most easily of fibres, whether of muscle or of interosseous membrane, by working the edge of the rugine into the *acute* angle which the fibres make with bone at their attachment.[1] Used in the opposite direction—towards the obtuse angle—the rugine tends to leave the bone and tear into muscle or membrane (Fig. 1). There is a two-way application of this principle when we expose the shaft of femur ; here the stripping angle opens proximally for adductors, distally for vasti. Then, too, on the fibula the muscles have a stripping angle opposite to that of interosseous membrane (pp. 294 and 296).

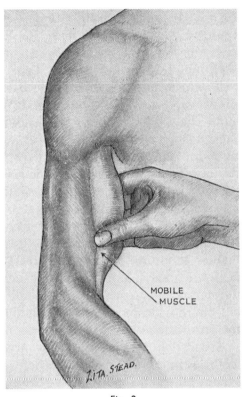

Fig. 2

Comparative muscle mobility

The biceps—fixed at either end—can easily be moved across the widely fastened breadth of brachialis. Thus, for exposure of the front of the humerus, the *fingers* can discover (in spite of fat or swelling) exactly where we should incise and where to find the part of brachialis that separates shaft from skin.

COMPARATIVE MUSCLE MOBILITY.[2]—We can make use before and during operation of the facility of moving certain muscles across their much more fixed companions. Lines of incision may

---

[1] Rooks, as members of the crow family, rank with " the most intelligent of birds." *They* use the stripping angle when they pluck twigs for nesting, but with a difference : standing below the upward slant they tug from the obtuse angle. (M. Burton, D.Sc., *Illustrated London News*, October 8, 1955.)

[2] *The Lancet*, 1940, **1**, 125.

thus be ascertained where fat, posture or swelling might cause disorientation ; and planes of cleavage, too, can be located by this means. Before we cut down on the front of the humeral shaft we first shall grasp and move the free biceps belly across the widely fixed attachment of brachialis fibres, and thus find out exactly where to split the portion of this latter muscle which separates the skin from bone (Fig. 2). Behind the humerus we move the long free head of triceps in relation to the lateral fixed head, and so find out exactly where to split the loose half-sleeve with which this pair of superficial elements covers the musculo-spiral nerve and deeper head (p. 18). A wad of three long bellies flanks the radius and must be mobilised before we clear its shaft. The fingers move these muscles to and fro *en masse* across the supinator and against the fixed extensor bellies. So we can feel out lines for skin incision and planes of cleavage, front and back : in front, when we approach the shaft of radius (p. 102) ; behind, in looking for the posterior interosseous nerve—the deep (terminal) branch of radial in Basle nomenclature (p. 115). The stiff edge, too, of lateral intermuscular septum (a structure vital to one femoral exposure) is recognised by moving the lax mass of biceps across its greater fixity (p. 219). Lastly, for access to ulnar bursa, mid-palmar space or deep terminal branch of ulnar nerve, finger and thumb locate and move abductor digiti quinti in the free margin of the hypothenar mass.

Separation of closely related structures.—We shall in general contrive to separate these structures cleanly if we begin their separation at the place where they begin to separate—a precept which Fiolle and Delmas stress throughout a book that is the breath of present-day exposure.[1] This principle has widespread application : it works, I find, as smoothly in the chest as in the limbs. The flimsy sacs of pleura tear unless we start divorcing them where they divorce themselves to clothe the apex of the lungs (p. 143). So on the limbs we look for places of divergence : a member of a bundle turns aside, or crowded bellies fan towards their tendons.

Sometimes, as we shall see, a pair of thumbs (well gloved, of course) laid lengthwise on a pair of bellies will open up a twisting plane of separation—technique that will be blamed by those who have not learnt to trust the hand, the quintessential root— in every sense—of surgery.

---

[1] J. Fiolle and J. Delmas, *Surgical Exposure of the Deep-seated Blood Vessels*, London, 1921.

THE CUTTING OF CUTANEOUS NERVES

So when the buckled girder
Lets down the grinding span,
The blame for loss, or murder,
Is laid upon the man.
Not on the Stuff—the Man !

—RUDYARD KIPLING.

Incisions must divide the *branches* of cutaneous nerves, but they should aim to cut as few as possible and should at least avoid the major stems. Once in a while painful neuroma follows their section or their injury, giving the patient little rest and sometimes ruining a life. These cases, though infrequent, are living accusations. We should endeavour not to swell their ranks.

Incisions will be planned accordingly. I have twice lately met with scars of operation on the knee, U-shaped and classical, giving rise to sharp and frequent pain, in one case lasting seven years—an extra reason for discarding crooked cuts. We can as easily excise the knee—or do whatever else we must—through an incision that is straight and *shorter* than the U. (A piece of string bent and unbent will illustrate the point.) Apart from nerves, however, the U that cuts the blood supply on either side of skin tends to produce a marginal necrosis.

In certain regions it will not be possible to heed these atraumatic counsels : a large exposure in the neck or shoulder *must* cut some large cutaneous nerves, rarely indeed with after-penalties, though I have seen two patients recently whose broken clavicles had injured branches from the neck, causing neuralgic pain. And often, in the fingers, trigger-spots arise from tiny twigs in necessary scars.

These then are counsels of perfection. Yet, if we look, we recognise abundant opportunities of sparing nerves, which those in daily contact with post-operative limbs will try to seize. Some, too, may find (as I believe) that these cutaneous disasters, though commoner in people with a certain temperament, can yet assail the balanced individual. To *all* of these unfortunates the pain is real, and little satisfaction can be got by blaming them for faults of therapy or chance.

Such lesions should be treated urgently before the pain takes root within the thalamus, thence to wear slowly out ; or else wear out the patient. For when the thalamus is sick no surgery can cure—except the guillotine.

Sometimes in early cases we succeed immediately. A procaine infiltration of the trigger-spot, if followed up at once by movement, may stop the pain; and even (rarely) after long duration. (This happened with the painful knee I mentioned, which was cured for months by two injections—till the patient fell and bruised the scar.) But failure, too, is common. Sometimes resection works a charm (it cured my two clavicular neuralgics) —or sympathectomy. They often fail. There is no rule whatever. Therefore (once more!) let us respect cutaneous nerves.

TECHNIQUE

I shall guard my asepsis as a girl should guard her virginity.
—A colleague, thirty years ago.

This modest note may find a welcome now that bones and joints will come the way of general surgeons—stirring perhaps unquiet memories; taboo and half-forgotten ritual; no-touch technique for knees, long instruments for femurs. But though the need for care is paramount, there *is* need also for simplicity. The common sense of Moynihan has left us safe and easy methods which retain the service of our best auxiliary, the hand, and let its well-gloved fingers touch both joint and bone. A twenty-year experience of these measures in general surgery and in major orthopædics has made me certain that a single ritual works well in either field.

The skin as enemy.—Moynihan would not permit the outer surface of a glove to touch the skin at all—either the hands of surgeons or the skin of patients: he branded contact as a fault, however well the hands were cleaned or skin prepared. And while for many years we all have learnt to don our gloves, touching their inner surface only, the gain is often lost by using them to handle patients' skin. If we avoid this fault throughout the operation, a sterile and undamaged glove remains as sterile as a metal tool, and may, I know, " explore a knee joint . . . with impunity " (Moynihan, *British Journal of Surgery*, 1920, **8**, 29).

But gloves (as L. G. Gunn once said of cats when sutures broke) " ain't what they used to be "; so it may now be wise to smear, in case of accident, some dettol cream upon the hands

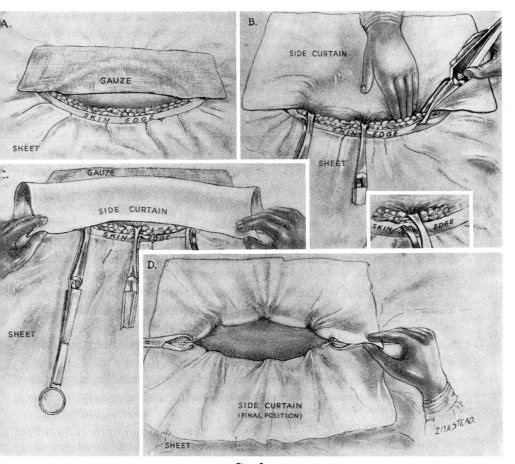

Fig. 3

Application of a side curtain. (A sterile sheet is already in place)

. Screen the patch of bare skin at one side of the wound with a piece of gauze.

. Lay the curtain flat on the gauze and bring the edge of the curtain to the *opposite* edge of the wound. Depress the edge of the curtain deep to the whole edge of the wound before applying clips. (That is vital ; otherwise skin will bulge between them.) Fix this depressed edge of curtain with clips so that one jaw of each clip fastens the cloth to subcutaneous tissue while the other bites directly on to the surface of the skin (see inset).

. Lift the free opposite edge of curtain, and cover the clips by turning the curtain over through two right angles. Discard the gauze, treating it as soiled, *having touched skin*. (The second curtain, applied in the same way, is screened from skin by the first and needs no gauze.)

. The two curtains in position. Terminal clips can be hidden at will, as shown on the right side.

before the gloves go on.[1] Or should the skin resent it, as does mine, wear *two* pair, using cream upon the first.

(This attitude to skin implies that we discard each knife used for dividing it—with other tools that touch—and then take fresh ones to continue.)

Masks.—The parts of these that screen the nose and mouth should be impermeable. The best are made entirely of cellophane (except for fittings on the face and ears) ; but pockets stitched to common gauze varieties of mask will hold thin sheets of cellophane and screen effectively.

Marking the skin for final closure, though not concerned directly with asepsis, allows of perfect apposition. The scratches of a fine *round*-bodied needle should cross proposed incisions ; a cutting needle is apt to leave a scar. These slight marks will help in closing any operation wound ; they are essential when the parts take new position during closure, a lesson sharply driven home by suturing an unscratched case of old luxation of the shoulder.

Side or wound curtains.—The use of these is almost universal, though they are often so applied that wads of naked skin bulge into view between the towel-clips. Fig. 3 and its legend show a technique due to my former colleagues, Richard Slattery and Faïd Yusry, and I shall only touch here on the value of Michel clips for fastening these curtains. *Clips have no handles,* a special virtue when one has to curtain neighbouring incisions, say on the foot.

LONG INCISIONS

Lines of cleavage and of crease.—A recent fashion teaches that most things good or bad about incisions must be linked with the so-called cleavage lines of Langer, which Dupuytren some twenty years before exploited by proving that a cobbler's awl, though circular in section, could leave deceptive *linear* wounds

---

[1] A friend whose skin was harbouring staphylococci has told me that use of dettol cream allowed him to complete his operating sessions with hands and *wrists* both negative to culture tests. In this connection, too, the observation made by L. A. Weed and Jessie L. Groves at Indiana University Medical Centre is relevant. One or more gloves were found perforated at the close of almost three-quarters of the operations performed— viz. after 3409 operations out of a total 4549 (*Surgery, Gynecology and Obstetrics*, 1942, **75,** 661). There is, however, still on many sides an unashamed solicitation of infection : the septic case (apart from all emergency) is often touched, or even dressed, with naked hands by persons who will presently affect aseptic ritual—a sight that stirs the gorge of those conditioned otherwise.

in skin—using the gist of his discovery to solve an actual 'who-dun-it.'

Aside from this, however, we now are told as follows : Surgical incisions made along Langer's lines heal with a minimum of scar tissue ; incisions crossing them heal with a broad or heaped-up scar. Thirdly, that where **crease** lines exist (*e.g.*, near joints), the cleavage lines usually coincide with the creases.

Alas ! (if one may credit the accepted charts) the cleavage lines that run behind the knees and at the front of elbows fail utterly to coincide with the crease lines of flexion : in fact, they cross them. But at the present time the making of a longitudinal cut directly in front of an elbow or behind the knee is frowned on or, in current slang, declared non-U—the sort of thing Jean Cocteau (D.Litt., Oxon., *Hon. Causa*, 1956) calls " *comme-il-ne-faut-pas.*" And so one sometimes wonders just how much the cleavage lines—at least in limbs—concern themselves with good, cosmetic healing.

Perhaps the flexor *crease* is after all a dominating factor ; for in the neck, when goitre surgeons cut circumferentially, they " kill two birds with one stone " : they follow there the ineluctable coincidence of cleavage lines with flexor creases—the latter latent or in being, on the neck. Not so the orthopædist who, in front of elbows and behind the knee, feels bound to let the lengthwise Langer lines go hang, and gives a crossway swerve to his incision at or near a flexor crease.

One of my growing bevy of detectives makes, I think, a comment apposite to this affair of crease and line : " Knowledge, like fruit, I guess, has to ripen before it's of any use."

For neurovascular bundles.—The use of wide approach for dealing thoroughly with nerves and vessels needs no defence, but tends to slip at times into oblivion. These neurovascular bundles are moored extensively along the limb by frequent offsets ; they are impossible to mobilise through short incisions, nor can they be explored. ' Closed ' lesions of the vessels as a rule in swollen, freshly injured limbs demand a long incision ; for often they are multiple and may occur in great variety, though signs are few and point to nothing certain but the need for intervention. Then, too, a neurovascular bundle—like that behind the knee—can bar the way to an objective and must be widely mobilised before we can retract it safely.

For bones.—The long incision is essential in exposing bones. I do not know of any principle of surgery less easy to instil ;

yet on its proper application depends success with compound fractures that reach us *early*—the rule to-day aside from stress of battle. In these fresh accidents a septic outcome has, I have found, been variously viewed by those concerned. To some it was a normal happening ; to some a case of surgical misfortune ; to some again it seemed the sign of slipshod treatment for which they felt a plain and personal responsibility. Of late the rediscovery of Pirogoff's great finding—so useful in its proper place—that septic limbs can stink their way to health in plaster, has innocently been the source of a defeatist question : What harm if early fractures suppurate ? The answer is : The curse of sepsis when it grips a bone ; or (on another plane of evil), the waste of time—and beds.

We can frustrate this curse, almost with certainty, by thorough early cleansing, in company with secondary measures ; so that an open fracture which has skin to cover it should normally be " simple " in a week, while those devoid of skin are rescued from the drag of suppuration. Incisions, therefore, must be long enough for us to find and clear away both dirt and damaged tissue.

If we have reason to suspect that dirt has reached the bone, then we must scrutinise the site of fracture—especially the central portion of the broken ends. For this too-frequently neglected step a cut three-quarters of the length of shaft will only just suffice, even with bones so near the surface as the tibia ; and thus, if dirt ingrains the ends, it can be lightly chiselled off. But if we do not look, it is impossible to *know* these broken ends have not been soiled ; and if we leave them soiled (whether from negligence or grim, extraneous necessity) we sabotage the operation. Bone, in the suspect case, will thus decide the length of our incisions : those long enough to let us bring the ends for scrutiny are long enough to let us cleanse the wound throughout.

A NOTE ON EARLY OPEN FRACTURE.—The background of a damaging remark made to me once by a surgeon, young, travelled, well-informed and capable, evoked these most unfashionable paragraphs. " Our generation," he said, " associates the treatment of compound fracture with a bad smell." This turned my thoughts again to Egypt where certain ancient Greeks, too faithfully disguised as seals, once lay in ambush and suffered terribly till rescued from the deadly stench.

These fractures were among the commonest emergencies of Cairo. Their treatment in my unit was carried out by colleagues who, since 1926, believed themselves at fault if they fell short of turning well over 90 per cent. of open lesions into clean or simple fractures. This work, I feel, deserves a record. For it seems clear to me that if some thirty years ago such high success could be achieved with soiled, subtropic fractures in patients often underfed or sapped by parasites, to-day with newer means and better nourishment the incidence of sepsis in early open fractures should be negligible—a thing I failed to note since leaving Egypt.

Our method in the Cairo unit was based on pages of Lejars'—remembered from a 1903 edition. It was enhanced by what I learnt in 1917-18 from Richard Stoney's notable results with bipp[1], dilute and harmless—another very grateful recollection.

We did not use a plaster case till 1931 for open fractures, but only splints or gutters, yet our success, considered in the light of absent sepsis and rapid union, was just as excellent without as with : it is the cleansing, not the plaster, that decides.

The cleansing of the wound and of the bone are dealt with in the text ; here I shall merely stress the fact that any slackness in preparing normal skin was always paid for by an upward trend of sepsis : our best results were got when wound and skin alike were cleaned with equal thoroughness. We learnt to treat the limb *en masse*—as if for sterile operation on a joint—and, using ether first, we painted all the skin with brilliant green—a 1 per cent. solution in 30 per cent. alcohol.

The need for mild antiseptics in the wound.—No matter how well we execute the task of cleansing a wound—not forgetting the routine but economic resection of its original damaged border—our cleansing is only macroscopic, and many dirty points remain unseen. It is, I believe, for this microscopic residue that mild antiseptics have their use in recent compound fracture. Those that served best in my time with the unit (1925-36) were : (1) the dilute non-toxic bipp of Stoney's formula—well rubbed in after sousing the cleansed wound with ether ; (2) a 1 per cent. aqueous solution of mercurochrome freely applied—combined, as we shall see, with bipp.

On not quite closing the wound.—In 1927—just when we felt most confident—I learnt from a septicæmic death in a long, completely successful series, never again to close the full length of these wounds ; and in our lines of suture we thenceforth left an opening opposite the site of fracture. Through this inch-wide gap a wick of sterile gauze or bandage impregnated with dilute bipp reached from bone to skin. If loss of deeper tissues left dead space, we used the wick to fill the cavity. This packing of the cavity with a loose bulk of heavily bipped wick, inimical to growth of organisms, is merely an example of the old and far too much forgotten Mikulicz device for drainage ; it leaves no breeding pools nor burrows for discharge to loiter in, but makes instead—all round the well-bipped pack—a film, unstagnant and unstinking, that flows directly to the surface.

We then covered the line of suture with an equally well-bipped pad, and the limb was put in plaster, leaving a long window opposite the pad. After forty-eight hours we withdrew the wick and renewed the pad.

(In thoracic non-tuberculous empyema complete drainage—unobtainable by tubes—can be got by using a Mikulicz " tampon." When mediastinal stability has been assessed a window is cut in the chest ; through this the centre of a square-yard of thinly bipped batiste is invaginated to form a sac whose lumen is then judiciously distended with wide bandage till the sac fills the whole empyema cavity. There is no pocketing ; pus drains from the film between sac and thorax along gutters in the gathered neck. The bandage is withdrawn a span at a time, beginning on the second day ; the sac remains until it comes away unforced and virtually of itself—this last a paramount condition for success. A thickly bipped dressing over the protruding neck prevents the sucking in of air (*Lancet*, 1944, **2**, 816).

I have sometimes wondered whether this means (which works so well in the abdomen) could not be used in the chest, with, say, pulmonectomies when bronchial sealing is precarious, or as a safety valve for questionable suture lines in the œsophagus. Apart, too, from drainage, surrounding tissues might profit by a sort of restful, splinted interlude, while moving structures worked against the semblance of accustomed pressure.)

Denuded fractures.—A wide destruction of the tissues is found in certain compound fractures and leaves exposed a length of bare and broken bone. The cleansing of such wounds when dirt-ingrained, by the slow process of picking up and cutting off each bit of damaged tissue takes more time than some of these patients can well stand.

The task compares in difficulty with piecemeal cleansing at low tide of rocks spread with seaweed ; when the tide flows, wide mats will rise on *pedicles* and lend themselves to clearance. Water from a tap at any place with clean supplies will serve to simulate the tide : under the stream the damaged tissues float on stalks, and these are then snipped off, in rapid contrast with the weary plucking of a sheet of scum.

The *force*, too, of the stream will help to clean the wound ; its whole might is brought to bear on every part in turn by narrowing the outflow from tap or tube. This simple method —far from original but little used—was put in hand for me by Faïd Yusry in 1931.

---

[1] For details of bipp, see footnote to p. 259.

Success began, I think, to smile on us one day in 1925 when I decided with my friend Handusa to rank the compound fractures with acute abdominal emergencies. That put their treatment in the able hands of five successive colleagues—Ahmed Handusa first, then Edward Sadek, Faïd Yusry, Lotfy Abdelsamie, Mohammed el Zeneini. When I see better results than theirs in open fractures on as large a scale with any other method I shall wish to try it.

For muscles.—We need a long incision, too, for mobilising certain muscles—the wad of bellies, notably, that screen the lateral face of radius. This wad takes origin above the elbow; the knife must therefore follow it and reach well up the *arm* to let us view the radius widely in the forearm.

OPENING DEEP FASCIA

Division of the fascial envelope needs something of the care we spend on dura mater; for otherwise we plough the muscles, wreck planes of cleavage, and even wound a shallow-lying popliteal nerve or radial vessel—in swollen limbs especially.

One useful method is to grasp the fascia with forceps and make a cut to introduce the tip of Mayo scissors. The tip keeps close against the fascia and opens slightly on the flat; it then alternately, in little steps, advances and divides. If it goes far enough to rip the envelope " in one," the contents, too, are ripped.

MEASUREMENTS

Those damned dots.—LORD RANDOLPH CHURCHILL.

Throughout this book a use is made of fingerbreadths, thumb-breadths and handbreadths [1]; sometimes of spans, which may be generous or otherwise. They have advantages: the means of measuring are always with us, and those I shall describe have stood the test of years. Their own variety appears to chime with the vagaries of anatomy that mock our text-book decimals—a consonance I always find amazing; for students, surgeons, patients and cadavers vary remarkably in size and shape.

---

[1] The hyphens are left out; they may be dropped in compound words (says Fowler) as soon as the novelty of the combination has worn off. And here this argument applies: Hippocrates employed the fingerbreadth, and this, no doubt, he " went an' took—the same as us."

SECTION I

EXPOSURES IN THE UPPER LIMB

. . . et ayme plus souvent à les saisir par quelque lustre inusité.—MONTAIGNE.

OUR first attack accords with the caprice of wounds. Choosing the arm we " pinch it to the bone " by an unwonted aspect and thus obtain the windfall of a type exposure.

This comes conveniently and well equipped to illustrate the Introduction. We find at once the means for wide inclusive access : a muscle we can move and steer by ; a V, a half-sleeve and seam, a bucket-handle ; useful mobilities and friendly dispositions. But terminology has seen to it that these auxiliaries (like persons in the fairy-tale) are neutralised and checked from full cooperation. They are, in fact, bewitched.

APPROACH TO THE WHOLE BACK OF THE HUMERAL SHAFT EXPOSING FROM BEHIND THE NEUROVASCULAR BUNDLES OF THE ARM

His opinion, in this matter, was, That there was a strange kind of magick bias, which good or bad names, as he called them, irresistibly impressed.
— TRISTRAM SHANDY.

The three heads of triceps.—A blight of terminology conceals the simple plan of triceps, a plan which is the key to this approach. And so we have the queer, ingrained confusion of a long head (unquestionably long but medial too) companioned by a head *called* " medial " or " inner " which has—in man at least—no title to the name. For the main bulk of so-called " medial head " springs, not as one might think, from medial parts of humerus, but (as Albinus notes) from the whole breadth : and, what is more, the head lies covered by its fellows. A curious example of nomenclature—amusing, if its " magick bias " were not a drag impressed on intervention.

When once we break that spell, the plan of triceps shows in full simplicity : two heads—the long which leaves the scapula, the lateral which springs from humerus—are *superficial*. And these

15

heads joining V-wise form a loose half-sleeve that shrouds the third
(Fig. 4). This third head, therefore,—miscalled the " inner " or
" medial "—is certainly the *deep* head of triceps.[1]

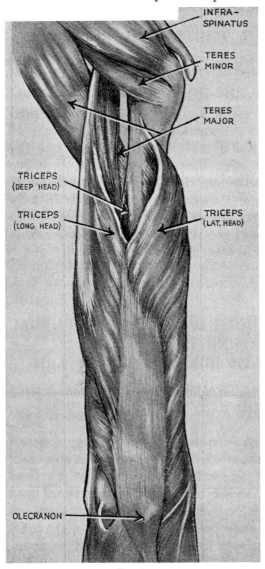

INFRA-
SPINATUS

TERES
MINOR

TERES
MAJOR

TRICEPS
(DEEP HEAD)

TRICEPS
(LONG HEAD)

TRICEPS
(LAT. HEAD)

OLECRANON

Fig. 4

The three heads of triceps

The superficial heads (the long and lateral) meet in a V ;
they spread and form a loose half-sleeve almost completely hiding the third and *deep* head of triceps (called
perversely ' medial ' or ' inner ').
The deltoid has been removed. Note how it would
slope across and cover the proximal part of the lateral
head.

Viewed in this way the
whole muscle becomes a
kind of wish-fulfilment :
the very details of
anatomy are on our side.

[1] Since that was written I
found my view already held
by a professional anatomist
who long ago had called the
head *deep*. Use of the term
medial head " is apt," he
wrote, " to give rise to some
misconception of its nature
and position " (T. H. Bryce
(1923), in Quain's *Elements
of Anatomy*, London, 11th
edition, vol. iv, Part II,
p. 124). No echo followed
this gentle understatement ;
but in an old number of the
Sunday Times I came (with
some surprise) on the appropriate remark : " If Dons,"
it quoted, " are not even
accurate, what the hell are
they ? "
   Albinus saw the facts
quite clearly ; the magnificent folio of *Tabulæ* from
Dobbin's great collection
shows the deep head dis-
played by the cutting away
of its two companions
" quibus subjacet " ; and
the note on Fig. 7, tab. XIX
(1747) adds : " Et initio suo
occupat amplitudinem ossis."
Albinus calls the deep head
brachialis externus, the
counterpart for him of our
plain brachialis—a muscle
which he qualifies *internus*.
(This seems confusing till
you let your arm hang naturally down ; then you will
see the force of his description.) So, for Albinus the
triceps has two layers : (1) a
superficial, bicipital layer
whose long head is our
long head and whose short
head is our lateral ; (2) a
deep layer.

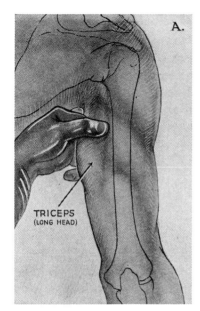

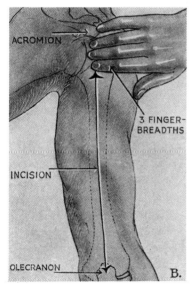

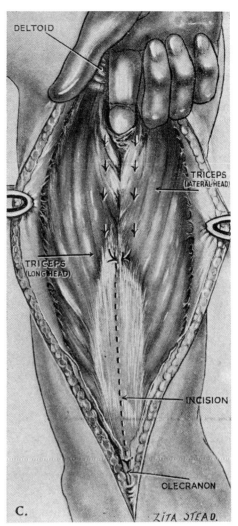

Fig. 5

A. **Finding the long head of triceps.**—This is your guide (1) for incising the skin ; (2) for finding the V-shaped opening of the half-sleeve. Grasp it where it goes from scapula to arm and move it on its stationary neighbours (deltoid and lateral head). Divide the skin and fascia close beside its outer edge ; the entrance to the sleeve lies *there*. (If you lose touch with longus you tend to lose your way between deltoid and lateral head.)

B. The **skin incision** begins beside the outer edge of the long head three fingerbreadths distal to the acromion. It goes down to olecranon.

C. **Opening the seam of the half-sleeve.**—Keep the finger close to the outer side of the long head and enter the V. Ease the loose sleeve off underlying structures. Begin the separation of long and lateral heads gently with the finger ; continue with the knife, dividing the oblique fibres of lateral head at their attachment to the tendinous lamina which is developed—as Albinus notes—by longus in the depth of triceps. This lamina looks forwards and out (see Fig. 6).

THE OPERATION

Finding the long head.—With the patient face-down we abduct the arm and look first for the long head of triceps, our guide in this approach.[1] Luckily the long head is far more mobile than the neighbouring deltoid and lateral head, and we need merely grasp and move it in order to distinguish it from either (Fig. 5, A).

Incision.—This follows the outer edge of the long head beginning three fingerbreadths below the acromial angle and going straight down to the olecranon (Fig. 5, B). When the skin has been divided, we shall again grasp and move the *proximal* part

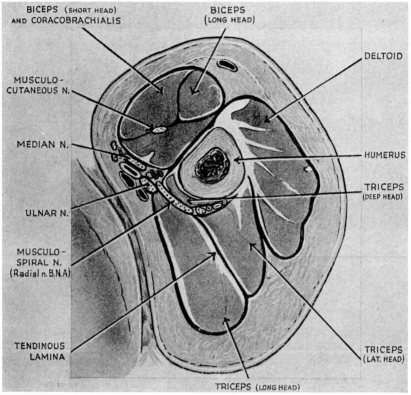

Fig. 6

The tendinous lamina developed by the long head

It marks the seam of the half-sleeve. Note, too, how the ulnar nerve lies at the sharp, anterior edge of the long head. This guiding edge is separated from the nerve by thin fascia. Note, too, the small tongue of deep head of triceps that always separates the musculospiral nerve from humerus (see legend to Fig. 9). This figure (taken from Poirier and Charpy, 2nd Edn., 1901, Vol. II, fasc. 1, p. 97) also shows the labile relation of the ulnar nerve, which here lies *lateral* to brachial vessels and median nerve—instead of medially. (See text, p. 22, and Fig. 7.)

---

[1] The V-shaped junction of the long and lateral heads may show as a depression on a thin subject with the arm abducted in the face-down posture.

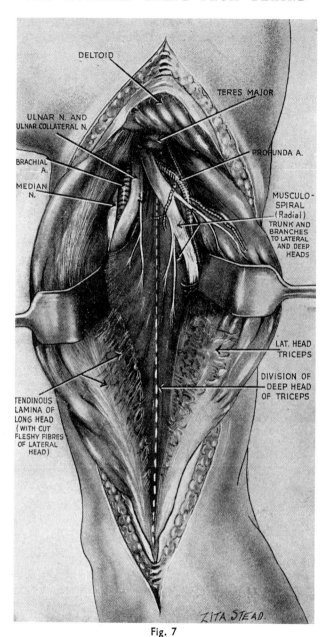

Fig. 7
The half-sleeve opened

The seam is ' ripped ' ; the two halves of the sleeve (the superficial heads—long and lateral) are separated, exposing the slanting neurovascular bundle. This consists of musculospiral nerve and profunda vessels ; it crosses the deep head, which clothes the humerus behind much as brachialis clothes it in front. Some four fingerbreadths of the main neurovascular bundle (ulnar and median nerves, brachial vessels) show in the space between long head and deep. Note the useful gap between the two parallel musculospiral twigs, leaving room to split the deep head. (The medial twig is the ulnar collateral.) Note and take care of the branch to the lateral head of triceps. (For the unusual lie of ulnar nerve, see p. 22.)

of the long head, so that we may open the deep fascia close to its outer side. Here the finger will enter the V-shaped meeting-place of long and lateral heads, and working down in contact with the long head will presently hook into the loose half-sleeve (Fig. 5, c). But we must be sure to keep in contact with the guiding belly ; the finger otherwise may open the wrong plane and lose its way between lateral head and overlying deltoid. That is the first pitfall.

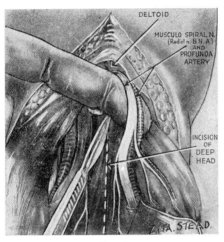

Fig. 8

Raise the oblique bundle like a bucket-handle, *working from below*, and lift it clear of the deep head. The deep head can then be split length-wise from end to end. (The branch to lateral head must be picked up with the main bundle ; it is likely to be cut if the bundle is mobilised from the proximal edge.)

Separation of the superficial heads (the long and lateral).— A finger hooked into the V-shaped opening lifts the sleeve from what lies under, and then begins to rip the seam that marks the meeting of these heads. But soon we need a knife (Fig. 5, c), for fleshy fibres of the lateral head slope down to join a shining lamina which the long head develops in the depth of triceps (Figs. 6 and 7).[1]

The bright face of this oblique ' intrinsic ' tendon is the plane for clean separation.

Opening the half-sleeve we find the large bundle consisting of musculospiral nerve (the radial of B.N.A.) and profunda vessels, a slanting band thinly divorced from bone by the deep head of triceps (Fig. 7). And if we raise the bundle gently like a bucket-handle and loop it back (Fig. 8), we then can pass the knife beneath, split the deep head lengthwise and reach almost the whole shaft from behind (Fig. 9, A).

Mobilising the musculospiral bundle.—Begin at the distal edge of the bundle on the medial side of the wound and work outwards. The lateral head of triceps receives a large nerve which runs a more transverse course than its parent trunk, and so is widely separate from the slanting bundle (Fig. 7). We must not

---

[1] This detail was familiar to Albinus : " It is impossible to show in this figure "—6 of tab. XIX—" how the long head develops (*efficiat*) a wide tendon on the side next (*a parte*) the lateral head, and how fibres of the lateral head reach it—just as on the *surface* of triceps (*extrinsecus*) fibres of the long head reach the lateral." (I have used our term " the lateral " for the head Albinus calls " the short.")

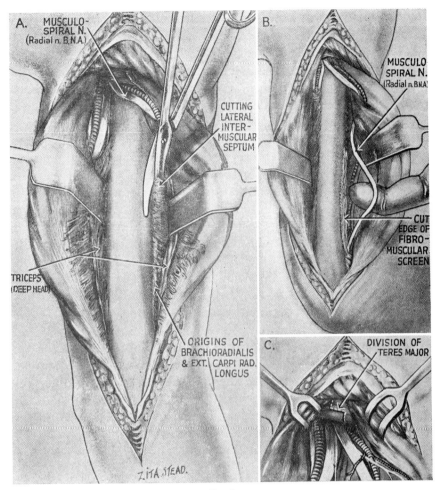

Fig. 9

A, B, and C. The humeral shaft exposed from behind with the musculospiral (radial) nerve

The two halves of the deep head of triceps have been peeled off the bone and retracted, exposing the lateral intermuscular septum. This retraction brings the small tongue of deep head, which always parts musculospiral from bone, round *behind* the nerve (B and Fig. 6).

For *distal* extension of the musculospiral exposure (A and B), divide the lateral septum plus the thin attachments of brachioradialis and extensor carpi radialis longus on its anterior face ; all three of these together screen the nerve.

For a more *proximal* extension (C), divide the flat band of teres major plus latissimus tendon. (Note the Z-shaped cut for sound repair.) Adduct the arm to relax the musculospiral which can then be drawn out like a loop (as in B).

fail to loop the branch and bundle up together (Fig. 8), for if we overlook the branch, it will most probably be cut—a frequent fault in making this exposure. (An ascending leash from profunda vessels may cross the field obliquely and go deep to deltoid (Figs. 7 and 10); sometimes it is large.)

Splitting the deep head.—Even the nerves to this part of triceps befriend our purpose : *the inner half* of the deep head is supplied by the fine ulnar collateral, a musculospiral (radial) twig that is often closely bound to the ulnar trunk and was long mistaken for a true ulnar branch (Fig. 7). This twig arises high in the axilla and enters the deep head two handbreadths distal to the acromion. *The outer half* has a stronger parallel twig (which also innervates the anconeus). It arises either with the branch to the lateral head or independently, and like the ulnar collateral enters the deep head two handbreadths below the acromion; thence it runs in the posteromedial part of the belly. Thus we can split the deep head between two longitudinal branches (Figs. 7 and 8). But the knife should keep close to the more lateral of these and aim for the olecranon; otherwise we may injure the ulnar nerve which sometimes bends outwards before reaching the elbow.[1]

It was noticed by the friendly critic of a first reprint that in Fig. 7 the ulnar nerve near the top of the wound is shown as lying *lateral* to brachial artery and median nerve. That was the true position in the specimen when the drawing was made. The reason for this lay, I believe, in the presence of a common type of ulnar collateral branch of radial nerve that fellow-travels briefly, or (to quote Professor Last) ' hitch-hikes ' in the substance of the ulnar trunk.

Anticipating Fig. 8, the radial nerve (plus the profunda brachii vessels) had been tentatively looped with a finger *before* Fig. 7 was completed, and so had pulled upon its ulnar collateral branch, which thus drew the ulnar trunk out to a lateral position—where it awaited the artist. My friend T. P. Garry has therefore called this neural arrangement " an error of retraction." (The orthodox medial position of the median trunk at the lower part of the segment seen in Fig. 7 supports this explanation.)

Labile relationship.—A quite different condition is apparent in Fig. 6 (which is an accurate copy of one made for the text-book of Poirier and Charpy some fifty years before my Fig. 7). Here,

---

[1] *This curve is dangerous.* I have seen the ulnar trunk divided during the exposure; but fortunately, so far, in the dead.

too, the ulnar nerve lies *lateral* to the median—*and* to the brachial veins and artery. But Poirier's specimen comes from an undissected cadaver, hardened, as the figure shows, while the arm lay pressed against the thorax. This pressure, in virtue of the natural mobility of main neurovascular structures at midarm level, seems to explain the anomalous relations of Fig. 6. Such relations, which come with diffuse pressure through skin and go with its relief, are *labile* relations. I have found them at midarm level in cadavers with orthodox neural patterns.

The posterior approach to the humeral shaft resembles that for exposing the anterior, homologous face of the femur There, too, a loose half-sleeve of muscle covers a deep head crossed by a neurovascular bundle ; there, too, we rip a seam, loop the bundle and split the deep head to reach bone.

EXTENDING THE POSTERIOR VIEW OF THE MUSCULOSPIRAL (OR RADIAL) NERVE.[1]—When the outer half of the deep head is fully raised from the back of the humerus the lateral intermuscular septum comes into view and—in company with the flat thin origins of brachioradialis and extensor carpi radialis longus— screens off the musculospiral nerve which goes in front. Divide this fibromuscular screen as close as possible to bone and so avoid the twigs to muscle (Fig. 9, A) ; then relax the nerve by adducting the arm (Fig. 9, B). That will let us deal with three more inches of musculospiral trunk, a surplus gain which often saves the nuisance of making fresh incision to find and liberate the nerve in front.

At the proximal part of the wound a similar length of musculospiral can be won by dividing the compound band of latissimus and teres major tendons, after easing the ulnar and musculospiral nerves safely away from its anterior face. A Z-shaped section of this band (Fig. 9, c)—made tense by abducting the arm—will favour strong repair.

THE MAIN NEUROVASCULAR BUNDLE OF THE ARM SEEN FROM THE BACK.—The brachial vessels and median nerve are easily explored in this posterior approach, for when we separate the

---

[1] " Musculospiral " appears again as an alternative. The recent imposition of " radial " on stem and branch alike has robbed the word of meaning for those acclimatised to both the previous terminologies. And some (who weathered each) would willingly agree with Pater that since " all progress of the mind consists for the most part in differentiation . . . it is surely the stupidest of losses to confuse things which right reason has put asunder, to lose the sense of achieved distinctions."

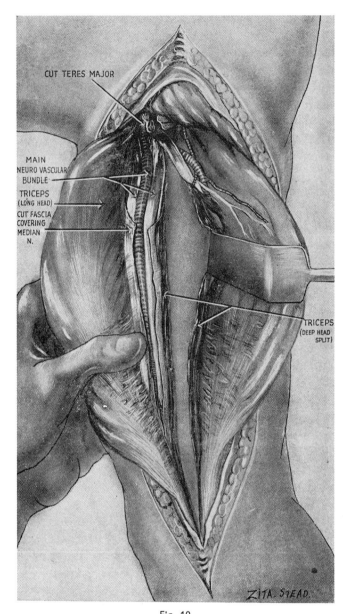

CUT TERES MAJOR

MAIN
NEURO VASCULAR
BUNDLE

TRICEPS
(LONG HEAD)

CUT FASCIA
COVERING
MEDIAN
N.

TRICEPS
(DEEP HEAD
SPLIT)

ZITA STEAD

Fig. 10

**The posterior exposure of humerus extended to the main
neurovascular bundle of the arm**

Separate the long head from the deep, and thus enlarge the upper space through which
the bundle is already visible ; a screen of fascia must also be divided. Grasp the arm as
in the figure (but through towels).   Work the bundle up into the wound, using your
finger-tips to bring it round the inner side of the deep head. (The median nerve sometimes
sticks to the front of the brachial artery.)   Access is easy and room sufficient to explore
the bundle and recognise its frequent abnormalities (high division of the artery, etc.)—a
further merit of the long incision.

long head of triceps fully from the lateral, some 4 in. of main
bundle are seen in the upper part of the field (Fig. 7).   But
farther down the arm the bundle is first veiled by a sheet of
fascia and afterwards concealed by the deep head of triceps, in
front of which it rests.   Turn then to this deep head and separate
the long head from it right down the arm.   Through the covering
towels grasp and gently squeeze the inner side of the arm in
such a way that the tips of the fingers will bring the bundle round
the inner side of the deep head and up into the wound.   Thus
we can deal from behind with the great anterior nerves and
vessels (Fig. 10).

APPROACH TO THE FRONT OF HUMERUS
WITH EXTENSIONS TO ITS JOINTS
TO THE FOREARM AXILLA AND ROOT OF NECK

During a surgical exposure important neurovascular structures are spared in one of two ways : either we seek them
out for protection, or else avoid them completely.   So, in
our access to the back of humerus we find the musculospiral nerve
and loop it clear, whereas with *frontal* intervention on the shaft,
the nerve will—if we wish—remain concealed and undisturbed.
And this exposure of the front of humerus provides, as we
shall see, a base for exploration of the parts at either end—
the joints, axilla, neck, and forearm.

ANATOMY

The *proximal* part of the bone is concealed in front by deltoid
fibres coming from the lesser curve of clavicle (Fig. 11);   the
muscle forms a thick unyielding cowl which gives when pulled
aside a grudging revelation of bone and shoulder joint;   and that
will often be the last successful thing it does.   So, for a *wide*
approach we mobilise the cowl in front and turn it harmlessly
away.
Clothing the *distal* reach of shaft are longitudinal fibres of
brachialis belly whose outer flank, left free of biceps, comes to the

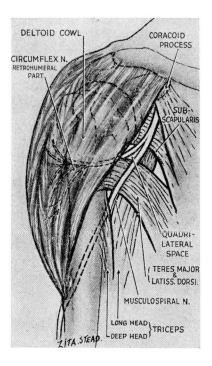

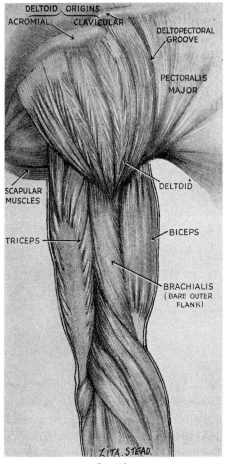

Fig. 12

The wide, bare *outer* flank of brachialis alone separates skin from shaft in the distal half of the arm (see also Fig. 13).

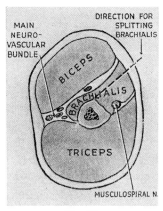

Fig. 13

Fig. 13

Cross-section through mid-third of arm, showing the outer flank of brachialis which is bare of biceps. This flank is split in the direction of the pointer to expose the distal half of humerus in front.   The cut slopes in to reach the *middle line* of shaft.   The musculo-spiral is safe.

surface in surprising width (Fig. 12). Here, then,—on the outer side of the arm—a single muscle (with its fascial coat) separates skin from bone; and here we shall attack the shaft through this uncovered flank of brachialis (Fig. 13).

The musculospiral (or radial) nerve.—The solid V of deltoid insertion fits down into a hollow V of brachialis, behind whose rearward limb lies the musculospiral nerve (Fig. 14); thus, we detach the limb (or separate its fibres) to find the nerve infallibly—a fingerbreadth below the deltoid eminence. But that is as we wish: the nerve need not be seen at all.

The *cutaneous trunk of musculocutaneous* curves forward at the outer edge of biceps just where the belly joins the tendon of insertion (Fig. 15). One of the outer cutaneous filaments is likely to be cut in the upper third of the forearm, though care will leave it running like a thread across the wound. (Main musculocutaneous branches to muscle are high up under cover of the inner part of biceps belly.)

The *cephalic vein* which follows the outer border of biceps and the inner border of deltoid enters the deep fascia in the lower third of the arm. It receives two or more lateral tributaries which must be divided. A humeral branch of the thoracoacromial artery accompanies the vein in the deltopectoral groove, and gives twigs to both muscles; the knife, therefore, cutting down on bone, should keep clear of this vascular gutter (Fig. 15) and go instead through fibres of the deltoid that form its outer lip.

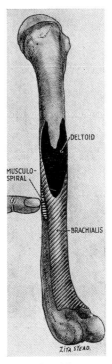

Fig. 14

Anterolateral view of the humerus showing how the solid V of deltoid insertion fits into the hollow V of brachialis. The musculospiral (radial) nerve lies behind the outer limb of brachialis V and can be found a fingerbreadth below the apex of the deltoid eminence (see also Fig. 23).

From these facts it appears that our incision to expose the front of humerus will skirt the outer side of the cephalic vein—below, where it follows the outer edge of biceps; above, in the deltopectoral groove. So we shall keep the knife a modest fingerbreadth *lateral* to the course we map for the vessel (Fig. 15). In the distal reach, however, no mere line will always guide the surgeon; fat or swelling may affect disorientation, and I have made (and often seen) the slip of

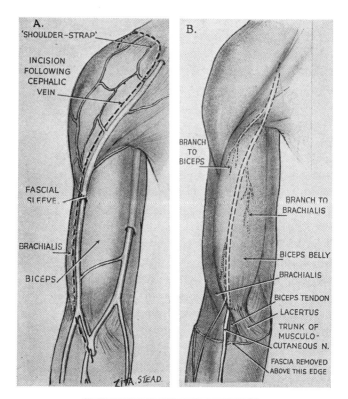

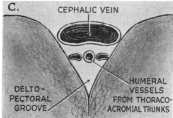

Fig. 15

A. The cephalic vein skirts the outer edge of biceps and the inner
edge of deltoid. Incisions to expose the front of humerus follow
the vein along its outer side. The broken line *above* the deltopectoral groove maps out the arching part, or ' shoulder-strap.'

B. Note how the chief cutaneous trunk of musculocutaneous appears
where biceps belly joins with biceps tendon.

C. Cross-section showing that the deltopectoral groove is a
vascular gutter. We shall avoid it and cut lengthwise through its
deltoid lip to reach the bone.

cutting through the biceps belly in mistake for brachialis flank.

We therefore grasp the front of the lax anæsthetised arm (Fig. 16) and move the free biceps belly across the fixed mass of brachialis. *Then* we can locate the outer edge of biceps and with it the cephalic.

We shall see, in a moment, how to find and follow the course of the deltopectoral groove in exposing the proximal part of humerus.

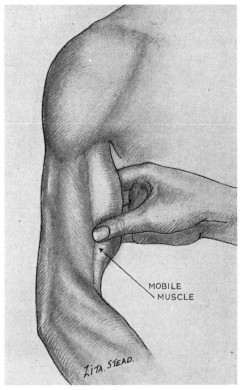

Fig. 16

Find the edge of biceps by moving its mobile belly across the fixed mass of brachialis. With this guide we can (1) place our skin incision for the distal part of the shaft a fingerbreadth from biceps ; (2) avoid the cephalic vein ; and (3) find the flank of brachialis, which (with its fascial coats) alone separates skin from shaft. This flank we shall split, directing the cut to the *midline* of humerus (see Fig. 13).

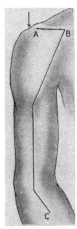

Fig. 17

The incision originally described for humeral exposure. The crooked proximal part (designed to give room to mobilise the clavicular origin of deltoid) is now replaced by a 'shoulder-strap' (see Fig. 18). The figure is retained to show the useful 'step-down' at the arrow which marks the acromioclavicular joint.

THE PROXIMAL PART OF HUMERUS AND THE SHOULDER JOINT

The incision I once used for this exposure was acutely angled at the outer third of the clavicle in order to give plenty of room : first, for mobilising the deltoïd cowl and turning it out of the way ; then, at the close of intervention, to allow easy fastening of the cowl back into place (Fig. 17).[1]   But crooked cuts in skin have three

[1] *British Journal of Surgery,* 1924, **12,** 84.

faults : they are troublesome to fit with side-curtains ; they are troublesome to close, and thirdly, they compromise healing. For many years, therefore, I have used incisions that cross the shoulder archwise from front to back (see *Irish Journal of Medical Science*, 1927, p. 634).

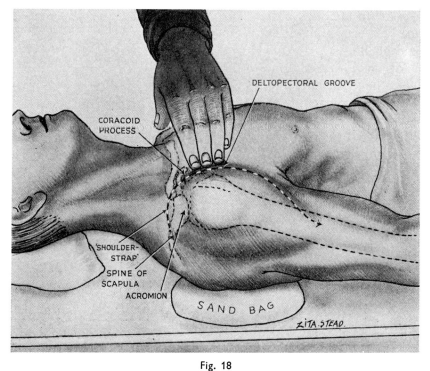

Fig. 18

Position and shoulder-strap incision for exposing the proximal part of humerus

Make the *back* of the shoulder accessible to the knife by putting a flat sandbag 5 in. square by 2 in. thick under the lower part of scapula on the side of operation. The bag must *not* obscure the scapular spine. Note how the coracoid tip is thrust into prominence. The knife goes through skin only, from deltoid eminence to scapular spine ; it follows the direction of deltopectoral groove and crosses the coracoid before arching over the shoulder. *To find the deltopectoral groove* the hand lies flat on the chest and slides out over the lax front of pectoralis major. The tips of the fingers strike the firm, oblique edge of deltoid ; the groove lies deep to them.

Position.—Care is required to make the *back* of the shoulder accessible to the knife. The patient lies with a flat sand-bag, 5 in. square by 2 in. thick, under the *lower* part of the scapula on the side of operation. The bag lifts the shoulder sufficiently to show the scapular spine, and also thrusts the tip of the coracoid process forward into helpful prominence (Fig. 18).

The shoulder-strap incision.[1]—
If we confine exposure either to
the joint or the proximal part of
humerus, the 'shoulder-strap'
descends no farther than the distal
end of deltoid; so we shall first
locate the deltopectoral groove,
whose course the knife will follow.
Sliding the fingers out towards the
limb across the hollow face of pectoralis we touch a firm obliquity of
deltoid edge (Fig. 18). The groove
is there, felt by the finger-tips.
The knife—which cuts no deeper
than subcutaneous fat—will follow
up the groove to reach the tip of
coracoid; then it will cut straight
on over the shoulder down to the
level of the spine of scapula—or,
of course, in reverse, according to
the side of the limb, or manual
convenience (Fig. 18).

Open the deep fascia along the
whole length of groove close to
its outer edge and look for the
cephalic vein which occupies its
channel. The knife can then avoid
the groove (with all the vessels
it contains) and split instead its
deltoid margin lengthwise from end

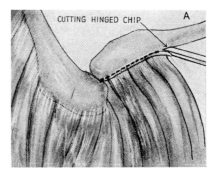

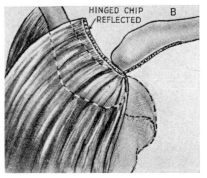

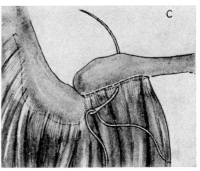

Fig. 19

Mobilising the front of deltoid

After reflecting skin, turn the deltoid out
on a hinged chip cut from the lesser curve
of clavicle, A and B. The deltoid origin
can be reconstructed with a single
ligature passed on a large curved needle,
C, and tied, D. Note how the chisel—
seated on its *bevel* to prevent undue
penetration—cuts out as far as the
acromioclavicular joint, marked by a
'step-down' (see Fig. 17).

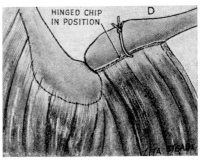

[1] I had ventured without hesitation to call this a shoulder-strap incision till I realised the
adjective came from a word used sometimes of bands running from tip to collar *along*
the shoulder. Let the term stand; my intention is plain to a majority: no woman will
question it.

to end.   This useful detail—due to G. A. Mason (*British Journal of Surgery*, 1929, **17,** 30)—divides a negligible strand of muscle from its nerve.   A small reflection of the shoulder skin gives access to the piece of deltoid that springs from the outer third of clavicle.

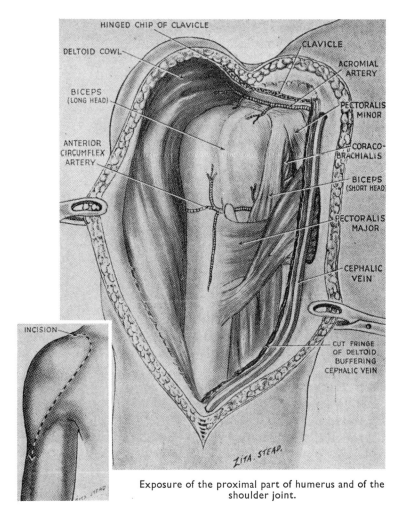

Exposure of the proximal part of humerus and of the shoulder joint.

Mobilising the front of the deltoid.—Divide the fascia and periosteum on the upper face of this outer third near the front of the bone.   Then detach a mere shaving of the edge that carries the deltoid origin.   If you are right-handed stand ' below ' the level of the patient's shoulder on his right side ; ' above ' it on his left.[1] Use a chisel and cut out as far as the acromioclavicular joint

---

[1] Or, if you prefer, let your stance in respect of the right shoulder ,be caudad ; of the left, cephalad.

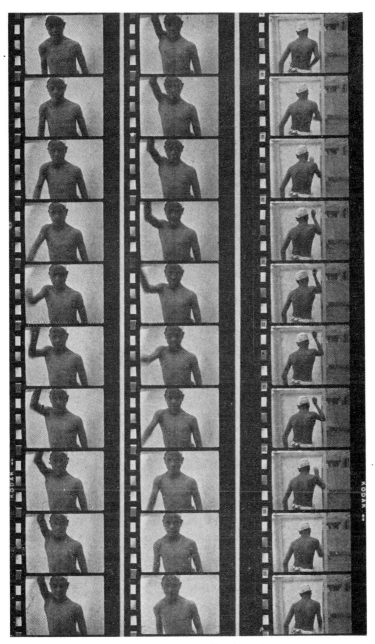

Fig. 21

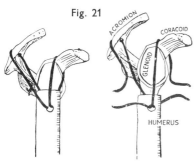

ACROMION
CORACOID
GLENOID
HUMERUS

To show the function of a limb after the deltoid has been mobilised and reconstituted. In this case the proximal fifth of humerus was resected for tumour, and the shaft slung with fascial strips to the scapula (see inset). Ten years later the function remained excellent. The left and middle columns are consecutive pictures from a film ; the patient, who worked in brass, raises his right arm, keeps it raised, and then lowers it. The right-hand column shows a complete hammering movement.

(Figs. 19 and 20). It is very easy to cut deep into clavicle and so remove too much bone. Seat the tool therefore on its *bevel*, and use it—like the blade of a carpenter's plane—to separate the edge only (Fig. 19 A).

The front part of the deltoid cowl can now be turned out on a hinged piece of clavicle, like a curtain on a rod. But the wide prospect we gain in this way is disappointing at first sight if we forget the spread of bursa that remains to mask (and be removed from) our objectives (Fig. 20).

After dealing with bone or joint a single suture passed through the muscle and round the clavicle with a large curved needle will lash the small piece of bone back into place and so reconstitute the deltoid origin (Fig. 19).[1] (The bony chip which carries deltoid need by no means be unbroken; I have often cut instead a band of mere contiguous flakes; and these united quickly with the clavicle, leaving the deltoid function quite intact.)

THE DISTAL PART OF THE HUMERUS (BELOW THE DELTOID LEVEL)

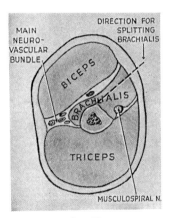

Fig 22

Cross-section through mid-third of arm, showing the outer flank of brachialis which is bare of biceps. This flank is split in the direction of the pointer to expose the distal half of humerus in front. The cut slopes in to reach the *middle line* of shaft. The musculospiral is safe.

Guiding our incision by testing for comparative mobility (Fig. 16), we keep the knife a slender fingerbreadth lateral to the edge of biceps, and so respect the vein; then we continue four fingerbreadths into the upper third of the forearm, curving a little in towards the middle line. Here we must open deep fascia with extra care, especially in swollen forearms. The swelling seems to thrust the radial vessels (which are, I notice, often slit in normal limbs) still farther into danger. Surgeons, too, will take a pride in rescuing the lateral cutaneous twig of musculocutaneous which runs in surface fat (Fig. 15). A longitudinal cut is then directed through the bare outer flank of brachialis, which we identify again by moving biceps

---

[1] I still describe this way of mobilising and reconstituting the deltoid origin, which served me well through twenty years in dealing with the following conditions: old subcoracoid luxations; osteoclastoma of the humeral head treated by resecting the proximal fifth

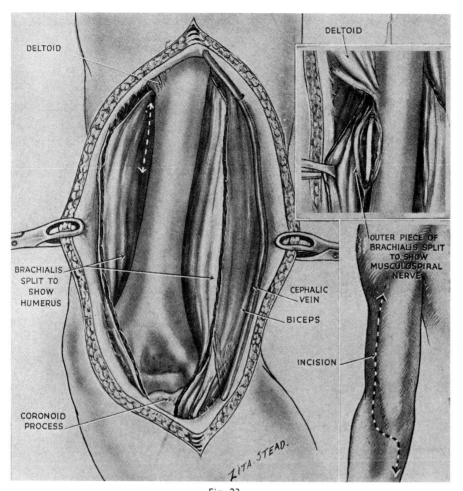

Fig. 23
Distal exposure of the humerus
A. The skin incision. B. When we have split brachialis as in Fig. 22, a partial flexion of the elbow transforms the split into a wide and shallow wound. If exploration of the elbow joint is not required, check the cut two fingerbreadths above the epicondyles. Musculospiral meanwhile is safe and out of sight. Should you wish to find the nerve, a touch with Mayo scissors parts the screen of brachialis one fingerbreadth below the deltoid eminence (B and C).

of the humerus and suspending the rest with fascia to coracoid process and acromion (see Fig. 21, from the *Irish Journal of Medical Science*, Oct. 1927, reproduced here through the courtesy of my friend the Editor, Mr. W. D. Doolin); recent subglenoid luxations of the shoulder with fractures comminuting the proximal parts of humerus. In every case exposure was completely satisfactory; in none did the chip fail to unite with clavicle, and none has required removal of wire, thread or catgut.

I have often wondered, however, if a subperiosteal detachment of deltoid would be compatible with the sound function I got after cutting the chip. And I had the fortune to hear from the late Lt.-Col. H. A. Brittain, R.A.M.C., that excellent results will follow. More sutures must be used to tie the muscle back in place than when it swings out on a rod; but that is no objection.

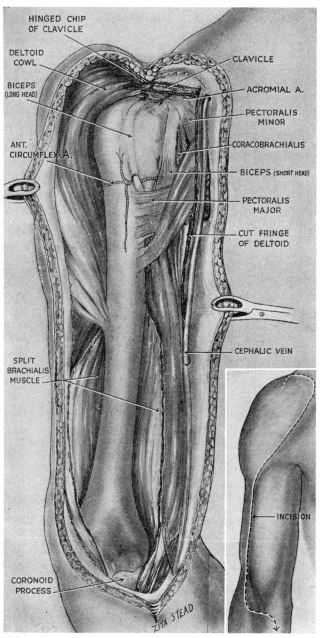

Fig. 24

Complete anterior exposure of the humerus, embracing shoulder and elbow joints, is obtained by combining the proximal and distal exposures in one procedure. The inset shows the full incision. The flexor crease at the elbow lies two fingerbreadths below the epicondylar level. The incision crosses just below the crease. Musculospiral does not appear unless we wish (see Fig. 23).

over it; the knife enters the flank a fingerbreadth lateral to the biceps edge and goes obliquely in to reach the front of the bone *at the middle line*—a vital emphasis (Fig. 22). (I have only once seen the nerve injured in scores of humeral exposures—then by a glancing, misdirected cut, wide of the ample target.) The outer strip of brachialis, thus separated, forms a buffer protecting the musculospiral (or radial) nerve from the rugine. The nerve is not seen if the front only of humeral shaft is exposed; the back, too, can be cleared safely while the nerve is concealed. But (should the surgeon wish) the musculospiral, in adults, is always found one fingerbreadth distal to the deltoid eminence by gentle blunt dissection through the buffering slip of brachialis (Fig. 23). Light pressure on this buffer removes the nerve sufficiently from contact with the shaft to give a rugine access. (This facultative finding of the nerve was plain in the original account (*loc. cit.*), but has been missed in later adaptations.)

The brachialis may be split to just within two fingerbreadths of the epicondyles without entering the elbow joint. Watch for sharp bleeding from a vein divided in the upper fibres. The bone, seen through the split, lies, in extension of the limb, deep and unworkable. Flexion of the elbow to a right angle transforms this appearance, relaxing the muscles and leaving the bone widely accessible in a shallow wound (Fig. 23).[1]

The elbow joint.—This joint can be opened—and even excised from in front—by a further splitting of brachialis. The tip of the coronoid process and the trochlea are at once visible; the capitulum and head of radius appear with adequate retraction.

After a distal approach, extension of the elbow before suturing the fascia will close of itself the wide wound in brachialis.

The whole front of humerus can be laid bare by combining the proximal and distal approach (Fig. 24); and we can, of course, expose any segment by using shorter lengths of the full-length incision. But these should not be short.

If, therefore, it is possible to reach objectives (sequestra are the commonest example) *without* hinging back the deltoid, we need not hinge it back,—a sentence one would like to think superfluous.

---

[1] For a continuation of distal exposure of humerus into antecubital fossa see p. 90.

EXPOSURE OF THE PROXIMAL PART OF HUMERUS COMBINED WITH AXILLO-CERVICAL EXTENSIONS TO NERVES AND VESSELS

Some score years ago with D. Bowie, F.R.C.S., then surgical specialist to Cairo Command, I saw a case of fracture-dislocation of the shoulder showing complete brachial palsy. We had thus to explore the bone, the joint and proximal parts of all the brachial nerves. The shoulder-strap incision described above (Fig. 18), combined with detachment of a clavicular chip (Fig. 19), served well; bone and joint were dealt with, and, after dividing the tendon of pectoralis major, each nerve was seen and fortunately found intact. The following account will give a sort of formula for multiple procedures of the kind.

AXILLARY EXTENSION OF THE PROXIMAL APPROACH TO HUMERUS.—The shoulder joint and upper part of humerus are first exposed (see p. 29). Then, when the deltoid is turned back, divide the tendon of pectoralis major close to its insertion and draw the muscle inwards (Fig. 25). The loose fascia now seen spreading between the divergent coracoid origins of pectoralis minor and coracobrachialis covers the main neurovascular bundle of the axilla. Open the fascia near the coracobrachial belly avoiding the musculocutaneous nerve which enters a medial *groove* on that muscle two fingerbreadths below the coracoid; farther down, the nerve tunnels through the muscle belly.[1]

When we have opened the loose axillary fascia it is quite easy to take the wrong path—even after careful warning—and be lured by the inviting space between bone and the composite band formed by short head of biceps plus coracobrachialis (Fig. 25). Resist that lure and keep dissection *medial* to the band. The nerves lie there in easily remembered grouping round the vessels (Fig. 25).

Some special points deserve a reference. The *median nerve* can as a rule be found, even with eyes shut, by Farabeuf's simple expedient—drawing the pulp of a finger across the main axillary bundle towards coracobrachialis; the nerve comes with the finger and leaves the artery bare (Fig. 25). The circumflex and musculo-

---

[1] Pictures in text-books of anatomy show the musculocutaneous dissected out of the coracobrachial groove; they therefore stress a relation of nerve to muscle which begins only at the *tunnel*. That, I think, is why we learn to expect the musculocutaneous in a third-stage axillary ligation, and why we seldom find it: the nerve has sunk into the groove and left the median to skirt the lateral edge of neurovascular bundle.

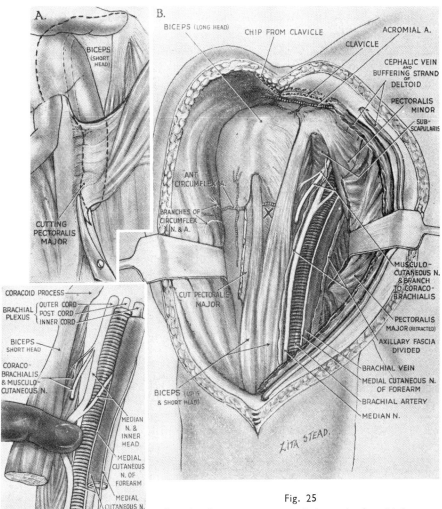

Fig. 25

Proximal exposure extended to the brachial nerves

A. The pectoralis major divided. B. The resulting exposure. X marks the pitfall to avoid when defining the neurovascular bundle—the tempting much-frequented interval between short head of biceps and humerus. (The bundle is, of course, medial to the common mass comprising biceps head and coracobrachialis.) C shows the relation of nerves to the double-barrelled lie of vein and artery in the axilla : the medial cutaneous nerve of forearm occupies the groove that demarcates the barrels in front ; the hinder groove conceals the ulnar nerve ; median overlies the outer border of the artery and is accompanied by musculo-cutaneous, while medial cutaneous of the arm is on the inner border of the vein. C also shows Farabeuf's ' blindfold ' method of locating the axillary part of median nerve.

spiral nerves spring from the hinder cord ; they thus lie deeper than the rest and come less easily to hand.

The circumflex nerve.—This nerve, considered for a surgical exposure, has here two parts—axillary and retrohumeral (Fig. 26).

The *axillary portion* which suffers most from injury lies deep ; and having failed on more than one occasion to find it quickly, I learnt at length to recognise it blindfold—defining in the first place with a finger the thick mass of main neurovascular bundle.

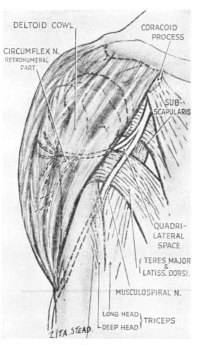

Fig. 26

The posterior cord forks into circumflex and musculospiral nerves. Each nerve has an axillary and a retrohumeral segment. The quadrilateral space is seen.

LOCATION OF THE AXILLARY PART OF CIRCUMFLEX BY TOUCH. —Stand behind the top of the patient's shoulder and use your right index for his left side, your left for his right. Place the tip of the finger on the tip of the cora- coid ; aim into the angle formed by the divergence of pectoralis minor and coracobrachialis. Slide the finger obliquely—down, in and back—across the coracoid tip as far as the proximal interphalan- geal joint. The tip of the finger penetrates soft areolar tissue above the level of the bundle, and, slanting down behind it, stops against the front of the subscapu- laris (Fig. 27). Now turn your index and hook the distal phalanx gently out towards the arm ; the thick strand thus caught by the pulp of the finger is the circumflex bundle : the nerve lies next the finger ; in front of the nerve are the posterior circumflex vessels.

But when we find this portion of the circumflex we have achieved a mere location : it lies as yet too deep, and seems too short, for useful intervention. Not till the clavicle is cut at the responsive point (p. 44), letting the limb fall outwards, will a workable length of nerve come near enough to the surface for convenience.

The *retrohumeral part of the circumflex* disappears through the quadrilateral space above the thumbwide band of latissimus and teres major tendons (Fig. 26). A finger easily enters the distal part of this space and follows the transverse course of the bundle round behind the humerus ; it lies in a loose zone of cleavage between deltoid and surgical neck.

EXPOSURE OF THE RETROHUMERAL PART OF CIRCUMFLEX.—This portion of the nerve is only seen by further mobilising deltoid—first distally as far as the insertion ; then at the proximal attachment.

Separation of the acromial origin of deltoid.—Leaving a strand to buffer the cephalic vein (pp. 27 and 31) the whole deltoid hood is mobilised without division of its fibres, first by detaching the hinged

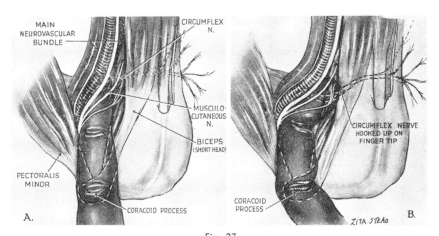

Fig. 27

Locating the axillary part of the circumflex nerve by touch

A. The index finger (the left for the right side—as in this figure—and *vice versa*) slides from above the patient's shoulder, on its palmar aspect, *across* the coracoid tip, *into* the angle between pectoralis minor and coracobrachialis, *behind* the main neurovascular bundle, viz. down, in and back. Stop the finger when its proximal' interphalangeal joint covers the tip of coracoid. The distal phalanx has then reached subscapularis—the soft mass in front of scapula.

B. Now turn the finger out towards the arm. The distal phalanx hooks the nerve.

clavicular chip completely, and then by cutting off with a chisel the deltoid edge of acromion (Fig. 28). Adopt the stance employed for slicing off the deltoid chip (p. 32)—' below ' the patient's right shoulder ; ' above ' his left. And once it bites into the bone, seat the chisel on its bevel (as in Fig. 19) and take the merest shaving from acromion, *except* at the acromial angle. Cut this angle off obliquely in such a way that when replaced it will fit firmly on the scapula. The whole bony margin—acromial plus clavicular—looks like a bent and sprawling U with one limb broken (Fig. 28, c). This separation is by no means difficult, but does demand most careful study of skeletal contour (Fig. 28) and gentle guidance of a *sharp* chisel. The very wide exposure thus obtained (Fig. 29) should also find a use in the rare case where mere *clavicular* detachment gives insufficient access to the shoulder, and where as well we have the chance of saving deltoid function.

The final restoration is extremely simple, for to secure it we need only tie back into place the chip first cut from clavicle. A single ligature will thus reconstitute the origin of deltoid—in front, behind and at the side.

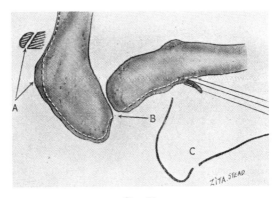

Fig. 28

Separation of the deltoid origin extended to acromion

A. The acromial angle ; the broken line marks the direction of the cut seen from above. The sagittal section shows in diagram the *slope* of the cut which lets the separated angle fit back later like a cap. B. The 'difficult' corner between the bones—where it is easy to drive the chisel *through* acromion instead of round its edge. C. The outline of the cut seen from above—a sprawling U with one limb broken. (The chips from clavicle and acromion are linked across the joint by ligament so that a single suture round the clavicle reconstitutes the deltoid origin.)

The musculospiral nerve.—The musculospiral runs obliquely in front of a useful landmark, the composite teres-latissimus tendon which crosses the field four fingerbreadths below the coracoid tip. The nerve lies, remember, like the circumflex, *behind* the main neurovascular bundle, shut off from it and bound by thin transparent fascia, so that when we draw the bundle inwards the musculospiral is often left unmoved and visible (Fig. 30).

The vascular tether.—But first we may have to sever a short leash of vessels that ties the bundle to the coracobrachial belly, near the latissimus tendon. A finger travelling down the belly catches the leash which comes either from brachial or profunda vessels ; and since the leash is short these last are easily hooked

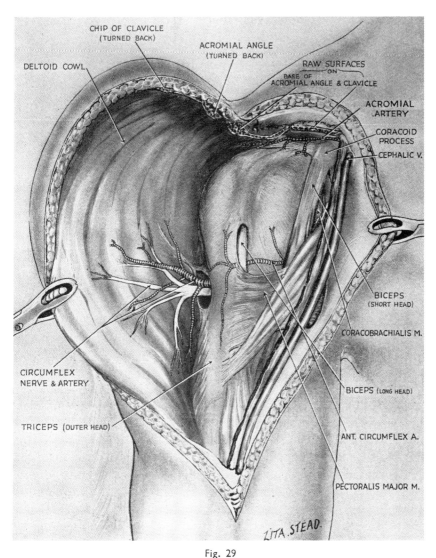

Fig. 29

Subtotal detachment of deltoid

Exposure of the retrohumeral part of circumflex obtained by detachment of the clavicular *plus* the acromial origins of deltoid. The wide, incidental, view of shoulder joint—front, side, and back—suggests further use for this subtotal deltoid separation. *One* ligature (placed as in Fig. 19, C) restores and clamps both origins.

up with it (Fig. 30). We shall do well, therefore, to separate and view the structures caught by the finger before dividing the leash, sparing of course the large profunda.

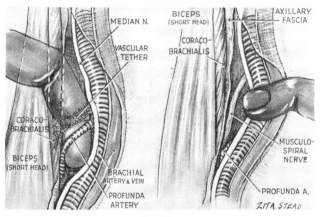

Fig. 30

A vascular tether binding the main bundle to coracobrachialis may need division before the bundle can be drawn aside to expose the musculospiral nerve. A finger hooked down the medial face of coracobrachialis picks up the tether—and sometimes the large profunda vessels with it. So look before you cut, and spare profunda.

THE CORDS OF BRACHIAL PLEXUS.—The cords from which the nerves arise are thoroughly exposed if the narrow, coracoid end of pectoralis minor is cut across.

EXTENDING THE EXPOSURE FROM THE AXILLA TO THE NECK.—For this the clavicle must be divided. The site made use of by Fiolle and Delmas affords a real seat of election, three fingerbreadths lateral to the sternal end (Fig. 31, Part 1). Division of the bone too far in threatens the subclavian vein which lies so dangerously close to the medial inch of clavicle ; on the other hand, a section too far out leaves an inner piece of shaft whose overlap conceals our main objectives. The ' seat of election ' corresponds in general to the outermost edge of the sternomastoid origin—a place to remember ; for there the external jugular vein penetrates deep fascia ; there, on a deeper level, we shall find the outer edge of scalenus anterior underlying that of sternomastoid—the two as if about to coincide in Euclid's mind.

When the clavicle is sectioned we can use the weight of the limb —some 7 or 8 pounds in the adult—to lever the outer fragment from in front of the plexus.

Position and incision.—The field is opened by turning the

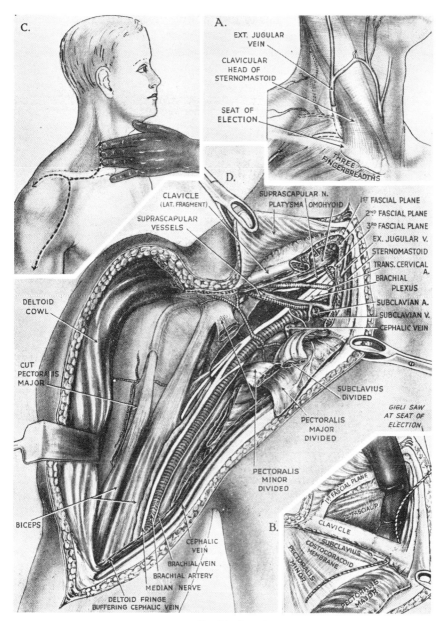

Fig. 31, Part 1

Exposure of nerves and vessels continued from axilla into neck by cutting through the clavicle

A and B. Seat of election for dividing clavicle, three fingerbreadths from the sternal end. It borders generally on the outer edge of sternomastoid—an edge which if displaced directly back would ' coincide ' with that of scalenus. Note the relation of external jugular.

C. Incision for *unforeseen* extension from joint and axilla to neck, going in from the ' strap ' to a fingerbreadth beyond the ' seat ', and then up sternomastoid—a useful makeshift (*cf.* Fig. 31, Part 2).

D. The view after (1) dividing pectoralis major close to clavicle ; (2) dividing pectoralis minor ; (3) dividing clavicle itself ; (4) drawing the limb clear of the table so that its *weight* will swing aside the outer fragment. This last manœuvre levers up the final tether (belly of subclavius). Cut through it, taking care to guard the sometimes formidable suprascapulars.

patient's head and neck away, and pulling on the hand to bring his shoulder down. Then comes the question of incision. Supposing, for example, we have used a ' shoulder-strap ' and bared the joint, only to find that we must *add* an exploration of the root of neck,

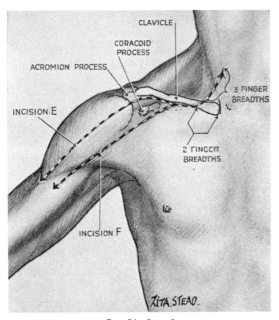

Fig. 31, Part 2

Skin incision for planned axillo-cervical approach

E. *For exposing axilla plus shoulder joint plus root of neck,* abduct the arm to straighten your cut. Divide skin length-wise over deltoid, aiming a thumbwidth *lateral* to the tip of coracoid. Curve the cut in along the lower edge of clavicle, and up, two fingerbreadths from sternum. F. *For simple axillo-cervical approach* again abduct the arm. By-pass the joint with an incision curved like E, but aimed a thumbwidth *medial* to coracoid.
Incision E affords inclusive access to the joint (Fig. 19). Incision E or F leaves room for opening the pectoralis lid to the axilla ; then for dividing moorings of the clavicle—a barrier which, cut across, not only swings aside but lets the shoulder girdle turn and offer up the contents of axilla on the scapula, as on a plate.

the requisite incision goes inward from the ' strap '—a second-best though workable procedure (Fig. 31, Part 1). But if we *plan* combined exposure—whether of shoulder joint and neck with axilla, or merely of axilla with neck—then we shall make a single cut, placing it farther in or out, to let us by-pass or include the joint (Fig. 31, Part 2). Reflect skin sufficiently to show three things : the site for dividing clavicle ; the origin of pectoralis major lateral to that site ; the lower fourth of sternomastoid.

Add—to expose the shoulder joint—the outer third of clavicle.

Division of pectoralis major and clavicle.—After severing the muscle near its humeral attachment we must divide it from the clavicle as far inwards as the place for bone section, so that presently the lateral fragment (which blocks our view of nerves and vessels) lies ready to be swung aside.

We now turn to the neck and open the most superficial of the three layers of deep cervical fascia close to this ' seat of election.' A finger introduced from above completes the isolation of the clavicle at the right spot. The instrument of choice for dividing the bone is a Gigli saw.[1]

Then, if we bring the limb well over the edge of the table, its weight will lever up the outer piece of clavicle and stretch the belly of subclavius. This we must divide without dividing vessels —variously termed the transverse scapular [2] or suprascapular— whose long *retroclavicular* course (stressed by the Baron Boyer in Napoleon's time) runs close behind subclavius. Many to-day, I notice, find their site and magnitude surprising. But John Bell, who lived his anatomy, often saw the artery (which frequently springs from the third stage of subclavian) " large, very long, tortuous like the splenic artery, and almost equalling it in size " (Fig. 31, D, Part 1). The vein may bulk still larger.

Section of the clavicle allows rotation of the scapula, which brings structures of axilla *forwards*, and, notably, the deep-seated circumflex nerve.

Before proceeding to the neck let us improve acquaintance with the *layers* of cervical fascia and (like an expert " digging up the past ") enlist their help as guides.

THE DEEP FASCIAL PLANES ABOVE THE CLAVICLE

Three are found here. The first is an *investing layer* which gives a sheath to trapezius and sternomastoid, and cloaks the

---

[1] By this I do not mean the futile things, of late in regular supply, which cut slowly and broke quickly—even with careful punctilio in the matter of angulation. I mean the tough Gigli saws (chosen with characteristic flair) that form part of the neurosurgeon's armoury. They cost a trifle more ; they cut fast, and for two years I watched class after class bend them double and pass them on intact.

[2] ' Transverse scapular ' (B.N.A.) : a factitious, ' portmanteau ' title caught from the well-named transverse cervical vessels that lie contiguously. ' Transverse ' they certainly are—in the neck ; ' scapular,' certainly in destination. But certainly not ' transverse scapular ' : they have a lengthwise course along the bone.

intervening triangle. Deep to this layer is a mass of fat and glands mingled with terminal twigs of transverse cervical and supra-scapular vessels.

Next comes a loose, *intermediate layer* of deep fascia which loops round the posterior belly of omohyoid and, like a mesentery,

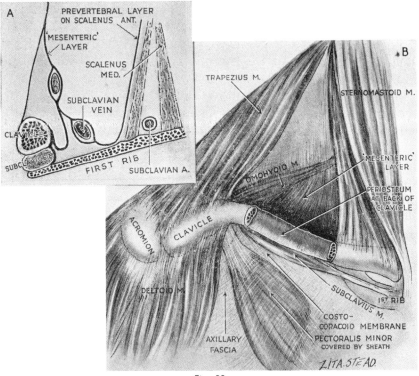

Fig. 32

The three planes of deep fascia above the clavicle. The diagram A (after Paulet) shows the three layers in sagittal section. Note how the ' mesenteric ' layer, which contains the omohyoid, dips behind the clavicle. B shows the continuity of the ' mesenteric ' layer—through the medium of the clavicular periosteum—with the sheath of subclavius (as seen in A), and thence with costocoracoid membrane, and sheath of pectoralis minor.

holds the muscle to the back of clavicle. Here the fascia blends with periosteum through which it is continuous with the hinder layer of subclavius sheath, and that descends towards the chest to form the costocoracoid (or clavipectoral) membrane which gives a covering to pectoralis minor (Fig. 32).[1]

It will thus be clear that when we divide the clavicle we open

---

[1] My appreciation of a fibrous sheet spreading (beyond both) from omohyoid to pectoralis minor, and crossed but not broken by the adhering clavicle, is due to an admirable speci-men made by my friend Major E. E. Dunlop, D.A.D.M.S., Royal Australian Army Medical Corps.

this second, 'mesenteric' layer—unless, of course, we first shell the bone out of its periosteum. The omohyoid belly may lie far down, behind the clavicle, or rise some fingerbreadths above it on a long 'mesentery'; it is a guide of great worth—a bathymetric muscle that measures the *depth* we have attained—and (like the posterior belly of digastric) flags the subjacent presence of all the neurovascular structures of chief account in its own part of the neck. Deep to the 'mesenteric' layer is a second complex of fat and glands, containing this time the main trunks of the transverse cervical and suprascapular vessels.

The third and last layer of deep fascia is the *prevertebral*; it spreads like a tight sheath of dull cellophane over the front of the scalene mass, binding on to these muscles the mesh of brachial plexus, the subclavian artery, and the phrenic nerve. (The nerve may travel *in* the fascial layer.) Deep to this layer there is *no* mass of fat and glands.[1] (It will be noticed that mention has not been made of the subclavian vein which lies sunk in this region, divorced from its artery by scalenus anterior. It is closely bound to the innermost part of the clavicle but is far enough away at the point of section to be avoided easily by hugging the bone.)

THE CERVICAL EXPOSURE RESUMED.—With these facts grasped we may proceed in all confidence, recognising and dealing with each stratum in turn—the three fascial layers; the two fatty screens. We shall divulse the fat and spare the vascular twigs by means of Mayo scissors, opening the fascial layers with the same respect we have for peritoneum, or—in the case of the last layer, the prevertebral—for dura mater; and with no less assurance. (The belly of the omohyoid may be severed or drawn aside, as is convenient.)

THE MEDIAL EXTENSION THROUGH STERNOMASTOID.—Should we wish to carry our exposure in across the neck, we must divide the clavicular head of sternomastoid—an act that calls for circumspection: the internal jugular vein is often fixed in fat to the deep face of the muscle. Old periadenitis—as over the carotid fork—may felt the structures too closely for 'blunt' separation, making it

---

[1] *Deep juxtaclavicular fascial layers of neck.*—These three may be remembered as layers in a club sandwich arranged thus : (1) *investing layer of deep fascia*; (2) complex of fat, glands, and terminal twigs of transverse cervical and suprascapular vessels; (3) *intermediate* ('*mesenteric*') *layer of deep fascia* enclosing the posterior belly of omohyoid; (4) complex of fat, glands, main branches and tributaries of transverse cervical and suprascapular vessels; (5) *prevertebral* ('*cellophane*') *layer of deep fascia*. (This last is really a lateral, *prescalenic* extension of the true prevertebral fascia. The true prevertebral fascia clothes longus capitis and longus colli.)

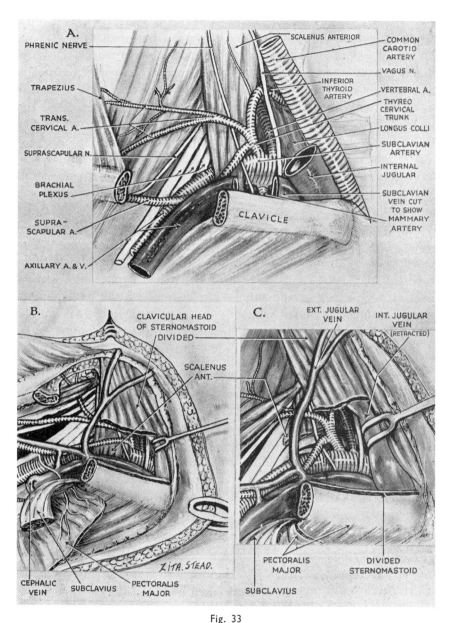

Fig. 33

The axillo-cervical exposure extended medially

The upper figure, A, is to remind us of anatomy. Sternomastoid has been entirely removed. B. Divide the clavicular head of sternomastoid *surgically* (see text), respecting external and internal jugular veins ; scalenus comes to view. Isolate scalenus *as you would an artery*, releasing phrenic nerve and vessels crossing it. C. Divide scalenus near the first rib. Note that its costal end withdraws and lets the two subclavian trunks touch in their second stage. Note how the lowest trunk of brachial plexus is ensconced between scalenus medius and subclavian artery. The posterior belly of omohyoid is not labelled in B and C. In B it is partly hidden by the distal piece of clavicle whose cut face shows how the weight of the limb has rotated the shoulder girdle.

(Clavicle, as a rule, hides the subclavian vein ; here the vein is high.)

most dangerous to slide a finger under and pick up this head of sternomastoid for mass division. It is wiser, therefore (after dividing the ' safe ' lateral fingerbreadth), to cut gradually through the front of the head, and use a finger to displace the deepest fibres from the vein.

Occasion may be found for a further safeguard, using the suprasternal space of Burns and Grüber's diverticulum.

BURNS' SPACE AND ITS DIVERTICULA.—Two accounts of this space are currently accepted. Merkel's, which prevails in our own text-books,[1] supposes a suprasternal cleavage of the investing layer of deep cervical fascia—an arrangement which. if actual, would offer no surgical advantage.

The second and fruitful view is favoured by French anatomists, though for reasons that seem less cogent than the little-finger test I shall describe. The French regard the space as an enclosure whose boundaries are formed by adhesions occurring between two fascial layers at the cavity's *margin*—the investing layer (1) uniting there with (2) the intermediate or ' mesenteric ' (p. 48). From this central space of Burns a short *cul-de-sac*, the diverticulum of Grüber, projects transversely on either side, extending for about an inch along and behind the upper face of clavicle.

If the first or ' cleavage ' view of Burns' space were correct, we should expect the fascia forming a Grüber's diverticulum to behave like investing fascia, in which event it would ensheathe the lower end of sternomastoid. *It does not do so*—the diverticulum lies in a plane *behind* the sternal foot of the muscle, and may even reach out behind the foot of its clavicular attachment.

According to the second or ' adhesion ' view the back wall of Burns' space, and so of Grüber's diverticulum, is formed by the *second* layer of deep cervical fascia—the intermediate or ' mesenteric ' layer which is the special sheath of infrahyoid muscles (Figs. 34 and 37). When, therefore, we open the central space of Burns, the little finger passed into it and out along a Grüber's diverticulum will, first, occupy the short diverticular lumen and there lie sandwiched between the sternal foot of sternomastoid in front and the infrahyoid ' strap ' muscles posteriorly. Then, guided by the lumen, the finger can break gently onward through the blind end of the *cul-de-sac* and slide past the clavicular foot of sternomastoid. Moving close behind this foot

---

[1] T. H. Bryce, however, supports the second view (Quain's *Elements of Anatomy*, *Myology*, 1923, p. 64).

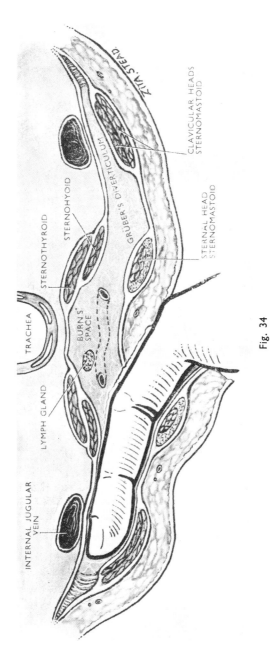

Fig. 34

A finger passed from the central space of Burns along or beyond the diverticulum of Grüber has in front of it the sternomastoid ; behind it, the sternohyoid and sternothyroid muscles. The finger-tip separates the clavicular part of sternomastoid from the internal jugular vein, making an excellent safeguard when the muscle is divided. (The junction between the two anterior jugular veins lying in the central space of Burns is not labelled.) Note how the intermediate (mesenteric) layer of deep cervical fascia—which ensheathes the strap muscles (Fig. 37)—forms the back wall of Burns' space.

it opens a safe path in front of the internal jugular vein, and in front, too, of any fringe of infrahyoid belly that may spread to cover the vessel. For this reason the diverticulum of Burns' space can be used as a safeguard when dividing the clavicular foot of sternomastoid. And let no one scorn its aid : help of this kind is by no means superfluous ; I have twice seen an internal jugular vein severed along with the covering muscle by a single cut— magnificent commando work but not surgery.

The transverse part of the anterior jugular vein which may occupy Grüber's diverticulum is easily spared.

The subclavian artery in continuity.—Section of the clavicular head of sternomastoid gives a good view of scalenus anterior with a glimpse of phrenic nerve (still under its cellophane fascia) sloping down and in across the muscle. Then, if we first free the nerve and its small companion vessels, we can isolate the scalene muscle as we should isolate a great longitudinal artery ; and after cutting through the belly close above the rib all three stages of subclavian trunk are seen in continuity (Fig. 33, c). Most of the branches, too, are visible, or can be brought to light by gentle blunt dissection. The vertebral artery with the vein in front of it disappears up into the apex of the deep angular space between the divided scalene muscle and the longus colli clothing the vertebral column. (Fig. 33, A, shows the origins of subclavian branches. Note the thyrocervical trunk rising and branching beside the inner scalene edge, directly opposite internal mammary.)

EXPOSURE OF CERVICAL STRUCTURES BY STERNOMASTOID EVERSION

If Fiolle and Delmas had done nothing else for surgical exposure, their short supplemental cut which turns the ordinary straight incision along the front edge of sternomastoid into a ' hockey-stick ' entitles them to fame. This supplement crosses and cuts down on the root of the mastoid process (Figs. 35 and 41) and so allows us to detach and evert the upper irretractile part of sternomastoid.

There was one flaw in this jewel : its authors advised a separation of the mastoid tip in order to mobilise the muscular attachment. But the attachment of sternomastoid climbs much too high on the mastoid process to be separated by cutting through the tip ; it is also difficult to divide the bone cleanly, and the chisel is liable to smash a cellular process and leave it oozing. Mastoid

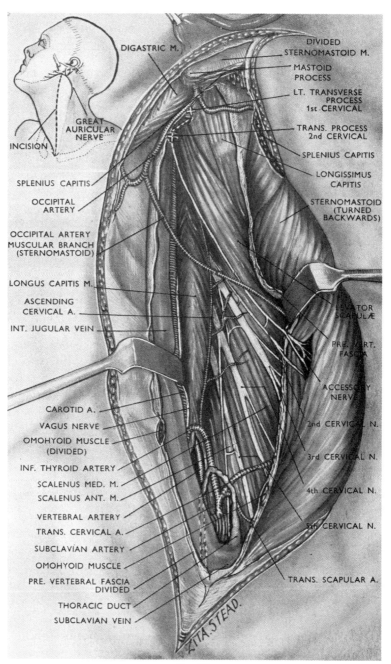

Labels on figure:

DIGASTRIC M.
GREAT AURICULAR NERVE
INCISION
SPLENIUS CAPITIS
OCCIPITAL ARTERY
OCCIPITAL ARTERY MUSCULAR BRANCH (STERNOMASTOID)
LONGUS CAPITIS M.
ASCENDING CERVICAL A.
INT. JUGULAR VEIN
CAROTID A.
VAGUS NERVE
OMOHYOID MUSCLE (DIVIDED)
INF. THYROID ARTERY
SCALENUS MED. M.
SCALENUS ANT. M.
VERTEBRAL ARTERY
TRANS. CERVICAL A.
SUBCLAVIAN ARTERY
OMOHYOID MUSCLE
PRE. VERTEBRAL FASCIA DIVIDED
THORACIC DUCT
SUBCLAVIAN VEIN

DIVIDED STERNOMASTOID M.
MASTOID PROCESS
LT. TRANSVERSE PROCESS 1st CERVICAL
TRANS. PROCESS 2nd CERVICAL
SPLENIUS CAPITIS
LONGISSIMUS CAPITIS
STERNOMASTOID (TURNED BACKWARDS)
LEVATOR SCAPULÆ
PRE. VERT. FASCIA
ACCESSORY NERVE
2nd CERVICAL N.
3rd CERVICAL N.
4th CERVICAL N.
5th CERVICAL N.
TRANS. SCAPULAR A.

ZITA STEAD.

Fig. 35

The cervical part of the exposure got by sternomastoid eversion. (A) Accessory and second cervical nerves enter an interval between superficial and deep parts of sternomastoid (see Fig. 53).
At the root of neck the two arched structures of the left side are seen—thoracic duct and inferior thyroid artery ; also the vertebral artery, forming the shaft of the broad arrow made by longus colli medially and scalenus anterior laterally. The inset shows how the great auricular nerve is jeopardised (see footnote, p. 56, for McCollum's observation).

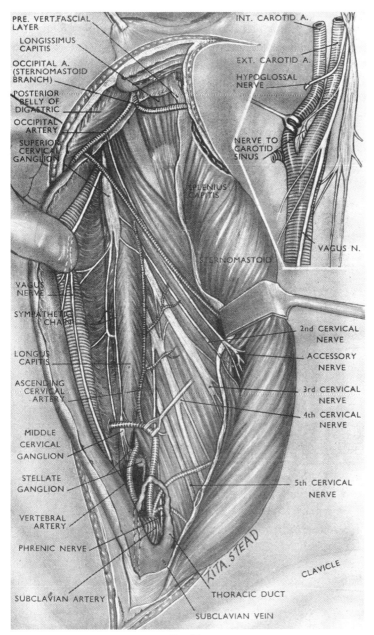

PRE. VERT.FASCIAL LAYER
LONGISSIMUS CAPITIS
OCCIPITAL A. (STERNOMASTOID BRANCH)
POSTERIOR BELLY OF DIGASTRIC
OCCIPITAL ARTERY
SUPERIOR CERVICAL GANGLION
SPLENIUS CAPITIS
VAGUS NERVE
SYMPATHETIC CHAIN
LONGUS CAPITIS
ASCENDING CERVICAL ARTERY
MIDDLE CERVICAL GANGLION
STELLATE GANGLION
VERTEBRAL ARTERY
PHRENIC NERVE
SUBCLAVIAN ARTERY

INT. CAROTID A.
EXT. CAROTID A.
HYPOGLOSSAL NERVE
NERVE TO CAROTID SINUS
VAGUS N.
STERNOMASTOID
2nd CERVICAL NERVE
ACCESSORY NERVE
3rd CERVICAL NERVE
4th CERVICAL NERVE
5th CERVICAL NERVE
CLAVICLE
ZITA.STEAD
THORACIC DUCT
SUBCLAVIAN VEIN

Fig. 36

The cervical part of the exposure got by sternomastoid eversion. (B)
The carotid bundle is displaced medially showing the sympathetic trunk
in the neck. A glimpse of the stellate ganglion is seen behind the
vertebral artery. The inset shows vagal and sympathetic twigs to carotid
sinus. The internal carotid artery hides the essential glossopharyngeal
branch. (The last $\frac{1}{4}$ inch of the thoracic duct often looks blue because of
venous reflux.)

section, in fact, is not only unlovely but useless. On the other hand, when the borders of the skin incision on the mastoid are reflected nothing is easier than to peel off the fibres of sternomastoid together with those of splenius.

When this detachment is accomplished and the upper part of sternomastoid has been everted well beyond a right angle, a superb approach begins to open, not only for the surgeon but for students of anatomy, giving to both at a most trivial cost in structure the freedom of the neck.

The special interest of Fiolle and Delmas lay, however, in the carotid bundle ; but when there is need for further exposure we must secure a much more complete eversion of sternomastoid than they required for their limited objective. The skin incision continues down along the anterior edge of sternomastoid to reach the sternum. Then after dividing the investing layer of deep fascia together with two cutaneous nerves (anterior cervical and great auricular [1]), plus the transverse part of the anterior jugular vein, a single obstacle remains to stop eversion of the whole muscle and prevent displacement inward of the carotid bundle.

The omohyoid check.—Opposite the sixth cervical vertebra the omohyoid crosses deep to the sternomastoid sheath and super-ficial to the internal jugular vein which overlaps the carotid trunk. The tendon of the muscle is fastened to the deep face of the sheath, which here unites with the ' mesenteric ' layer of deep cervical fascia—a fascia that wraps the omohyoid as though it were gut and moors it loosely to the clavicle (p. 48 and Fig. 32). This ' mesenteric ' layer also clothes and links the bellies of the other muscles of the infrahyoid group, and with them represents in man and other mammals the single fleshy layer in the seal and certain reptiles (Fig. 37). The ' mesenteric ' fascial layer is thus what French anatomists have called *une aponévrose déshabitée*, a forsaken muscle sheath. It shows at birth a trace of fleshy fibre and may retain through life a few striped shreds that cling like creeper to the internal jugular vein. The jugulo-omohyoid lymph gland, too, lying where the muscle crosses the vein, can become a focus of infective induration stemming from an ulcer at the tongue's tip, or spreading from nearby glands. Care is thus required when we free and divide this omohyoid check. With

---

[1] Mr. S. McCollum, Surgeon to the Adelaide Hospital, Dublin, tells me that his *men* patients who shave complain of the anæsthetic area produced in front of the angle of the mandible by section of the great auricular nerve. It should not be impossible (in the absence of dense adhesions) to save the nerve and free it far enough to leave sternomastoid ' on the leash ' but mobile.

that done we can evert the *whole* sternomastoid through roughly
two right angles ; then we can reach and deal with every structure
of surgical importance in the neck (Figs. 35 and 36). A catalogue

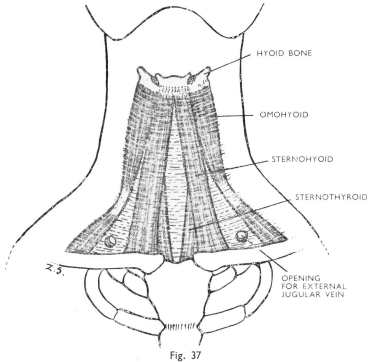

HYOID BONE

OMOHYOID

STERNOHYOID

STERNOTHYROID

OPENING
FOR EXTERNAL
JUGULAR VEIN

Fig. 37

The infrahyoid ' strap ' muscles ensheathed by the second (or ' mesenteric ')
layer of deep cervical fascia. These muscles form a continuous layer in the seal,
and in Uromastix, the spiny-tailed lizard of Egyptian deserts. In man there are
gaps where the fascia is no longer occupied by muscle, forming the *aponévrose
déshabitée* of French anatomists who agree that it is *this* fascia which forms the
back wall of Burns' space (see Fig. 34). T. H. Bryce (Quain's *Anatomy*, 11th Edn.,
vol. IV, p. 64) also holds the French view against the consensus of British opinion
which relates the space to cleavage of the first, or peripheral, layer of deep
cervical fascia.

of possible objectives would therefore be as tedious as the recital
of an index, and I shall merely name and deal with two :—

1. The vertebral artery in two parts of its second stage, and
   in its first.

2. The posterior rami of C1, C2, C3, C4.

The vertebral artery followed down on either side will lead
us past the stellate ganglion, behind and past the arch of the
thoracic duct on the left side. Down beyond this in the absence
of adhesive lesions dissection with the finger can—without tearing
a venule—expose the whole length of the left subclavian artery

to where it springs from the aorta, or, on the right side the tight twisted fork of the innominate artery ; then the trunk itself, and with it part of the aortic arch.

THE VERTEBRAL ARTERY

EXPOSURE OF THE TOP SEGMENT OF THE SECOND STAGE [1]

This stage begins as a rule at the foramen in the sixth cervical transverse process and ends as the vessel leaves the upper rim of the foramen in the atlas vertebra (Fig. 38). *I* begin topsy-turvily by dealing first with the all-but-final part of the *second* stage of this artery : its ' seat of election,' gauged by ease of access, lies at the top of the neck, near where the upper end of sternomastoid can be detached and everted from the mastoid process.

During the lapse of twenty years this method existed only as a glass-jar specimen at the Dublin Royal College, and as pages in a book—a cure, in fact, for which there was no disease. But there is a saying, older much than Homer (who quotes it twice), that new, valid material " will *of itself* lure and exploit its man." [2] And, after twenty years, the exposure was most courteously

---

[1] The substance of the following pages was written over thirty years ago and was later published in *Exposures of Long Bones and Other Surgical Methods*, Wright, 1927. On receiving my copy of the *Journal of Bone and Joint Surgery* for February 1956 I learnt for the first time (from a paper by Jefferson *et al.*, p. 114) that Drüner (1917) in *Zentralblatt für Chirurgie*, **44,** 67, had published a method of tying this same second-stage segment of the vertebral artery, which Sir Geoffrey agrees to regard as ' the site of election.'

The comment, however, that " Henry's operation is not strikingly different from Drüner's " would certainly have weight if the *objective* and not the approach is to be the test of an exposure ; then all exposures would be alike—whether the femur, for example, were reached from the front, the side, or the back.

In the present circumstance (unless my German fails me), Drüner incises from the mastoid process downwards at the hinder edge of sternomastoid—" abwärts zum Hinterrande des Kopfdrehers (St. cl. m.) "—thereby threatening, rather than avoiding (as he claims), injury to the accessory nerve. Happily for me the wiser hands and heads of Fiolle and Delmas were there to lead my own approach down to the *front* of sternomastoid.

The whole drift of Drüner's access is different—use, for example, of a lesser occipital nerve as guide to the artery, instead of a plain trust in bony points. Indeed, I might make quite a list of variants if I could for a moment forget the heart-felt "Ha-ow pahltry ! " of a bored Yankee.

Applicability is, after all, what matters in a method ; and perhaps it is unreasonable to think that the rumour of virtual identity, with so august a background and so long a start, can be overtaken by fact.

[2] *Odyssey*, XVI, 294, and XIX, 13. In pre-Homeric days the new thing was iron—iron in the Bronze Age.

acknowledged and recurringly employed by Dr D. C. Elkin, then a colonel in the U.S. Army Medical Service (*Annals of Surgery*, 1946, **124**, 934). Nearer home, Mr Harvey Jackson, F.R.C.S., tells me he has used it on four occasions.

Prior to 1925, ligations of the vertebral, other than in the first stage, had been performed where the artery lies in its third stage upon the atlas arch. Even in the cadaver the passage of a needle round this atlantal portion of the vessel tears the large venous plexus which envelops it; and, whatever method of exposure is used, the vessel remains deeply placed in a limited field.

Injury to the venous plexus, with serious loss of blood, occurred in the two cases in which ligation of the third stage has been recorded,[1] and it seemed desirable to describe a simple *overt* method of tying the second stage of the artery, particularly as forcible hæmorrhage from the cephalic end of the vessel has occurred in cases where the vertebral was injured.

Actually, the question of tying this part of the vertebral arose in relation to a case of large innominate aneurysm which the late Sir F. Conway Dwyer was treating in 1925 at the Richmond Hospital, Dublin. His initial ligation of the right subclavian and carotid stems had resulted in a slight immediate diminution of the aneurysmal swelling, too small, however, for Dwyer's satisfaction. It was therefore proposed to tie the vertebral artery, but X-rays showed the aneurysm extending from the aortic arch to the seventh cervical transverse process—almost completely covering the access to the *first* stage of the vertebral artery. I therefore ventured (I was young once) to suggest the following method of tying the second stage—needlessly, for the patient's aneurysm five weeks later had shrunk sufficiently to quash the thought of intervention, much to my callow and unchristian disappointment.

ANATOMY

In the adult skeleton the breadth of the examining thumb lies comfortably between the transverse process of the atlas and that of the axis vertebra; $\frac{3}{4}$ in. of the vertebral artery is available in this interval. Elsewhere in the neck the intertransverse spaces are comparatively small and are less easily identified. The second

---

[1] R. Lauenstein, *Zentralb. f. Chir.*, 1918, **45**, 149 ; and E. Schemmel, *ibid.*, 1918, **45**, 871.

stage of the vertebral is thus most readily exposed between the
atlas and axis (Fig. 38).

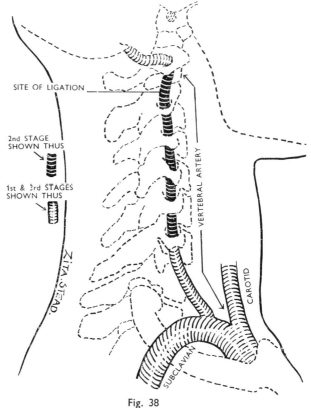

SITE OF LIGATION

2nd STAGE
SHOWN THUS

1st & 3rd STAGES
SHOWN THUS

VERTEBRAL ARTERY

CAROTID

SUBCLAVIAN

ZITA-STEAD.

Fig. 38

The vertebral artery in the neck showing the second stage and the
site for ligature.

Under the cutaneous, platysmal, and fascial coverings of the
neck, five structures must be dealt with at successive depths :—

1. The *sternomastoid muscle*.

2. The *spinal accessory nerve*, which enters the muscle two
   (or sometimes three) fingerbreadths below the tip of the
   mastoid process, running as a rule in a layer of fat and
   often obscured by lymphatic glands (Fig. 42).

3. The dense and dubiously named *prevertebral fascia* lying
   deep to the fat.[1]

---

[1] The term ' prevertebral' applied to this fascia though acceptable to morphologists
because they know it covers muscle supplied by *anterior* rami may raise some doubt
in surgeons who deal with what they see.   For levator scapulæ, which springs from the
transverse processes of atlas and axis and from *posterior* tubercles of those of C3 and C4,
lies " at the back and side of neck " (Gray), for the most part *behind* the vertebræ.

4. The stout and quite separate first slip of the *levator scapulæ muscle* arising from the tip of the transverse process of the atlas (Fig. 43).

5. The thin flat first tendon of splenius cervicis lying deep to the levator slip.

Deep to structures 4 and 5 is the first intertransverse space, bounded in front and behind by an intertransverse muscle, and containing the part of the vertebral artery to be tied (Fig. 38).

The posterior intertransverse muscle is as a rule very feebly developed and does not screen the artery. The *anterior intertransverse muscle*, too, in itself does not conceal the vessel. It is often, however, continuous laterally with the first slip of the splenius cervicis (Fig. 39) which lies deep to that of levator scapulæ and so, too, must be cut in order to open the first intertransverse space. The weak fibres of intertransverse muscle are easily divulsed.

The *internal jugular vein* (Fig. 42) is in danger during the definition of the spinal accessory if the dissection is carried *in front of* the tips of the transverse processes.

The *anterior ramus of the second cervical nerve* crosses the vertebral artery transversely and is fixed and flattened out against it by the tight translucent sheath that clothes the vessel.

BONY LANDMARKS.—The first deep guide in this ligation is the tip of the long transverse process of the atlas (Fig. 40). It should be unmistakable when the sternomastoid

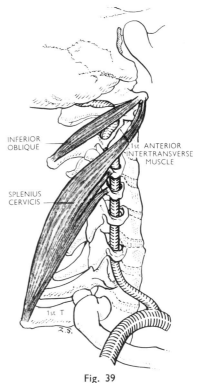

Fig. 39

The head, in this figure, faces ' half left,' as if for operation on the right side of the neck. Inferior oblique partly masks the top segment of the second stage of the vertebral artery in the thumb-wide first intertransverse space.

The first anterior intertransverse muscle often blends, as in the figure, with splenius cervicis whose highest tendon goes to the tip of the transverse process of atlas where it is covered by the highest tendon of levator scapulæ. Failure to recall this superposition of a nearly finger-thick and well-defined levator origin upon a thin and flattened splenius tendon explains why the surgeon, after easily surrounding and dividing the levator piece, so often thinks he has merely cut through part of it. So, for complete clearance of the first intertransverse space, divide levator and splenial attachments to the transverse process of atlas ; disrupt the anterior intertransverse muscle.

has been mobilised, and is felt one fingerbreadth below and one in front of the mastoid tip.

The transverse process of the axis, on the other hand, is much shorter, and may be confused with a bony eminence behind and below it which consists of the articular process of the axis and that of the third cervical vertebra. During the operation this joint becomes surprisingly prominent when the head is turned away.

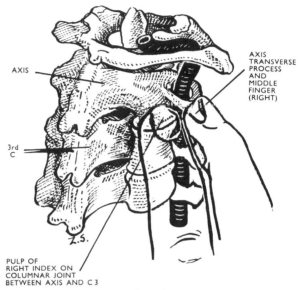

Fig. 40

Find the thumb-wide space between the transverse processes of atlas and of axis. Mark the tip of each process with recognisable forceps for easy reference throughout the operation. When the patient's head is turned away from the surgeon, the columnar joint between axis and the third cervical vertebra becomes prominent and may then be mistaken for the transverse process of axis. The figure shows how, on the *right* side, when the pulp of the *right* index finger touches the articular prominence, the adjacent middle-finger tip will touch the tip of the transverse process of axis. (Left fingers are used on the left side.)

These two bony points may be distinguished in the following way : On the right side, when the right index finger-tip of the surgeon, *pointing to the patient's head*, rests on the projecting joint, the tip of the middle finger alongside (and touching the index) rest precisely on the transverse process of the axis (Fig. 40).

THE OPERATION

Posture.—The patient lies on his back with the neck extended and the chin turned away from the vessel to be tied. This,

of course, moves our main landmark : the tip of the atlas transverse process turns with the chin and lies in front of that of
axis.

Incision (Fig. 41).—The skin, platysma, and deep fascia are
divided along the anterior border of the sternomastoid from the
cricoid level to the skull. The knife then turns back across the
base of the mastoid and cuts to the bone, dividing the sterno-

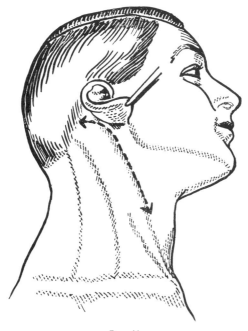

Fig. 41

Draw the lobule of the ear forward. Divide skin,
platysma, and fascia along the anterior border of
sternomastoid from the cricoid level to the skull.
Cut backwards to the bone across the base of the
mastoid, dividing the attachment which the
process gives to sternomastoid and splenius capitis.

mastoid insertion with the mastoid part of the splenius capitis.

Mobilise the sternomastoid and turn it down and out through
two right angles with the mastoid part of splenius (Fig. 42).[1]

Define the spinal accessory nerve, which enters the sternomastoid two (or three) fingerbreadths below the mastoid tip. In
doing this avoid the internal jugular vein by keeping the dissection
posterior to the tips of the transverse processes.

[1] This detachment and eversion of the mastoid end of the muscle is invaluable *as a first
step* in the ordinary removal of cervical glands in malignant cases.

Feel the deep guide, *i.e.*, the tip of the transverse process of the atlas. Pick up and divide the thick ' prevertebral ' fascia obliquely downwards from this bony point, parallel with the spinal accessory

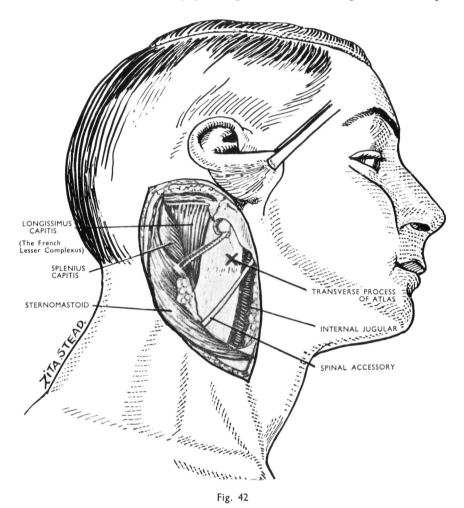

LONGISSIMUS
CAPITIS

(The French
Lesser Complexus)

SPLENIUS
CAPITIS

STERNOMASTOID

ZITA STEAD.

TRANSVERSE PROCESS
OF ATLAS

INTERNAL JUGULAR

SPINAL ACCESSORY

Fig. 42

Mobilise the cut fibres of sternomastoid and splenius. Turn them down and out through two right angles, exposing a layer of fat in which the accessory nerve runs obliquely. Define the nerve, and from the tip (X) of the transverse process of atlas—your deep guide— cut through the fat, above and parallel to the nerve. A thick fascia, questionably termed ' prevertebral,' is thus exposed ; divide it along the same line as the fat. Locate the tip of the cervical transverse processes and work *behind* them to avoid injuring the internal jugular vein.

(Fig. 43). The stout, and quite separate, origin of the levator scapulæ from the atlas transverse process is thus exposed. Define it just below the atlas in the same way as a vessel is defined : use an aneurysm needle and divide the muscle upon it. A few shreds of muscle disturbed by the needle will often remain (anterior intertransverse fibres); divulse these. Raise and divide the thin first tendon of splenius cervicis on the needle.

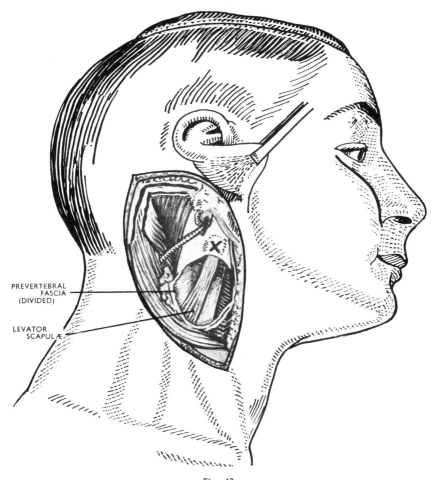

Fig. 43

Division of the so-called prevertebral fascia exposes the topmost and quite separate slip of levator scapulæ.

The vertebral artery is then seen passing up, forwards, and out in the space between axis and atlas. It is crossed here at variable heights by the anterior ramus of the second cervical nerve, and this irregular location, together with the squeezing of the ramus by the tough perivascular sheath, may retard its detection. The nerve swells surprisingly once the sheath is opened.

The simplicity of the operation depends on a lively and constant regard for two bony points—the ipsilateral tips of the transverse processes of atlas and axis : *In all positions of the head the line joining their tips overlies and is parallel with the relevant*

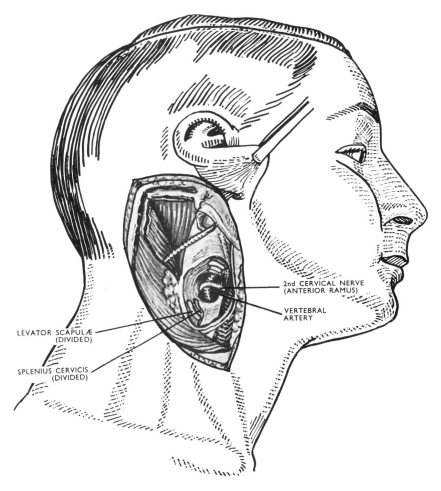

Fig. 44

Pass an aneurysm needle around the slip of levator scapulæ *as if it were an artery*. Deep to it lies the topmost slip of splenius cervicis (Figs. 39 and 50) ; divide this, too, and divulse adherent shreds of anterior intertransverse muscle. The vertebral artery, crossed by the anterior ramus of the second cervical nerve, is then exposed in the thumbwide intertransverse space between atlas and axis. The nerve is so tightly bound to the vessel that it may be difficult to see till the tough, thin sheath is opened.

piece of vertebral artery. A Michel clip fastened over each bony point keeps them in view.

THE VERTEBRAL ARTERY

EXPOSURE OF THE SECOND STAGE FROM C2 TO C6

This portion of the artery lies in the channel formed alternately by tunnels that pierce cervical transverse processes and the spaces that separate them. The vessel can be exposed in continuity if we resect appropriate parts of *costal* elements of vertebræ from C2 to C6, after a full sternomastoid eversion.

Two prevertebral muscles—longus colli and longus capitis—lie immediately in front of these costal objectives, and must be mobilised and drawn outwards. To reach these muscles, say on the right side, displace the right carotid bundle leftwards, and with it the larynx and pharynx after dividing the short sagittal mooring that links the common sheath of the cervical viscera to prevertebral fascia (Fig. 45). Then deal with longus colli.

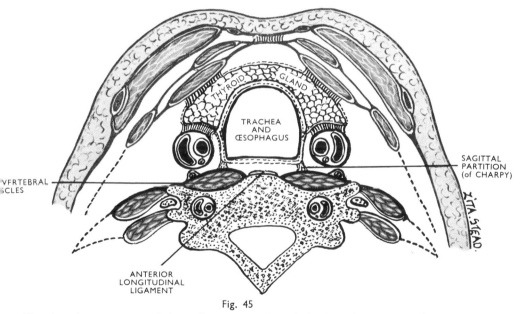

Fig. 45

The visceral compartment of the neck containing thyroid gland, trachea, and œsophagus. At a higher level of section the compartment contains larynx and pharynx. The figure shows (1) how the sagittal partitions of Charpy—which are easily disrupted or stretched— moor the viscera, but very loosely, to prevertebral fascia and bound the retrovisceral space ; it also shows (2) how the retrovisceral space will allow of visceral displacement when one of the sagittal partitions bounding it is either broken or stretched ;   (3) how there is a relative solidity between the cervical viscera which permits of *en masse* movement not only vertically as in swallowing, but also *transversely*, thus allowing exposure of the interval between right and left prevertebral muscles. The figure shows that there is sufficient union between the carotid bundle and the visceral compartment to let the bundle share in the *en masse* sideways movement ; and (4) how the median part of the anterior longitudinal ligament lies uncovered between prevertebral muscle fibres on either side. We can thus work from *there* when we detach longus colli from the vertebral bodies (See also Fig. 46).

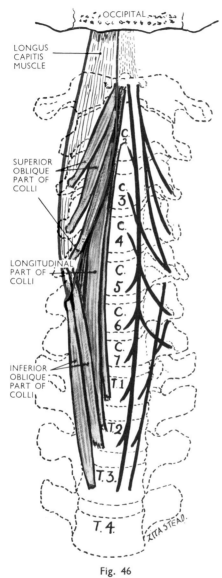

Fig. 46

The three parts of longus colli (in black) : longus capitis (in red) seen from in front

The longitudinal part of colli and the 'red muscle' (capitis) sandwich the upper oblique part of colli. When, therefore, we detach the deep longitudinal part of colli from the vertebral *bodies*, the whole sandwich—longitudinal part of colli, the upper (intervening) part of colli, and longus capitis—can be turned out towards the anterior tubercles ; for these tubercles are now the sole remaining attachments of its relevant parts.

The ' vertical ' part of colli (Fig. 46).—This part (whose fibres curve gently and are vertical to nothing) is the key to the position : it is the most medial and deepest component of a tripartite muscle ; it lies behind two *oblique* components, an upper and a lower. The *lower* oblique is the smallest and most variable of the three[1] ; it slopes up and out from bodies of T3, T2, T1 to anterior tubercles of C6 and C5. The *upper oblique component* slopes up and in from anterior tubercles of C6, C5, C4, and C3 to the lateral face of the tubercle on the anterior arch of atlas.

Important and powerful additions pass with an upward and inward slant from costal elements of C5, C6, C7 to join the deep ' vertical ' part and seem to determine the actual outward curve of its fibres. The gently curving ' vertical ' fibres are attached only to vertebral *bodies*—the lower moiety from T3 to C5, the upper from the anterior tubercle of atlas to C4. (As the state of longus colli attachments escapes concise description, I give an orthodox account.)

[1] According to the high authority of Le Double, longus colli is "the most variable of all muscles in the human economy"—a remark which applies in chief to the number of its attachments. The basic tripartite *plan* of colli is, however, as constant as anything in myology.

The crucial disc.—The transition, therefore, of ' vertical ' fibres from so-called origin to so-called insertion (or better, from upper to lower moiety) takes place at the disc between C4 and C5. For that reason the infinitesimal ' stripping angle ' (p. 5) which the longitudinal fibres of colli make with vertebral bodies opens downwards above the disc and upwards below it. A rugine, therefore, introduced medially at the level of this crucial disc will best detach the ' vertical ' part of colli by working *into* those unseen but important angles—upwards above the disc, downwards below it.

Fortunately for our purpose in these pages, a midline fusion of right and left ' colli ' (normal in herbivoræ, where the two form a single muscle) is very rare in man, so that, except near atlas, a thumbwide space separates them and leaves the vertebral bodies clothed only by anterior longitudinal ligaments. The presence of this interspace holds a special benefit : it shortens the distance through which we need to shift larynx and pharynx in order to make the medial border of colli accessible for detachment.

Very rarely longus capitis will fuse with its fellow across the middle line and cover the interspace between the two colli muscles —a rub to test the art of surgery.

Longus capitis (formerly rectus capitis anticus major).—This, which is the only other muscle immediately concerning us, covers all but the inner edge of the *upper oblique* part of longus colli. The longus capitis is the more anterior, more lateral, and more bulky of the two prevertebral muscles ; it forms with the ' vertical ' fibres of longus colli a sandwich whose ' filling ' is the upper *oblique* part of colli (Fig. 46). (Capitis often springs, as shown here in *red*, from C3 to C6 ; it may also join with the lower oblique part of colli and thus get origin from thoracic *bodies*.)

When, therefore, we detach and displace the ' vertical ' part of longus colli outwards, that muscle will carry off with it the two bellies that lie on its anterior face—(1) its own oblique upper belly, and (2) the major part of longus capitis. This clearance of muscle attachments from the front of a body and a transverse cervical process must reach to and *stop* at the medial side of the relevant anterior tubercle. A path is thus cleared to costal processes from C3 to C6.

If, however, we wish to include in our exposure the vascular segment encircled by the foramen transversarium of C2 we must divide the topmost tendon of the upper *oblique* part of colli—a part that is *not* covered by capitis and reaches (with ' vertical ' fibres) to the tubercle on the anterior arch of atlas (Fig. 46).

The groove marking the relevant piece of costal process.— Displacement of the prevertebral muscles lays bare a shallow longitudinal groove on the front of each transverse process from C3 to C6—a groove just wide enough to lodge the tip of a little finger (Fig. 47).

The groove is bounded *laterally* by the anterior tubercle whose apparent size is magnified by scalene attachments ; *medially* by a flatter prominence, more diffuse in character, which *looks* as if the rib-head of a plastic costal rudiment had spread against and stuck to the side of its own vertebral body. Each rib-head thickening has an upward projection or apophysis, semilunar in shape, whose ' free ' upper border is like the curved edge of a trimmed finger-nail, and about as long. The semilunar apophysis overlaps the lateral side of the intervertebral disc next above it and bounds the so-called ' unco-vertebral ' joint [1] of Trolard.

Each groove, from C2 to C6, exactly covers and (except for a part of vertebral vein and sympathetic nerves) lies next the vertebral artery as it goes through a foramen. The bone forming the floor of the groove is about as thick as the toe-nail of a big toe. It is most safely resected by using a rongeur forceps whose blunt nose has the same width as the groove which it must span, grasp, and bite through from upper to lower edge provided it bite shallowly and with great caution (Fig. 47).

The anterior rami of cervical nerves lie opposite the groove but *behind* the artery. Immediately lateral to the groove, however, the rami curve so sharply forward round the artery that if the anterior tubercle of a transverse process is removed, the numerically corresponding ramus just below it is likely to be hurt.

The special case at C2.—The foramen transversarium of axis is unlike those from C3 to C7 in two respects : (1) it is not bounded in front by a thin grooved scale of bone but by an ungrooved bar about $\frac{1}{5}$ in. in diameter ; (2) its direction is not vertically upward, but slopes up and out, making an angle of some 45 degrees with the transverse plane of the neck. The slope of the artery corresponds to that of the foramen.

---

[1] Poirier (*Traité d'Anatomie Humaine*, 2ème Edn., 1899, T.I., p. 794) states that these joints were " dimly perceived " by Barkow, well studied by Luschka in 1858, and named by Trolard of Algiers in 1892—not very happily, however, for uncus means a hook, while these apophyses are not hooked like claws but concave like fingernails on their deep aspect. Unguiculo-central or, better, costo-central, might denote the joints they bound, for they are in series with thoracic articulations between rib heads and vertebral bodies.

Before dividing this bony bar locate the single tubercle of the transverse process of axis. Using a rongeur, divide the bone from in front at the inner side of the tubercle. Cut piecemeal and posteromedially. The length of the oblique cut will be $\frac{1}{4}$ in.

The venous accompaniment of the vertebral artery.[1]—The vertebral vein while in its second (transversarial-intertransverse) stage is fed chiefly from cervical vertebræ, each a capacious reservoir. Serial sections show that the semilunar outline of this

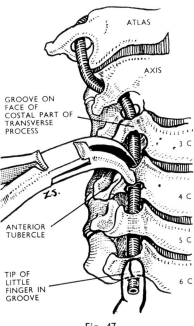

ATLAS

AXIS

GROOVE ON FACE OF COSTAL PART OF TRANSVERSE PROCESS

3 C

4 C

5 C

6 C

ANTERIOR TUBERCLE

TIP OF LITTLE FINGER IN GROOVE

Fig. 47

The costal face of each cervical transverse process, except the first and second, shows a longitudinal groove. The groove just fits the tip of a little finger. It is bounded laterally by the anterior tubercle of the process ; medially by a low, placenta-shaped thickening, such as the head and ligaments of a recessive rib might make in fusing with the relevant vertebral body. (The free, upper edge of the thickening helps to form a Luschka's joint.)

Resection of the grooved part of the costal face—which has the thickness of a big-toe nail—reveals a transversarial segment of the vertebral artery. The anterior ramus of a cervical nerve lies directly behind each of these arterial segments.

[1] A network called the suboccipital venous plexus permeates the mass of fat in front of the complexus ; it is largely made up of tributaries from adjacent muscle. The plexus is at once a link and a source. *As a link*, it unites three deep cervical veins—vertebral, profunda cervicis, and (when present) posterior jugular—with the collar-like plexus on the atlas ring, immediately below foramen magnum. Here the basilar sinus joins with the occipital sinus. The vertical depth of the collar thus formed is supplemented by the topmost reach of veins that have either just been lining the inner face of the spinal canal or else have coated the outer face of cervical vertebræ.

As a source, the suboccipital plexus is the principal origin of the three deep veins already mentioned. The vertebral and posterior jugular have a common origin on the atlas arch ; the deep cervical vein arises more laterally nearer the mastoid process. At the root of the neck deep cervical and posterior jugular each pass forward between the transverse process of C7 and the neck of first rib ; the deep cervical joins the vertebral vein, which it often exceeds in size, while posterior jugular (like the vertebral) enters the innominate. *Posterior* jugular, like profunda cervicis, lies behind the cervical transverse processes, but more medially, and like profunda, it, too, enters the innominate vein after passing between the neck of the first rib and the transverse process of C7. The small *anterior* vertebral vein, which begins as a plexus round cervical transverse processes, enters the lower end of the vertebral, and an *accessory* vertebral vein may leave the foramen in the transverse process of C7 and join the innominate. If these facts are not anticipated the multiplicity of veins close to the stellate ganglion may cause surprise.

All these veins anastomose among themselves so freely that they are often able to deplete the cranial cavity when the anterior, external and internal jugular veins are blocked by strangulation, leaving the face congested and the brain blanched (Charpy).

vein embraces the lateral curve of the arterial wall, and that though single above, the vein is apt to duplicate below and to give downward branches that have special bony channels formed by subdivisions of some or other of the transversarial foramina.

At each intertransverse space of the neck the main vertebral vein receives an influx brought by some twenty to sixty tributaries that pass out with spinal nerves through each intervertebral foramen—a fact that might seem to make approach to them less attractive than one directed to segments that are bone-encircled. Also it is worth noting that while the vertebral artery is relatively free in its osteofibrous canal, the principal vein (whose task, apart from draining spinal cord and nerves, is to drain bone) is *fixed* : to bone in transversarial foramina ; to fibrous tissue in the intertransverse spaces.

Experience shows, however, that although it is impossible to expose any part of the second stage of the vertebral artery without wounding the vein or its tributaries, *styptic* hæmostasis, with muscle shreds or otherwise, is easily obtained in the narrow track of the vertebrals.

The risk of air embolism.—This accident seems *not* to have happened in man in connection with the surgery of vertebral vessels but is none the less worth considering. The main vertebral vein is, we saw, bound to bone or fibrous tissue so that its lumen when cut into is likely to gape. Air embolism by way of vertebral veins is therefore not impossible ; it was, in fact, as François Franck proved, a special cause of death in dogs whose cranial diploe was opened ; for the vertebral vein of dogs has far more importance than their tiny internal jugular, and is, in them, the chief path by which blood returns from head and neck. It may be that in man the restricted size and semilunar shape of the vertebral vein are safeguards. But time alone will show whether a prophylactic ligature of the lowest or ' free ' stage of the vertebral vein, in prelude to exposure of the second stage of the artery, would be a wise and justifiable procedure—or just ' plain yellow.' In such matters Hegel's advice is good : " Obey your conscience, but remember that you may have the conscience of an ass."

THE VERTEBRAL ARTERY

THE FIRST STAGE, WITH RELATED STRUCTURES

After we have mobilised the lower part of sternomastoid and turned it out through two right angles (p. 56), we must displace the carotid bundle inwards. For this nothing could serve us better than the complete absence of lateral branches or tributaries stemming from or entering the common carotid portion of the bundle : *its vascular ties are on one side only*—a fact in daily use, which though unique in the anatomy of large vessels is not, so far as I know, mentioned as worth notice.[1]

It happens, too, that both posterior branches of the *external* carotid have a lengthwise course in the neck and so will not hamper the medial movement of the bundle.

These opposite displacements of bundle and sternomastoid reveal an arched disposal, single on the right, double on the left.

THE ARCHED STRUCTURES (Fig. 35)

On the left side the thoracic duct curves out behind the carotid sheath ; somewhat higher up, but on a deeper plane, the inferior thyroid artery curves in. On the right, the right lymphatic duct is surgically negligible, and only the *thyroid* arch needs attention.

The arch of the thoracic duct.—On the left side, the top of this lymphatic arch lies two or three fingerbreadths below the carotid tubercle of Chassaignac. This tubercle which projects forward from the transverse process of the sixth cervical vertebra is often small and in most persons owes its prominence and palpability less to its own size than to the rather sharp recession of the seventh process in the region where the forward curve of bodies of cervical vertebræ begins to blend with the backward curve described by the upper dorsal bodies.

Find this arch, which runs in a potentially tough blend of fat and small lymph glands, at the place where it nears the junction of internal jugular with subclavian to end—by a blue $\frac{1}{4}$-in.—in either. It will then be seen that when sternomastoid has been

---

[1] *Farabeuf's triangle.*—This is another useful and neglected feature of carotid anatomy which forms an admirable rallying point in the neck. The triangle is bounded laterally and *behind* by the internal jugular vein ; *in front*, by the stem of the common facial vein (which often conforms to the term thyro-lingual-facial) ; *above*, by the forward curving of the hypoglossal nerve which is the base of the triangle. The *floor* of the triangle is formed by the carotid bifurcation and is roughly bisected by the descendens hypoglossi nerve.

turned outwards (after dividing omohyoid and the anterior jugular vein), all closely related structures, *excepting* the carotid bundle, lie on planes immediately behind this arched portion of thoracic duct. When found and mobilised the ductal arch can for the moment be pushed down behind the clavicle.

The arch of the inferior thyroid artery, and the thyrocervical trunk from which it rises, are next dealt with. The arch lies about a fingerbreadth below the carotid tubercle, and the trunk is often held laterally by two transverse branches—the suprascapular behind the clavicle and, higher up, the transverse cervical. If these vessels prevent displacement of the arch, tie and divide them. Open the prevertebral fascia close along the *medial* side of the phrenic nerve which shows through this covering, taking care not to injure scalenus anterior. Catch the medial lip of the divided fascia and use it to envelop and retract the thyroid arch which it will thus draw inwards. With the arch goes the close-linked middle sympathetic cervical ganglion. The ascending cervical artery and possibly the anterior vertebral vein (which it is important not to slit lengthwise) are also rolled cigarette-like in the fascial wrap. The phrenic nerve remains *in situ*.

The broad arrow of the vertebrals.—This cigarette-rolling retraction exposes the angle formed below the carotid tubercle by the almost vertical edge of longus cervicis meeting the outward slant of scalenus anterior. Below the tubercle the vertebral vessels divide the angle and thus form the shaft of a kind of broad arrow. Near the tubercle the vessels are covered by an overlap of muscle, but, after the fascia has been rolled off, they lie bare some three fingerbreadths below that landmark. At this level the vertebral vein is anterior to the artery, but lower down it moves out and *forward,* going thus in front of the finger-thick subclavian artery to reach the back of the innominate or the subclavian vein.

Thus, merely by turning the lower part of sternomastoid out through two right angles, and the dividing prevertebral or more accurately prescalene fascia—using the fascia to draw aside arched intervening vessels—we can expose the whole first stage of the right or left vertebral artery down to the origin of either from the first stage of the subclavian trunk.

THE FIRST STAGE OF THE SUBCLAVIAN ARTERY, ITS BRANCHES AND THE STELLATE GANGLION

These structures, we have seen, become visible while exposing the first part of the vertebral trunk by the method just described.

Of the other subclavian branches the whole thyrocervical trunk is already bare, while the costocervical trunk can be traced to the first rib where it divides into deep cervical and superior intercostal branches. The start of the internal mammary artery appears, with the phrenic nerve slanting behind it or in front. The cervical moiety of the stellate ganglion lies behind and between the paths of two arteries—the vertebral which goes upwards, the costocervical trunk which slants out. At the outer side of the vertebral artery the top of the ganglion gives off a short, usually threefold, band—the vertebral nerve of Cruveilhier—that enters the transverse process of the sixth cervical vertebra.

This cervical part of the stellate often slopes, surprisingly, out and down, and then continues with the first ganglion of the thoracic trunk—marked from it by a mere notch or waist. The part of stellate corresponding to the first thoracic ganglion lies in front of and frequently along the neck of the first rib, separated from the subclavian artery by the apex of lung and pleura, and by suprapleural membrane. Against the neck of this rib the ganglion is often felt as a rubbery thickening by the pulp of a finger passed down through the thoracic inlet so that it will find and touch the *outer* side of a small bony lump which marks where the head of the first rib joins the first thoracic vertebra. If then we tie and divide the costocervical trunk and depress the pleural dome over which the trunk has curved and acted as a mooring, the arch of the subclavian artery can be coaxed forward *and in* towards the vertebral artery, exposing completely the part of the stellate ganglion that lies behind the arch, sandwiched—now that pleura is depressed—between the arch and the catapult fork of the eighth cervical and first thoracic nerves, whose handle crosses the first rib as the lowest trunk of brachial plexus. Striping the front of the ganglion (and thus included in the sandwich) is the highest posterior or intercostal vein which may hook forward below the subclavian artery to reach the vertebral vein or the innominate.

THE LEFT SUBCLAVIAN ARTERY

Apart, however, from dividing any branch, finger dissection through sound tissue will isolate the *left* subclavian artery and leave it free and visible for easy access down to its origin from the aorta, whose arch is felt and seen in the depth of the thorax (Fig. 48).

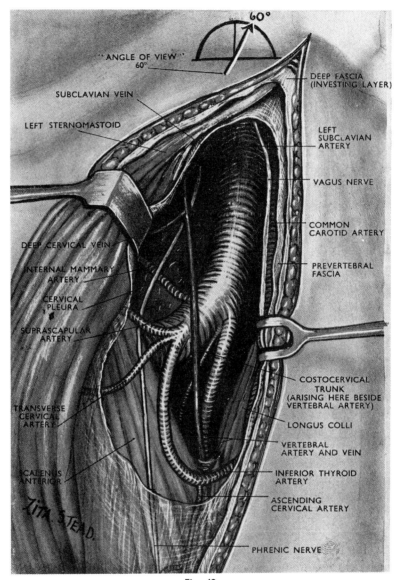

Fig. 48

The root of the neck after full eversion of the left sternomastoid

The surgeon standing at the *left* of the patient's neck looks along the arrow which makes an angle of 60 degrees with a transverse plane passing through the carotid tubercle of Chassaignac on the sixth cervical vertebra.

Note.—The thoracic duct has been thrust down out of view behind the clavicle. The jugular vein is omitted to simplify the picture.

The aortic arch could be felt and glimpsed at the base of the subclavian trunk, and it is easy—again in the absence of impassable adhesions—to tie the subclavian at that spot.

The previous medial displacement of the carotid bundle has removed the vagus nerve from our path ; the phrenic falls away with light pressure. (Throughout this procedure the thoracic ductal arch has lain where we thrust it, down behind the clavicle —crumpled but in no way injured.)

Before they are disturbed the left phrenic and vagus nerves *cross each other at the level where the arch* of the subclavian artery begins, the phrenic passing anteromedial to the vagus. The nerves thereafter keep this relation as they go apart to reach the left or ventrolateral side of the aortic arch.

THE WHOLE SUBCLAVIAN TRUNK

Our exposure can, of course, be extended to the third stage of the right or left subclavian artery (p. 53) ; and all three stages are seen in continuity when scalenus anterior is divided after safeguarding the phrenic nerve.

A plethora of veins.—The profunda vein passes between the neck of the first rib and the seventh cervical transverse process, receiving on its way a vein from the upper one or two intercostal spaces ; then it lies over the top of the pleural dome and loops forward from the pleura below the subclavian arch to reach the lower end of the vertebral vein, which terminates in the innominate. When, however, as in this present exposure, the pleural dome has been depressed, the profunda vein, carrying its superior cervical tributary, falls back against the front of the thoracic part of the stellate ganglion where it lies *medial* to its fellow-artery. Beside it, too, may lie a posterior jugular vein (p. 71). This, when it is present, ends in the innominate behind the vertebral, with which it sometimes joins.

THE INNOMINATE ARTERY

On the *right* side the lower part of our everted sternomastoid approach will reach the innominate bifurcation behind the upper part of the sternoclavicular joint.[1]

And there, again, in sound tissues mere finger dissection can

---

[1] Those who take anatomy from text-book figures instead of from the body may be surprised to find the right subclavian artery rising quite so closely up the back of right carotid, recalling otherwise the less immediate relationship of ulnar to radial artery at the normal forking of the brachial trunk—a feature that is constantly misdrawn. For artists are allowed (or are they urged ?) to show the whole fork flat, as if it all lay in a single frontal plane of the extended supine limb.

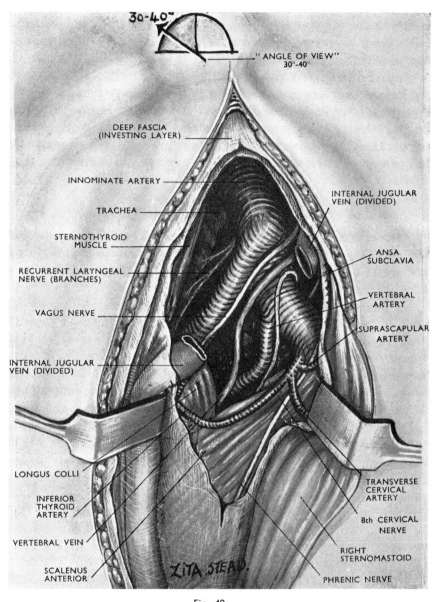

30-40°

"ANGLE OF VIEW"
30°-40°

DEEP FASCIA
(INVESTING LAYER)

INNOMINATE ARTERY

TRACHEA

STERNOTHYROID
MUSCLE

RECURRENT LARYNGEAL
NERVE (BRANCHES)

VAGUS NERVE

INTERNAL JUGULAR
VEIN (DIVIDED)

INTERNAL JUGULAR
VEIN (DIVIDED)

ANSA
SUBCLAVIA

VERTEBRAL
ARTERY

SUPRASCAPULAR
ARTERY

LONGUS COLLI

INFERIOR
THYROID
ARTERY

VERTEBRAL VEIN

SCALENUS
ANTERIOR

TRANSVERSE
CERVICAL
ARTERY

8th CERVICAL
NERVE

RIGHT
STERNOMASTOID

PHRENIC NERVE

ZITA STEAD.

Fig. 49

The root of the neck after full eversion of the right sternomastoid

The surgeon standing at the *right* of the patient's neck looks along the arrow which makes an angle of 30 to 40 degrees with a transverse plane at the carotid tubercle of Chassaignac on the sixth cervical vertebra. The right ansa subclavia, which was here a single band like that found normally on the left side, is often divided into from two to six parts. The aortic arch can be glimpsed and felt, and—in the absence of intervening aneurysm or adhesive lesions—the innominate artery can be tied where it arises.

(To simplify the picture, structures are viewed through a gap in the internal jugular instead of by retracting that vessel.)

carry the exposure of this large vessel down to the aortic arch (Fig. 49). The easy path for the finger is by the medial side of the *carotid* between that trunk and the trachea ; for passing down along the right subclavian the finger may be caught in one or other of three neural loops that clasp the artery : ansa subclavia, the right recurrent laryngeal nerve, or, farthest out along the first stage of the vessel, the loop of strands that join the phrenic to the upper end of stellate ganglion.

It is, of course, obvious that these deep, aortotropic descents into the chest are only possible in the absence of local adhesive invasion, and for the moment their precise application escapes me. But, for my part, it would be ungrateful, and indeed unwise, on that account to damn these excursions as useless. I have therefore described them, letting them wait their season : " In the long lapse of time there is nothing that may not happen."

ARTERIAL VARIETIES AT THE ROOT OF THE NECK

In the preceding paragraphs I have described arrangements which Quain (who was wise in these matters) refers to as ' usual ' —writing the word between inverted commas. In that spirit I have dealt, for example, with the arches at the root of the neck, but with full awareness of their wide range of variation.

My own experience in that region reminds me of the dangerous jest made by a Berlin comedian before the last war. " *We* all know," he said, " that 99 per cent. of the German people are strong for the Fuehrer, but wherever I go—in bus or train or tram—I meet the 1 per cent." I shall therefore be content to indicate departures from the ' usual,' neglecting their percentage happening, since figures that proclaim infrequent incidence no more preclude the surgeon from meeting an example than they will save unlucky persons from death by lightning.

But departures from Quain's ' usual ' arrangements give least trouble when we know they exist ; then, a wide access lets us see and deal with them.

They can be grouped (by the help of a little mythology) under six headings, which ' explain ' their mode of origin as follows :—

1. **Absorption.**—If we imagine a fictitious process of this kind occurring, say, at the thyrocervical trunk, some or all of its three branches (suprascapular, transverse cervical, inferior thyroid) will then arise *directly* from the subclavian artery with the occasional addition of the ascending cervical.

2. **Fusion** with a neighbour may produce a *left* innominate artery, plus the ' usual ' right.

3. **Multiplication.**—Two right vertebrals may spring separately from the subclavian and unite higher up the neck—a natural extension of those *single* vertebral trunks which spring by more than one root.

4. **Deficiencies.**—These create the need for ' replacement ' variations—as when a superior thyroid branch supplies the *back* of the gland in the absence of an inferior thyroid artery ; or when the inferior thyroid comes, as a rare anomaly, from the common carotid ; just as either the deep branch of the transverse cervical or the suprascapular artery may spring (as they often do) directly from the third stage of subclavian.

5. **Transposition.**—A left innominate artery often arises from an aorta arching to the *right*.

6. **Embryological Shift.**—A right subclavian springing from the descending (dorsal) aorta may cross up to the right behind the œsophagus. (I met one once associated with a plunging goitre.)

Displacement of the sternal end of sternomastoid.—If access to the lower end of the wound is cramped by the presence of an enlarged thyroid gland, more freedom can be got by mobilising the sternal tendon of sternomastoid—cutting through skin and fascia at its medial edge and slipping the tendon, *which is flat and finger-wide when relaxed*,[1] outwards across and past the knob-like medial end of clavicle. (It is easy to do this without injuring the sternoclavicular ligaments.)

A LATERAL APPROACH TO THE FIRST, SECOND, AND THIRD POSTERIOR CERVICAL RAMI

Exposure of this group of nerves is simplified by an exact use of the method I shall presently describe—a method based on bony points and on a gleam of fat which in the wilderness of nuchal muscle takes the eyes like a pool. Dissecting binoculars give the deep parts of the operation a final clarity.

---

[1] Like the proximal tendon of adductor longus and the distal tendon of biceps femoris. All three tendons become cord-like when taut, with a V-shaped cross-section.

OPERATIONS FOR SPASMODIC TORTICOLLIS

Unilateral section of these three rami plus section of the opposite accessory nerve was carried out in 1888 by two surgeons, Gardner of Adelaide and Keen of Philadelphia, for spasmodic torticollis. The aim of the operation is to paralyse each twitching muscle.

When, for example, spasms turn the face to *rightward* and throw the head back, then, *on the left side* we must paralyse the left sternomastoid and left trapezius by cutting the left accessory nerve plus branches of the left anterior rami from C2 and C3 in relation to sternomastoid, and for trapezius from C3 and C4.[1]

On the right side we must paralyse splenius capitis, longissimus capitis (the lesser complexus of the French), semispinalis capitis (our own complexus), together with the two right obliques plus the right recti posteriores of the head, by cutting right posterior rami of C1, C2, C3, and also (if the right trapezius is condemned) the ipsilateral nerve or nerves supplying it.

Binnie, by no means a timorous counsellor, characterised the procedure as " very complicated, and for most surgeons inadvisable " ; and the description he quotes of the operation, taken from R. Kennedy's (*British Medical Journal*, 3rd October, 1908), explains why it was not " a glittering success " : it left the surgeon deplorably unpiloted by landmarks.

Dandy (*Archives of Surgery*, 1930, **20,** 1021) made use of laminectomy to reach and cut the motor and sensory *roots* of C1, C2, C3 with, in addition, intrathecal section of both accessory cranial nerves. But even so he felt obliged to add a further section of each accessory nerve in the neck. His operation, dividing motor roots, must of course be followed by paralysis of unoffending muscles supplied by *anterior* rami.

Apart, however, from cases of spasmodic torticollis, the lateral approach by turning back the occipitomastoid attachments of

---

[1] There has been recurring doubt about the motor function of *anterior* ramal contributions that enter sternomastoid from C2 and C3. Claude Bernard in 1858 concluded that division of the spinal part of the accessory knocked out sternomastoid as a ' muscle of orientation,' leaving it to act merely as a respiratory muscle, and then only during deep inspiration. According to Sternberg (1898) the sternomastoid receives all its motor fibres from the accessory nerve, the role of the supply from anterior rami of C2 and C3 being purely sensory. More recently K. B. Corbin and his associates, Yee and Harrison, have proved that in rabbits, cats, and monkeys the cervical contributions to the innervation of sternomastoid and trapezius, coming from anterior rami of C2, C3, C4, and joining with the extracranial part of the accessory nerve, carry no motor fibres to those muscles but are entirely proprioceptive in function. " It seems," say the authors, " reasonable to conclude that a similar condition obtains in man." (*Journal of Comparative Neurology*, 1938, **69,** 315 ; 1939, **70,** 305 ; *Brain*, 1939, 191.)

sternomastoid and splenius has, I think, a special application for lesions with deep, central scarring like the following :—

A naval officer slipped on the companion-ladder of a destroyer

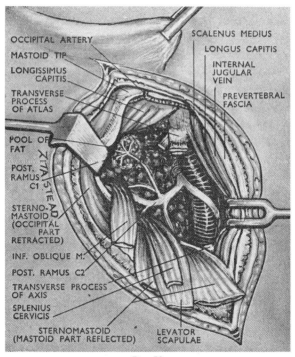

Fig. 50

The small pool of fat. (The parts are shown magnified by $1\frac{1}{2}$: the true length of the segment of vertebral artery is a thumbwidth)

The first stage of the exposure is similar to that for the seat of election of the vertebral artery in the thumbwide space between the transverse processes of atlas and axis. In addition the inferior oblique muscle has been detached from atlas and turned down and back, revealing the pool of fat that bathes the five-fold branching of the posterior ramus of C1. The trunk of C2 is seen dividing into anterior and posterior rami. (The anterior ramus—flattened and fixed against the vertebral artery—is not labelled.) At the tip of the atlas transverse process three muscles have been divided—levator scapulæ ; deep to it the upper slip of splenius cervicis ; and medial to both, the inferior oblique.
Longissimus capitis is the small complexus of the French.
The internal jugular vein is the sole hazard ; its medial retraction has exposed scalenus medius (which here reached atlas) together with longus capitis.

and fell on his head with the neck in acute flexion. During the ten years which elapsed before I examined him he had suffered from severe occipital neuralgia running to the vertex and requiring a heavy and increasing aspirin dosage for sedation. Below the occiput and to the left there could be felt a dense curled mass deep in the neck. This, I believe, was the detached and rolled up ligamentum nuchæ. The upper portion of the left complexus (semispinalis capitis)—the part supplied through the posterior rami of C1, C2, C3—was completely wasted, the motor twigs having apparently been wrenched out or broken during the extreme neck flexion, leaving the main sensory portion of the greater occipital (C2) to be caught and squeezed by scar.

ANATOMY AND THE OPERATION

To avoid repetition I shall unite structure with procedure in a single account. Detachment of sternomastoid as with exposures of the vertebral artery will be a first step, and the muscle (with the mastoid part of splenius capitis) will be mobilised and everted as far down as C6.

French textbooks simplify a rather cumbrous nomenclature : they use our old term complexus for semispinalis capitis, and call longissimus capitis complexus minor. These two ' complexi' pass from neck to skull without forming any attachment to the first three cervical vertebræ. So, since the skull base projects back at an angle from the spine, these muscles bridge the angle and subtend a space. This space, which is divided from its fellows by the midline partition of ligamentum nuchæ, forms *one half* of the suboccipital space : each half is encroached on (1) by a major mass of fat ; (2) by bellies of two posterior recti and two oblique muscles. Our three ramal objectives lie in the ipsilateral half space.

These objectives are the first posterior cervical ramus or suboccipital nerve, which is purely motor, save for an occasional sensory twig ; the second, whose medial branch is the greater occipital ; the third, whose medial branch is the third occipital. The greater and third occipitals are mainly but by no means entirely sensory.

A small downward extension of the exposure described below reveals the posterior ramus of C4. If, therefore, we expose the outer edge of the complexus mass, we can then find a path in front of it to all our main objectives. The *back* of both ' complexi' has already been uncovered at the upper end by the reflection of sternomastoid and splenius capitis ; the outer edge remains concealed by slips of levator scapulæ and splenius cervicis—both of which reach the transverse process of atlas.

The precomplexal fat.—With these slips turned down and back the edge of the complexus mass appears, and we are free to pass in front of it and enter the potential space. This space is filled with a major bulk of soft fat that bathes the second and third posterior rami together with a rich venous suboccipital plexus.

A separate and minor fat deposit that lies on a plane deep to the small muscles of the suboccipital triangle and therefore next the vertebræ, guides us to the suboccipital nerve.

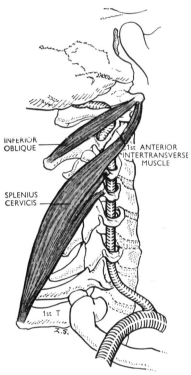

Fig. 52

The head, in this figure, faces ' half left,' as if for operation on the right side of the neck. Inferior oblique partly masks the top segment of the second stage of the vertebral artery in the thumbwide first intertransverse space.

The first anterior intertransverse muscle often blends, as in the figure, with splenius cervicis whose highest tendon goes to the tip of the transverse process of atlas where it is covered by the highest tendon of levator scapulæ. Failure to recall this superposition of a nearly finger-thick and well-defined levator origin upon a thin and flattened splenius tendon explains why the surgeon, after easily surrounding and dividing the levator piece, so often thinks he has merely cut through part of it. So, for complete clearance of the first intertransverse space, divide levator and spenial attachments to the transverse process of atlas ; disrupt the anterior intertransverse muscle.

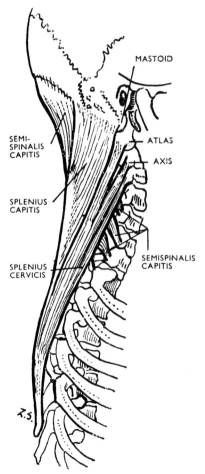

Fig. 51

Two covering muscles—sternomastoid and levator scapulæ—have been removed showing the underlying set.

The entry to an intertransverse space.—The slips or fascicles of levator scapulæ and splenius cervicis, together with those of longissimus cervicis and scalenus medius (which all go to posterior tubercles of transverse processes) cover the outer edge of the two ' complexi ' ; they also mask the entry to upper intertransverse spaces. The *names* of the fascicles, however, matter less than the ease of cutting them at their attachment to transverse-process tubercles. After they are cut, access can be got by divulsing intertransverse muscles. (This paragraph merely repeats and extends the procedure used in exposing the vertebral artery between axis and atlas, p. 64.)

Thus it is clear that if *lower* parts of splenius and the ' complexi '—supplied by C4 and C5—are also concerned in spasm, we must (since a cervical nerve corresponds numerically with the vertebra next below) open the *third and the fourth* intertransverse spaces to reach these rami. The third space will need for that a small retraction of the *anterior* ramus of C3 ; and the fourth and fifth the additional and less easy displacements of the corresponding rami of C4 and C5.

FALLACIOUS GUIDES.—It has long been the custom of text-books to repeat that we should begin by finding the thick posterior ramus of C2, and should then proceed to use it for locating the less thick rami of C1 and C3 by tracing the connecting loops that link them with C2.

Unfortunately, these connecting loops are hard to find. That to C1 may pass either in front of, or through, or behind the belly of inferior oblique, while the connection with the posterior ramus of C3 is equally elusive. Both loops break when strenuously sought.

FIXED LANDMARKS.—These posterior rami can be found *separately* by relating each to a fixed landmark.

The posterior ramus of C1 (the suboccipital nerve).—Find the belly of inferior oblique lying on the axis lamina deep to the complexus mass ; it goes from the axis spine to the end of the transverse process of atlas. Isolate it cleanly and divide its lateral attachment. Then, when the belly is turned *in* towards the spine of axis, the eye catches a gleam of fat among so many muscles—a pool no larger than a finger-tip, confined by membrane to the atlas arch. This fat is the required shield for the sub-occipital nerve and its companion vessels in a zone of restless concertina movement. It lies *deep* to where inferior oblique and rectus capitis major diverge as they go outwards from the axis spine (Fig. 50).

A very gentle dissection of this minor pool of fat with the lesser ball of a dental burnisher reveals a spray of motor nerves that stem from the posterior ramus of C1 and pass (1) to both obliques; (2) to the posterior recti; (3) to complexus. These nerves mingle with large, delicate veins (connected with the vertebræ), which then join the corresponding half of the sub-occipital venous plexus that lies in the *major* bulk of precomplexal fat.[1]

The posterior ramus of C2 parts from the anterior ramus one fingerbreadth medial to the tip of the second cervical transverse process. After this it floats in the major mass of fat in front of the ' complexi ' and seems surprisingly redundant till we recall the free excursion of the head. Apart from size there is a sharp (and useful) difference between the anterior and posterior ramus of C2 ; the posterior ramus is lax, mobile, and therefore fugitive ; the anterior is rigidly fixed to the top segment of the second stage of the vertebral artery. We can thus use the steadfast, easily located anterior ramus to guide us to its large and more elusive fellow.

Find first the top segment of the second ' vertebral ' stage (p. 58). Find on the outer face of this segment the part of the anterior ramus of C2 that hugs the artery. This part of the ramus often lies as much as a $\frac{1}{2}$ in. above the transversarial foramen of axis ; it is always tightly bound to the vessel by a tough, thin sheath of fascia, and may be squeezed so flat as to seem absent— unless the sheath is opened, when it swells surprisingly. Do not, however, liberate the anterior ramus and so lose the advantage of its fixation.

Then, having found the arterial segment of the anterior ramus, make the ball of the dental burnisher follow its lower edge *inwards* across the back of the artery ; the ball leaves the artery, dips forward and strikes bone near the atlanto-axial joint. Keep touch with bone and continue to move the ball inward *in the same transverse plane* through a mere $\frac{1}{4}$ in.—the fore-and-aft thickness of a little finger-tip. The ball will then engage the angle where the two rami part. Turn the ball in and down, and hook backward the lax posterior ramus. Divide it on the burnisher, controlling

---

[1] *Another means of finding the suboccipital nerve.*—Supposing that the minor pool were dissipated through rupture of its membrane by surgical activity, then—on the *right* side of the neck—put the pulp of the *left* index finger, pointing headwards, on the back of the tip of the transverse process of atlas. The pulp of the middle finger, thrust in alongside index towards the atlas arch, will touch the spot. (On the left side use the two corresponding fingers of the right hand.)

first the large companion offset from the vertebral artery. (The ball of the burnisher is a safeguard ; for if the instrument should stray too far inwards while the patient's head is turned away from the surgeon, the ball precludes the risk of breaking the thin posterior atlanto-axial membrane and entering the spinal canal. Used properly, however, the ball will always have the bulwark of the lateral atlanto-axial joint in front of it.)

Beyond the point of section the lax posterior ramus divides into two branches : (1) a slender lateral branch which is purely motor ; and (2) a stout medial branch, the greater occipital nerve, which is chiefly sensory though giving strong motor twigs.

The posterior ramus of C3 is found when the back part of the space between the second and the third transverse process has been opened by dividing tendinous fascicles attached to the tubercle of the second process, and cleared by removing the second posterior intertransverse muscle. Proceed inwards till you see the *back* of the column formed by articular apophyses of C2 and C3. The third posterior or cervical ramus winds backwards against the posterolateral surface of the *upper* articular apophysis of C3. (Soulié, in Poirier and Charpy's *Traité d'Anatomie Humaine*, 2ᵉ Edn., 1901, T. iii, fasc. 3, p. 887, gives the upper apophyseal relation to the posterior ramus of C3, but he makes the ramus lie in a *rainure*, a narrow groove or fissure, whereas it lies, as Wood Jones shows, on a smooth surface that is concave from above down ; and so does the posterior ramus of C4. On C5 the smooth surface may be replaced by a groove—a true *rainure*—and be absent on C6 and C7 (*Journal of Anatomy and Physiology*, 1912, **46**, 41).)

A posterior ramus is easily displaced while opening an inter-transverse space ; leaving its articular apophysis, it may lie like a bucket handle near one or other transverse process—a fact worth remembering before search becomes fevered. It is also worth remembering that though medial branches of cervical dorsal rami may send twigs to reach skin, they, like the lateral branches, always supply muscle. It is therefore important to resect both branches in order to procure sufficient nuchal palsy. The books, however, show reluctance in describing *where* exactly the dorsal ramus divides.

One of my former teachers, H. M. Johnston, found that in the cervical region the medial branches from the dorsal rami of the lower six cervical nerves (C3 to C8) are separated from the corresponding lateral branches by distinct ligamentous bands, each of which extends from the capsule surrounding the articular apophysis to the transverse process of the succeeding vertebra, *e.g.*, from the joint between C2 and C3 down and outwards to the transverse process of C3 (*Journal of Anatomy and Physiology*, 1909, **43**, 81). It follows therefore that a very proximal division of the dorsal ramus occurs in the neck, and that a very proximal neurectomy is needed to include the lateral with the medial branch.

So, if you find a dorsal nerve winding round the posterolateral face of a columnar articular process, trace it proximally—out and forwards—to ensure complete resection of the two branches.

The accessory nerve on the side opposite the ramal exposure.— Section of this nerve is best made in the way advised by Aird, through an incision in the skin-fold of the neck, 3 cm. (two fingerbreadths) below and behind the angle and lower border of the mandible. (The *other* accessory has been exposed already, with the rami.) After dividing the investing layer of deep fascia the accessory is found coursing obliquely down and back on the prevertebral sheet, often one or two fingerbreadths below the tip of the transverse process of atlas but seldom crossing it. The nerve lies either superficial or deep to the internal jugular vein, which it sometimes perforates.

It will, however, be remembered that the sternomastoid also receives fibres that usually come from the anterior ramus of C3 but sometimes from that of C2, or from both. (See footnote on p. 81.) These fibres often join with the accessory fibres through a loop-hole in the muscle that is best seen when the upper end of sternomastoid is detached and turned outward from the skull (Fig. 53).

The accessory nerve either (1) passes deep to the whole potential triceps (or rarely, quadriceps) arrangement of sternomastoid ; or (2) perforates the almost vertical fibres of the deep, cleidomastoid head of the muscle, and is covered by the two (or three) more oblique and superficial heads—the sternomastoid and cleido-occipital (Fig. 53), plus if it is present, the rare and slender sterno-occipital head. According to Farabeuf, the accessory never pierces a superficial head, nor does it insert itself *directly* between the single deep head and the two (or three) superficial heads, but only intervenes after passing through the deep head.

The need for treating the large functional element in spasmodic torticollis suggests the value of a placid interval obtainable by paralysing relevant nerves for a mere few months, instead of permanently, by resection. The interval can be got after crushing the nerves in continuity.

I learnt this useful thing the hard way in 1930 when in a moment of unwise compunction I elected to crush limb nerves in an *organic*

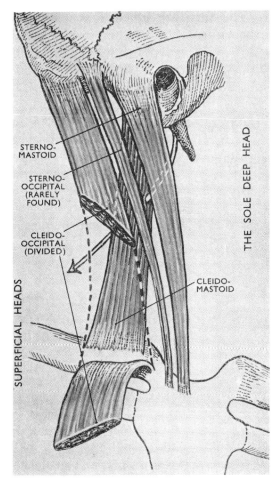

Fig. 53

The sternocleido (occipito) mastoid (after Maubrac and Charpy)

This muscle is commonly a triceps, the separation of whose heads varies in degree. It becomes quadriceps (as seen above) only when the rare sterno-occipital head is manifest. In either type all heads but one are superficial. The sole deep head is the cleidomastoid. The accessory nerve may lie deep to the deep head, or may pierce it—like the plastic arrow in the figure.

case with spastic paraplegia, and three months later was obliged to resect them when the full spasm returned.

Recently G. D. H. Shawe (*British Journal of Surgery*, 1955, **42**

474) has published work on the rabbit, which is perhaps relevant to my clinical reverse. He finds that on the average each axon central to a crushed point in a motor nerve gives three branches by 20 days. The level at which branching begins is about 6 mm. above the injury. Below the crush the number of fibres reached its maximum at 50 days. By 100 days many branches had disappeared, but the fibre content of the nerve was about 50 per cent. higher than normal and remained so for as long as it was studied (225 days). Curiously, if a nerve had been *severed* and sutured immediately, branching was of greater extent than after crushing, while the distal portion of the nerve contained *twice* the normal number of fibres even 200 days after the lesion.

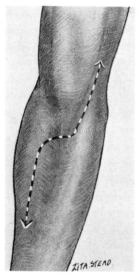

Fig. 54

Showing how the biceps tendon dips into the antecubital V

Beside and medial to biceps is the Fiolle and Delmas incision; it is designed solely for neurovascular structures. In order to expose these structures *in company with humerus* (and elbow joint) the upper part of our incision lies *lateral* to biceps (see Fig. 24).

THE DISTAL PART OF THE HUMERUS EXPOSED IN CONTINUITY WITH ANTECUBITAL STRUCTURES

What follows is a mere variant of the innocuous and beautiful exposure described by Fiolle and Delmas, which brings to light the least accessible part of the ulnar vessels and median nerve, and I shall first indicate *their* method. A skin incision medial to the biceps goes down beside the tendon, and then obliquely out to the junction of the lower and middle thirds of radius; nothing is cut except skin, superficial fascia and veins. The deep fascia is carefully opened.

In this region the biceps tendon dips into the wide part of a muscular V (Fig. 54), whose medial limb is the pronator teres flanked by flexor muscles; the lateral limb of the V is the brachioradialis with two other bellies that form a wad which can be grasped and moved below the elbow (p. 94). After dividing the tight surrounding sleeve of fascia the two limbs of the V part easily; if then the forearm is flexed and placed in full pronation, the muscles covering deep-lying 'difficult' portions of ulnar vessels and median nerve relax and give wide access to every antecubital structure.

Remembering this method we combine exposure of the humerus with easy exploration of the fossa, although the upper part of our incision is on the *outer* side of biceps and therefore opposite to that of Fiolle and Delmas.

THE OPERATION

With the patient's elbow extended and the forearm supine continue the lateral incision for the shaft of humerus (p. 34) beyond the antecubital fossa, curving it in to end two-thirds of the way down the ulna (Fig. 55, A). When we reflect the skin covering the tendon of biceps we shall find the stout band of bicipital fascia (lacertus fibrosus) that forms a sort of retinaculum over the median nerve and distal end of the brachial artery. Dividing the band we then proceed to rip the sleeve of fascia that constricts the antecubital V and cramps its limbs together. But once these limbs are free, a finger, dipping in between, can easily disrupt the loose connecting tissues which " break and disappear like soap-suds."

Find the origins of the radial and ulnar arteries close to the inner side of the biceps tendon. Look for the median nerve still farther in beyond them. Mobilise these neurovascular structures by gently opening Mayo scissors close alongside ; then put the forearm into full pronation and draw the limbs of the V apart. The whole complexion of the wound is suddenly transformed : a beggarly view becomes a wide prospect with every structure fortunately placed (Fig. 55, B).

The interosseous artery and its anterior interosseous branch.— These wide and deeply situated branches lie behind a double screen : the parent ulnar trunk lies on their origin, and it is masked in turn by the main radial vessels. These last are mobilised by cutting twigs that moor them to the muscles. A fan-like set (called ' radial recurrent ' from *upper* twigs that loop towards the elbow) is found at once : a finger moving down the outer face of biceps tendon will catch the loop and let us cut the fan. Then forceps on the severed stem rotate the radial artery and veins away towards the ulnar shaft, uncovering the ulnar artery and drawing it aside by gentle force transmitted through the parent brachial trunk (Fig. 55, c).

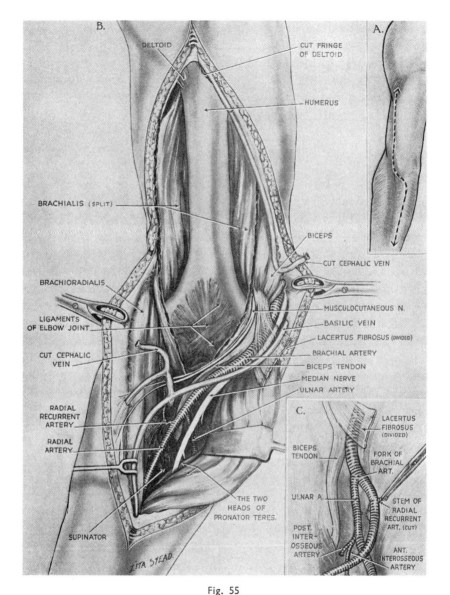

Fig. 55

Extension of distal humeral exposure to the antecubital fossa

A. The whole incision. This is made with the limb supine. (See legend to Fig. 24.) B. The exposure. The forearm is now *pronated*, relaxing the antecubital V so that retraction shows the deep part of the ulnar artery. C. Division of the stem of the vascular fan formed by the so-called 'radial recurrent' provides a handle for rotation and displacement of the brachial fork towards the ulnar shaft—a movement which uncovers interosseous vessels.

This simple movement inwards of radial and ulnar affords a full exposure of our interosseous objectives and yields a thorough view of veins and arteries that ramify within the fossa—a place whose depths should cease to give excuse for hæmostatic rooting.

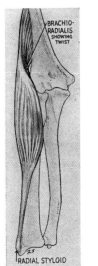 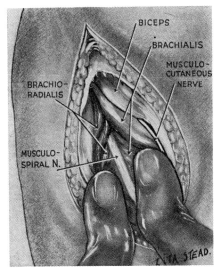

Fig. 56

Finding the distal end of the musculospiral (radial) nerve

A thumb on each muscle opens the spiral plane of cleavage between brachioradialis and brachialis as one would open a book. Inset, The twist of brachioradialis which is moulded to the tapering brachialis.

FINDING THE DISTAL END OF THE MUSCULOSPIRAL (OR RADIAL TRUNK.—There is sometimes delay in finding this part of the nerve It lies here in a peculiar *spiral* plane of cleavage between brachioradialis on the lateral side and brachialis on the medial; for where these bellies touch the brachialis tapers while its fellow twists. So, after dividing deep fascia do not use a knife to reach the nerve; instead place well-gloved thumbs, lengthwise and parallel, one on each belly, and open the plane—like a book on your knee. The nerve marks the place (Fig. 56).

THE FRONT OF THE FOREARM

ANATOMY

We shall consider the muscles first; their arrangement in respect of each other, and sometimes their intimate constitution, are clues to several exposures. So we shall make it easy for the mind to build the part like a model—and then take it to bits.

The mobile wad of three.—Let us first exclude three muscles we have met already (p. 90), which can be grasped with finger and thumb, and moved to and fro as a mobile wad just below the lateral epicondyle of the humerus (Fig. 57). They are, from before back, brachioradialis, and the long and short radial extensors of the wrist. These mobile bellies flank the radius on the outer side and ride at anchor on a fan-shaped leash of vessels from the radial trunks—a leash we must divide before we can retract the muscles outwards or the trunks in (pp. 91 and 99).

The rest.—The remaining muscles are arranged as three groups : (1) superficial ; (2) intermediate ; (3) deep.

The *superficial group* consists of four muscles, remembered by placing the *ball* of the opposite thumb on the front of the medial epicondyle, letting the thumb and *three* fingers point along the supine forearm (Fig. 58). The thumb lies obliquely and marks the course of the oblique pronator teres ; the index finger touches the tendon of flexor carpi radialis close by the radial pulse ; the middle finger takes the place of a frequent absentee—palmaris longus ; the ring finger covers the last muscle

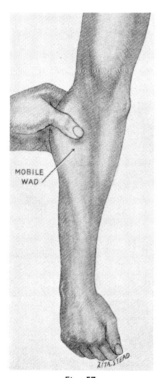

Fig. 57

Recognition of the mobile wad of three muscles below the lateral epicondyle of humerus

The muscles, from before back, are brachioradialis, long and short radial extensors. This wad can be moved *across* the part of radius clothed by supinator, *against* the neighbouring muscles. The anterior and posterior edges of the wad, defined in this way, serve as guides for making incisions and discovering planes of cleavage (see Figs. 65 and 77, A).

of the group, flexor carpi ulnaris. (The little finger plays no part

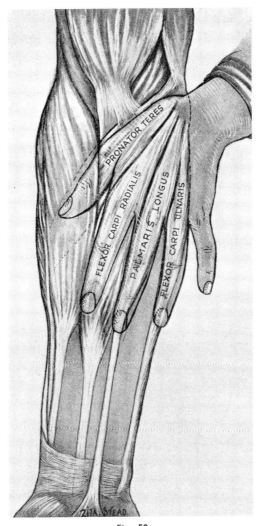

Fig. 58

A manual mnemonic for superficial muscles on the front of the forearm

Place the opposite hand on the front of the forearm as in the figure, with the thenar eminence covering the medial epicondyle. Thumb and fingers indicate the lie of superficial muscles ; the little finger plays no part. Note how pronator makes a bridge across the forearm.

in these manual mnemonics which we shall do well to practise first on our own forearms.)

The *intermediate group* has one muscle only—flexor digitorum

sublimis—but a muscle of some complexity, whose close and peculiar relations with the median nerve are of practical importance. Its tendons go behind the trans-
verse carpal ligament as if they had
'formed two deep'—a fact which be-
tokens the two-layered arrangement
of the fleshy parts. The *superficial*
portion of sublimis belonging to the
front-rank tendons—for ring and middle
finger—is a thin sheet that slants
across from humerus to radius bridging
the interval between the bones of the
forearm (Fig. 59). The median nerve
and the deep, 'difficult' portions of
the ulnar vessels diverge as they leave
the antecubital fossa and pass beneath
this bridge, whose arch—which gives
them entry—has varying relations
with the bridging belly of pronator
teres. Pronator either overspreads the

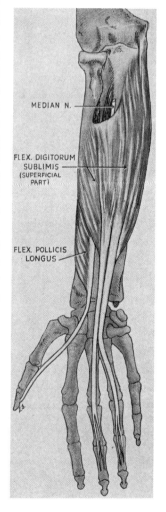

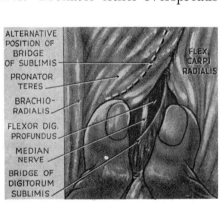

Fig. 59

The superficial part of sublimis

This part gives rise to the two front-rank tendons (for ring and middle finger). It
forms a bridge whose oblique entrance may have a high or low level in the
forearm and thus be either deep or distal to pronator teres. The median nerve
therefore runs either under a two-layered arch (formed by pronator plus sublimis),
or else must cross a gap between two separate spans. (See inset where flexor carpi
radialis has been retracted to show the median in the gap. The dotted line indicates
the proximal variety of sublimis arch.)

arch of the sublimis (forming a double-layered span), or else sublimis
lies more distally (so that the spans are separated by a gap)—a
point of some importance in looking for the median nerve (p. 106).

The *deep part of sublimis* is trigastric (Fig. 60) ; the two distal bellies correspond to the rear-rank tendons—for index and little

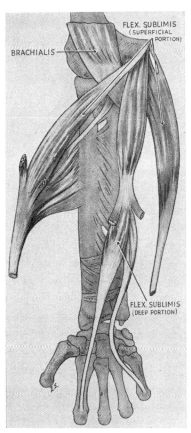

Fig. 60

**The deep part of sublimis
(after Poirier)**

The two distal bellies of the trigastric portion give tendons to little finger and index—the rear-rank tendons which enter the wrist behind those of the other two fingers. The median nerve is bound in satellite relation to the radial side of the deep part of sublimis.

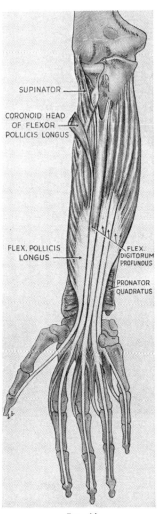

Fig. 61

**The deep anterior muscles
met in surgical exposure**

One lies lengthwise along each bone. One joins the proximal ends of the bones, one the distal. (The index tendon is the only tendon of profundus that separates in the forearm ; the others are conjoined till they reach the palm.)

finger ; the proximal belly springs from the common origin on the medial epicondyle of the humerus.

The satellite median.—After leaving the antecubital space the median nerve becomes a satellite of the deep part of sublimis, lying first to the radial side of the proximal belly ; then to the radial side of the intermediate tendon which is sometimes an obvious glistening thing, but often dull and cord-like enough to simulate the nerve itself. Below this level, fascia binds the median in a lateral groove between the front- and rear-rank tendons that go respectively to middle and index fingers. The nerve, therefore, stays with sublimis if we separate that muscle from profundus. We shall see (on p. 109) how to find the median near the wrist.

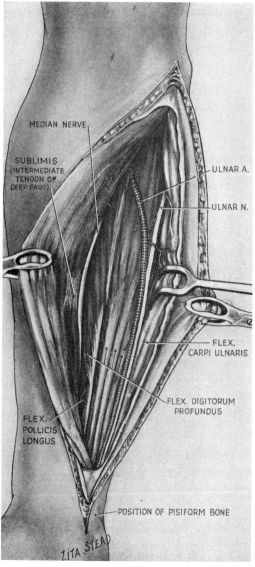

Loose tissue joins the single, intermediate, sublimis to the deep group, forming a plane of facile cleavage that is used with great advantage by McConnell (p. 107).

The *deep anterior group* consists of four muscles (Fig. 61): one lies along the length of each bone —the flexor of the thumb upon the radius, profundus digitorum on the ulna. The other muscles cross *between* the bones — the supinator near the elbow, the flat quadratus near the wrist. (I know I contravene morphology by classing supinator with anterior muscles, but here we meet the

Fig. 62

The ulnar neurovascular bundle belongs to the *deep* layer of muscles. Note how the bundle splits proximally. The median nerve sticks to sublimis.

supinator first in *front*; and this book deals in practice.) Note that the tendons of profundus digitorum—unlike the tendons of sublimis—lie in a single rank of four abreast.

The *ulnar nerve* comes to the front of forearm from behind the elbow. It is thus natural to find it fastened to a member of the *deep* group of forearm muscles—flexor digitorum profundus, a muscle one of whose origins wraps widely round the upper and inner two-thirds of the ulnar bone.

The *ulnar vessels* join the nerve at a sharp angle and then go down its radial side, forming with it a neurovascular bundle (Fig. 62) partitioned from the inner flank of forearm by the tendon of flexor carpi ulnaris. We have already noticed these vessels leaving the antecubital fossa (p. 96); we now see they do so by passing between the deep and intermediate groups of muscle.

The *radial artery* begins at the medial side of the biceps tendon; and so its oblique proximal part becomes a satellite of the oblique pronator teres which also has a medial origin : the artery is bound by fascia to the muscle, though books omit the fact and harp instead on the relation here of brachioradialis. That is why one sees despairing *outward* hunts in the proximal third of forearm to find a vessel which comes from the inner side. This artery, with its companion veins, is dangerously near the surface and may be slit in opening the fascial sleeve of swollen limbs.

The *tendon of biceps* is a major landmark, a vertical partition which divides the proximal portion of the antecubital V into a ' dangerous ' area on the medial side, a ' safe ' one on the lateral —provided of course the knife stays close to the tendon and does not wander out to threaten the end of the musculospiral nerve, the radial of Basle nomenclature.

The tendon leads through loose fat to the tuberosity of radius, a part of which is covered by the *bicipital bursa*—whose aid we shall enlist.

The radial leash, called " recurrent."—Crossing the ' safe ' lateral area of the antecubital fossa is a group of vessels called recurrent radial; only the most proximal deserve the name by running up the limb; the other members are important muscular twigs which spread out fanwise to the mobile wad of bellies that flank the radius (p. 91). The wad therefore is moored to the radial trunks by a fan-like vascular leash whose vessels—which rib the fan (Fig. 63)— seldom lie in a single plane but diverge in a set of layers two or three deep; *all* these must be divided to free the tethered muscles—unless we cut the stem from which they spread. A finger moving distally along the outer face of biceps tendon will feel the leash (which lies invisible in fat) and hook it up—a welcome guide in featureless surroundings.

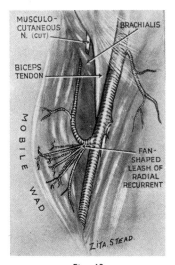

Fig. 63

The fan-like leash of vessels called ' radial recurrent '

(The veins are not shown.) Only the proximal rib of the fan is recurrent. The ribs are in several layers—two, three, or four deep. They are muscular branches which tie the mobile wad to the radial vessels.

The branch once called the radial branch of musculospiral, alias (in B.N.A.) the superficial terminal branch of radial, and now (in fitful text-books) lumped with the parent stem as ' radial '[1]—this branch, by any name you choose, clings to the mobile wad of muscles, the hinder one of which it may supply.[2] The satellite relation of the nerve and wad involves reciprocal divorce (and therefore easy severance) from close-adjoining radial vessels, which go for their part with pronator teres and then with flexor longus pollicis. (A way of finding the distal end of the parent trunk is described on p. 93.)

The *medial cutaneous nerve* of the forearm lies to the ulnar side of any elective incision we shall make on the front of the limb—excepting McConnell's (p. 107).

EXPOSURE OF THE WHOLE SHAFT OF RADIUS FROM IN FRONT WITH EXTENSIONS TO MEDIAN AND ULNAR NERVES

We have thus built a rough but working model of the front of forearm. Let us now take this apart sufficiently to see the whole length of radius.

First, we must still further mobilise the wad of three mobile muscles (brachioradialis, long and short radial wrist-extensors) so that we can draw them well away from the lateral face of radial shaft. We shall therefore use an incision that follows these muscles

---

[1] Impatient persons (like the *Queen of Hearts*) wish off the heads of *all* who are responsible. But *Alice* (duly coached and kindlier) might put our three nomenclatures in one portmanteau and call the slithy nerve the *radial branch of musculoradial.* (Its deeper fellow is, of course, the *muscular.*)

[2] C. R. Salsbury, *British Journal of Surgery,* 1938, **26**, 95.

right into the *arm*. Then, after opening deep fascia, we shall cut the fan-shaped vascular leash—the so-called radial recurrent—which holds them tethered to the main radial trunk. Lastly, we undo the supinator, whose *deep* fibres come across from ulna to grasp from behind—like fingers of a hand—the upper third of radial shaft. A second set of supinator fibres slopes down over these.

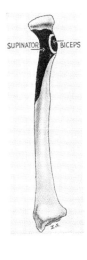 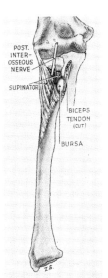

Fig. 64

Anatomical relationships at the upper part of the radius. The white crescent between the two black areas of attachment marks the site of the bicipital bursa and shows how it lies in a bay formed by the supinator edge. The surgeon is guided to the bursa and thus to the edge of the supinator —by the outer face of the biceps tendon (see insets to Figs. 67 and 68).

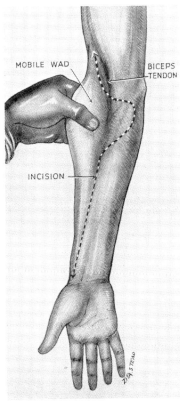

Fig. 65

Incision for anterior exposure of the radius

The knife follows the front edge of the upper part of the mobile wad (brachio-radialis, long and short radial wrist extensors), and then proceeds as in this figure.

The *posterior interosseous nerve* (deep terminal branch of radial, B.N.A.) penetrates the anterolateral face of the supinator muscle, and separates its two layers; the deeper layer fends the nerve from radius. The part of supinator edge that skirts the tuberosity of radius curves also round a bursa of the biceps, which lies next bone and lubricates the tendon (Figs. 64 and 67). At first loose fat swamps everything; but once we find and cut the fan-shaped leash the outer face of biceps tendon leads us to the bursa, which we divide to reach the tuberosity, thus leaving the rugine a place to come in contact with the bone. Then, starting at the *edge* of supinator, we find the muscle easy to detach.

THE OPERATION

Incision.—First, with the limb supine, feel out the mobile wad of three muscles and incise as in Fig. 65. The incision goes up a

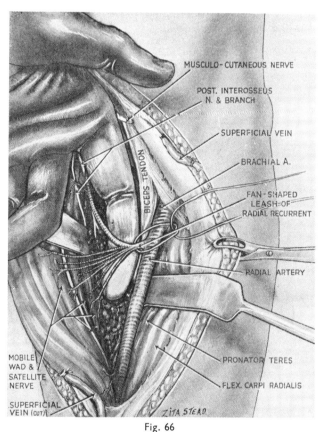

Fig. 66
Finding the fan-like leash

A finger slid lengthwise down the outer side of the biceps tendon feels the resistant loop of the recurrent proximal vessels. Be sure to catch up *all* the layers of the fan—two, three, or four—unless, as in the figure, you tie and cut instead the short single stem of the fan. Note that the radial branch of musculospiral (=superficial terminal branch of radial) is bound in satellite relation to the mobile wad.

handbreadth into the arm, keeping a fingerbreadth lateral to the edge of biceps (see p. 34); below, it reaches to the radial styloid. Divide and tie the large superficial vein that crosses the mid-third of radius, and may continue thence as the cephalic.

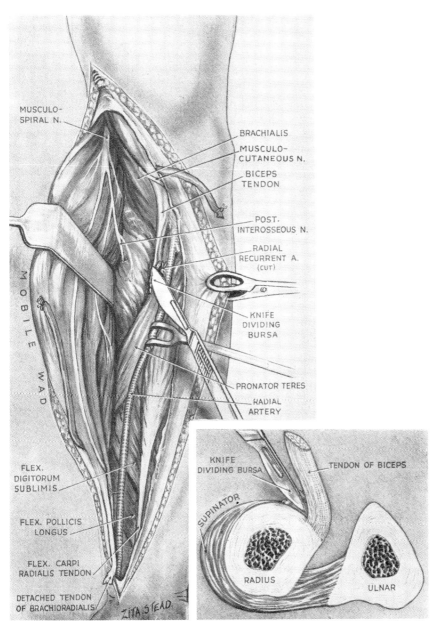

MUSCULO-
SPIRAL N.

BRACHIALIS

MUSCULO-
CUTANEOUS N.

BICEPS
TENDON

POST.
INTEROSSEOUS N.

RADIAL
RECURRENT A.
(CUT)

KNIFE
DIVIDING
BURSA

PRONATOR TERES

RADIAL
ARTERY

MOBILE WAD

FLEX.
DIGITORUM
SUBLIMIS

FLEX. POLLICIS
LONGUS

FLEX. CARPI
RADIALIS TENDON

DETACHED TENDON
OF BRACHIORADIALIS

KNIFE
DIVIDING BURSA

TENDON OF BICEPS

SUPINATOR

RADIUS

ULNAR

ZITA STEAD

Fig. 67

The fan-like leash has been cut ; the mobile wad is free for lateral retraction. The knife,
with the flat of its blade touching the ' safe ' outer face of biceps tendon, cuts through loose
fat ; it then cuts through the bicipital bursa to strike the tuberosity of radius at the edge
of the supinator insertion (see inset).

In this figure and the next, two points should be noted : (1) Fat which veils the front of
supinator is omitted in order to show the muscle. (In spite of fat the *lining* of the bursal
sac will glint when once the knife has cut into the cavity.) (2) The peculiar *curved* course
of the cutaneous part of the musculocutaneous nerve is due to its retraction inwards with
the skin. Note how the proximal part of the nerve appears at the junction of biceps tendon
with biceps belly—a sure guide to its discovery.

The deep guide.—First expose the biceps tendon by dividing deep fascia on its lateral side. Go on dividing this fascia throughout the wound with *blunt-nosed scissors*, thus taking care of the radial vessels. Pass the finger down through the swamp of fat, along the outer side of the guiding tendon till you meet the resistance of the recurrent vascular loop (Fig. 66). Remember that this loop is only the proximal rib of a fan-like spread of vessels that lie in several layers. Hook up *all* the layers of the fan gently on the finger; divide and tie them —or tie instead their narrow stem. Mobilise the wad of three long muscles which flanks the outer face of fore-

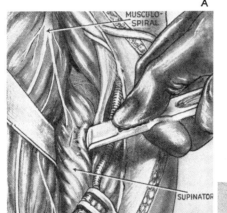

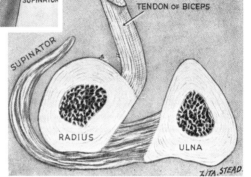

Fig. 68

The rugine working outwards from the site of the divided bursa begins to peel the grasp of supinator from the radial nerve. (In this figure the musculocutaneous nerve has no label.)

arm. Detach the flat tendon of brachioradialis from its hold on the base of the radial styloid. Flex the elbow through 90 degrees and retract the outer muscles widely to expose the supinator.

Return then to the biceps tendon. First make the tendon taut; then, keeping the flat of the knife close to its outer face, cut down upon the bone. The knife divides bicipital bursa and strikes the tuberosity of radius, which lies embraced within a bay formed by the supinator edge (Fig. 67). From this strategic point the rugine peels the supinator muscle off the bone (Fig. 68). The muscle is turned outwards, sandwiching within its substance the posterior interosseous nerve (deep terminal branch of radial, B.N.A.).

Lastly, a vital part of the exposure: put the forearm into full pronation; the radius then will be revealed from end to end (Fig. 69).

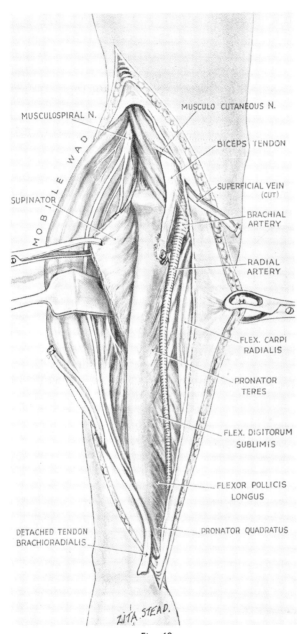

MUSCULOSPIRAL N.

MUSCULO CUTANEOUS N.

BICEPS TENDON

SUPERFICIAL VEIN
(CUT)

SUPINATOR

MOBILE WAD

BRACHIAL
ARTERY

RADIAL
ARTERY

FLEX. CARPI
RADIALIS

PRONATOR
TERES

FLEX. DIGITORUM
SUBLIMIS

FLEXOR POLLICIS
LONGUS

DETACHED TENDON
BRACHIORADIALIS

PRONATOR QUADRATUS

ZITA STEAD.

Fig. 69

The forearm remains supine till supinator is mobilised.
Complete the exposure by putting the forearm into full
pronation ; this will bring the bone to the surface, as in the
figure.

UNREDUCED ANTERIOR LUXATIONS OF THE RADIAL HEAD.—
These injuries are common where men fight with quarterstaffs.
A forearm guards the skull from a descending blow whose force,
breaking the ulna, drives the fragments on against the radius and
thrusts its head in front. Then, if a closed reduction fails, the upper
third of the complete exposure will serve for reposition or resection.

EXTENDING THE EXPOSURE OF RADIUS TO THE MEDIAN AND
ULNAR NERVES.—Should we wish to extend the exposure, we have
already seen how this is done for nerves and vessels of the ante-

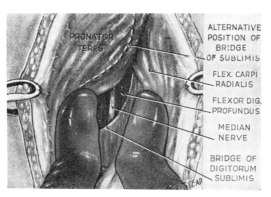

cubital region (p. 90):
an attack begun there
from   the   outer side
of humerus was carried
over to include them
all. Let us now with
equal ease spread our
exposure of the radial
shaft to embrace the
median and ulnar nerves
in the rest of the fore-
arm—the   distal   two-
thirds. If we begin our
approach to the bone
with a view to including
these nerves, we shall
of course make the
forearm portion of the

Fig. 70

Finding the median nerve distal to pronator teres.
—Begin to separate the belly of pronator teres from
that of flexor carpi radialis *where they diverge.* Use
the thumbs back to back to move the muscles harmlessly apart. A short length of median *may* appear
between pronator and sublimis, as in this figure. If
not, you must split the thin superficial part of sublimis
to see the nerve.

incision nearer the middle line than if radius were our sole
objective ; though in any forearm a *long* incision combined with
trivial skin-reflection will bring us where we wish.

Exposing the median nerve from in front.—We must first find
the plane of cleavage between pronator teres and flexor carpi
radialis (between thumb and index of the manual mnemonic in
Fig. 58). The *tendons* of these two muscles separate widely in the
distal third of forearm, the place, of course, from which to prise
apart the close-packed bellies—a thing most gently done with
two thumbs back to back (Fig. 70). And now a short, flat-looking
piece of median trunk will often show in the proximal part of the
separation ; it goes between the distal edge of pronator and the
proximal edge of the bridge-like portion of sublimis. This glimpse
of nerve (Fig. 70) is only possible when the sublimis bridge lies

farther down the limb than the more superficial span of pronator teres—leaving a gap for the nerve to cross (p. 96). But when one span lies level with the other and covers it, there is no gap nor glimpse at all : there is instead (between our separating thumbs) an unrevealing face—the thin bridge of sublimis, whose grain we now must split to see the nerve. We know already we shall find it bound by a transparent fascia to the deep, trigastric part of that two-layered muscle.

The ulnar nerve exposed from in front.—If we wish to include the ulnar in the anterior approach, we must open the plane between sublimis and the deep layer, relaxing sublimis by flexing the hand. Drawing the muscle forwards, we shall then see that the space is closed on the ulnar side by a shining band of tendon, the flexor carpi ulnaris ; beside it we shall find the ulnar nerve—bound, with the vessels, to deep flexor digitorum. Combined exposure of median and ulnar nerves is thus obtained as a by-product of the approach to radial shaft.

But, if our quarry in the forearm happens to be the distal two-thirds of median nerve, or the whole length of ulnar nerve—or both ; or if a *medial* wound determines our direction, then we can make use of an exposure that has the " simple elegance " which Horace praised, joined (this time) with fidelity.

McCONNELL'S COMBINED EXPOSURE OF MEDIAN AND ULNAR NERVES IN THE FOREARM [1]

Lay the forearm supine. Incise skin only—from *radial* edge of pisiform to medial epicondyle (Fig. 71). Open deep fascia along the radial side of flexor carpi ulnaris tendon, working up from the distal end of the wound. The ulnar nerve and vessels are found at once and traced in a *proximal* direction to the sharp angle where they part company, the line of the vessels turning outwards from the straight course of the nerve (Fig. 71). It is then easy to find the friendly plane of cleavage between sublimis mass and flexor profundus (Fig. 72). The median nerve, we know, lies in a shallow groove upon sublimis, to the radial side of its deep trigastric portion. So, when the plane is opened up, nerve and sublimis move (and stay) in company.

It is often easy to mistake the intermediate tendon of the deep trigastric moiety for the median nerve (Fig. 71), and I shall

[1] A. A. McConnell, *Dublin Journal of Medical Science*, 1920, p. 90.

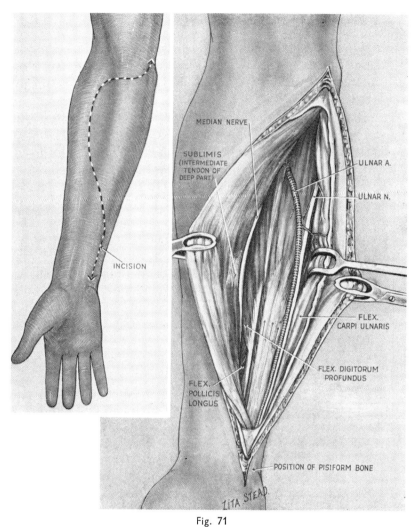

Fig. 71

McConnell's combined exposure of median nerve and ulnar neuro-
vascular bundle

Incision runs from medial epicondyle to pisiform. (See legend to Fig. 24.) The plane
between sublimis and profundus is opened up. Note how the median sticks to the
sublimis ' roof ' ; the ulnar bundle sticks to the profundus ' floor.' Note, too, the
intermediate tendon which sometimes simulates the median.

close with a double counsel : Do not too quickly rejoice at the first cord-like structure you may see—it is possibly a flexor tendon ; do not cut into the deep face of sublimis to look for the nerve ; you will only make a mess.

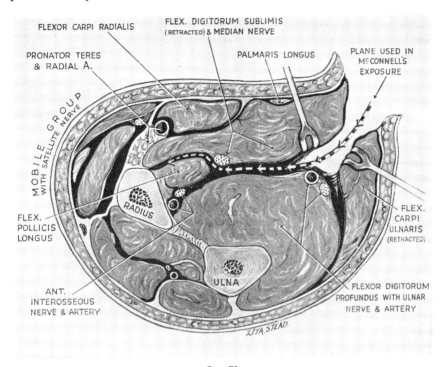

Fig. 72

Cross-section showing the plane of cleavage in McConnell's exposure

The plane is entered in front of flexor carpi ulnaris and in front of the ulnar bundle ; it lies between the intermediate layer of muscle (which consists only of sublimis) and the deep layer. The median nerve sticks to the ' roof ' ; the ulnar bundle to the ' floor.' (In practice entry is effected at a more distal and facile level—in front of the *tendon* of flexor carpi ulnaris.)

EXPOSURE OF THE MEDIAN NERVE ABOVE THE WRIST

The nerve just here is literally median, a fact to grasp if we would find it quickly ; for, despite tradition, palmaris longus is a mere decoy and has no value as a landmark. Out of 100 forearms, Tandler (that attractive person whose good work embraced both quick and dead) notes how the median lay behind or radial to palmaris tendon in 53 ; in 35, the nerve lay to its inner side ; in 12 he found no tendon. And I would add that when the median does lie close behind palmaris, the tendon often moves away once we retract deep fascia.

Other relations near the wrist.—The nerve—true satellite of the sublimis mass—keeps on one level and so comes near the surface at the wrist ; for the limb tapers as the bellies shrink, leaving the nerve bare of flesh and flanked by tendon. But even here the inner edge of median (still faithful to sublimis) weds the groove between the front-rank middle finger tendon and its rear-rank index-finger file. The groove is deepened by the pointed fleshy tongues that coat these tendons till they reach the wrist ; and up the groove a severed median may withdraw from sight.

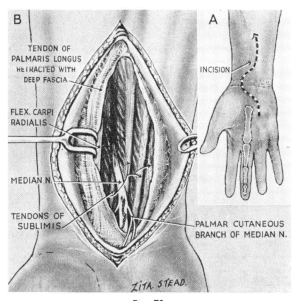

Fig. 73

Exposure of the median nerve close above the wrist

A. The axis-line incision reaching the distal ' bracelet.'
B. The exposure. Palmaris longus is retracted with deep fascia. The *fixed* relation of the nerve is to the middle-finger tendon of sublimis, in front of which it winds.

THE OPERATION

The axis line.—The certain guide (because the nerve is median) is the long axis of the middle metacarpal bone—produced, of course, into the forearm (Fig. 73). So make the knife continue that long axis up the limb. Begin incising at the distal ' bracelet ' which marks the forearm skin, and end the cut at least four fingerbreadths above. Use this line, too, for opening the deep fascia ; displace the chance obtrusion of palmaris tendon. The nerve is seen at once, marked often by a small meandering vessel.

Above, the median disappears beneath a pointed fleshy tongue of the sublimis ; below, and near the ' bracelets,' it gives a branch which overlies the parent trunk and goes to palmar skin. The main nerve leaves the wound beneath the bridge of transverse carpal ligament and, just before it vanishes from sight, lies on the *front* of the sublimis tendon for the middle finger (Fig. 73).

This exposure may, of course, continue, or be continued into, the *anterior* approach to median and ulnar nerves described on page 107.

THE BACK OF THE FOREARM

The arrangement of parts here is very simple.

The *mobile wad* is the same wad of three muscles we know already :—extensors (radial) long and short, brachioradialis—a boring refrain, but useful in practice ; nor should we scorn the metre which comes (with a past) from the very front of the chorus.

These three muscles are moved at will with finger and thumb, not only across the radial shaft (clothed by supinator), but also *against* the neighbouring mass of common extensor that lies more firmly bound. Presently their mobility will help us to find and rip a seam in the cloak covering the neuromuscular sandwich of supinator and posterior interosseous nerve.

The rest of the muscles.—Excluding the mobile wad, the muscles on the back of forearm lie in two layers—superficial and deep. We can now proceed, as we did in front, to make a manual mnemonic for the *surface layer*. But this time we must carry the ball of the opposite thumb round *behind* the forearm and place it on the back of the lateral epicondyle (Fig. 74). The oblique thumb again (but rather awkwardly) marks an oblique muscle—the anconeus. The index will press the belly of extensor carpi ulnaris against the ulnar shaft ; the middle finger marks extensor digiti quinti, while the ring finger lies on the rather fixed mass of common extensor. (The little finger is not used at all.)

The deep layer.—There is good reason to remember the arrangement of this layer (Fig. 75). All its tendons (excepting sometimes that of proprius) can be seen in one's own hand ; all go to thumb or index. They are four in number : abductor pollicis longus, extensor pollicis brevis, extensor pollicis longus, extensor indicis proprius.   Except for the first—the long abductor which springs from *both* bones—the tendons point towards their bone of origin.

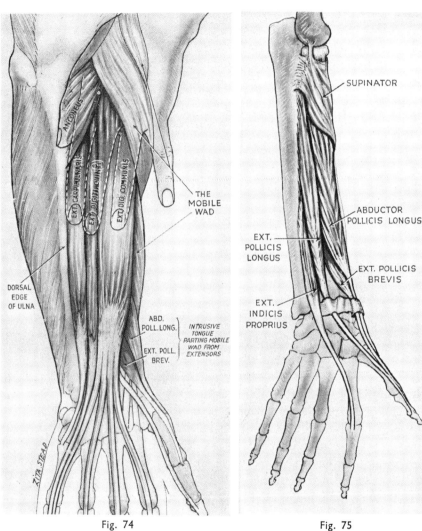

ANCONEUS

EXT. CARPI ULNARIS

EXT. DIGITI QUINTI

EXT. DIGI COMMUNIS

THE MOBILE WAD

DORSAL EDGE OF ULNA

ABD. POLL. LONG.

EXT. POLL. BREV.

INTRUSIVE TONGUE PARTING MOBILE WAD FROM EXTENSORS

ZITA STEAD

SUPINATOR

ABDUCTOR POLLICIS LONGUS

EXT. POLLICIS LONGUS

EXT. POLLICIS BREVIS

EXT. INDICIS PROPRIUS

Fig. 74	Fig. 75
Manual mnemonic for posterior superficial muscles of the forearm	**The deep posterior muscles**
The ball of the opposite thumb lies this time on the *back* of lateral epicondyle. The index finger feels the dorsal edge of ulnar shaft. (Again the little finger plays no part.)	These send their tendons to thumb or index. (Supinator also makes a wide posterior appearance. It has already been described and dealt with in the front of the limb.)

So the short thumb extensor comes from radius ; the long extensor and the proprius from ulna.   (The bellies of two muscles of the thumb, the long abductor and short extensor, thrust out a common fleshy tongue between the mobile wad of three and the more fixed extensor of the fingers—a tongue which helps to emphasise the parting we shall presently exploit.) [1]

We have seen (p. 101) how the posterior interosseous nerve (the deep terminal branch of musculospiral) enters the antero-lateral face of supinator and slopes obliquely down across the striped grain of that muscle. The nerve can be found on the *back* of radial shaft at a quite definite point—three fingerbreadths distal to the head of radius (Fig. 76). I would stress the fact that this measurement must be made neither on the outer side of the bone, nor on its posterolateral face, but on the back only.

EXPOSURE OF THE POSTERIOR INTER-OSSEOUS NERVE (THE DEEP TERMINAL BRANCH OF THE MUSCULOSPIRAL) FROM BEHIND

This nerve, they say, is difficult to find. The fault, however, is not in the *nerve.* Its faithful rendezvous upon the back of radius (like that kept by the parent trunk in skirting round the humerus) is just another of those ' certainties ' on which it is unfair to bet.

THE OPERATION

Incision.—The knife should aim to go between extensor carpi radialis brevis and extensor digitorum communis (Stookey and

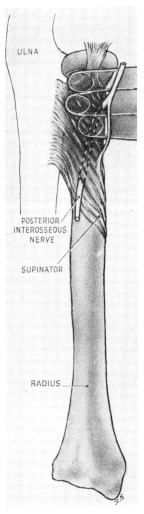

Fig. 76

The three-finger method of locating the posterior interosseous nerve (deep terminal branch of musculospiral)

The test must be applied at the *back* of radius. The edge of the proximal finger-tip fits the curve where head joins neck. Sandwiched in fibres of supinator, the nerve crosses the back of radius deep to the pulp of the distal finger-tip.

[1] The site of separation is further marked by a pit which can be felt in the *prone* forearm just proximal to the bulge of the intrusive ' tongue,' a handbreadth above the wrist. The finger-tip receives a sharp impression of the shaft of radius, unpadded at the bottom of the pit by tendon or by belly.

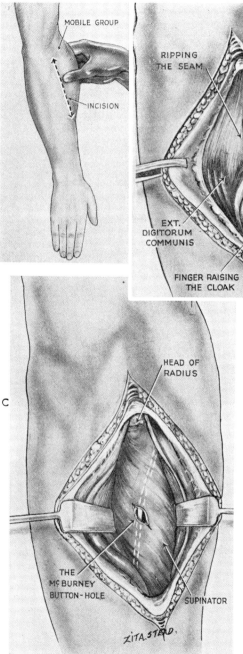

Fig. 77

Exposure of the posterior interosseous nerve

A. The skin incision. Grasp the mobile wad and move it sideways to locate the seam of union with the fixed extensor mass. Divide skin along the hinder margin of the wad.

B. Split the cloak that covers supinator. Begin *distally*—near where the cloak is split already by an oblique tongue of thumb muscles (long abductor, short extensor, Fig. 74).

C. A small McBurney button-hole, three fingerbreadths distal to the *back* of the head of radius (see Fig. 76), reveals the nerve within the supinator sandwich. Start from the buttonhole with Mayo scissors and cut the surface layer to expose the nerve.

Guild, 1919).[1]   With the patient's forearm prone the line for separating these is found at once by grasping with a thumb and finger the wad that lies just distal to the outer epicondyle. This wad (whose hindmost belly *is* extensor carpi radialis brevis) moves readily against the much less mobile mass of the communis. We therefore easily locate the *hinder* margin of the wad and trace it with a knife (at first through skin) a generous handbreadth down the limb, from outer epicondyle (Fig. 77, A).

When we have opened deep fascia—beginning distally—we verify once more the plane between the zones of different mobility, and take advantage of their distal parting to separate them cleanly. This pair of bellies covers supinator with a loose cloak, ripped easily in two where it divides but toughly fused above within a fibrous hood. A finger, therefore, working from below, will help to raise the cloak for clean division (Fig. 77, B). Then we shall see the striped (and sometimes flashy) supinator belly. The nerve (sandwiched, remember, in the muscle) slopes *across* the stripe. Measure then with the tips of three fingers—side by side and touching— from the *back* of the neck of radius ; the posterior interosseous nerve lies on the *back* of shaft deep to the distal finger (Figs. 76 and 77, C). And here a small McBurney cut, splitting the supinator grain, will let us glimpse the flat and whitish shape of our objective ; and then, if we transect the grain, we shall expose the nerve. A word of caution : the sandwich is *thin*, so do not nick the nerve with your McBurney (Fig. 77, C).

EXPOSURE OF THE HEAD AND NECK
OF RADIUS FROM BEHIND

It has been said that any cut made behind the proximal end of radius will expose the head and neck of the bone safely, provided that it stops before we wound the posterior interosseous nerve. This statement is soundly based : extensor digitorum communis takes origin within a hood of tough fibrous tissue that lies behind the radial head and yields no plane of cleavage. We shall accordingly divide the skin and then cut down on bone, using three fingers to locate the nerve (Fig. 76), and cutting only to the second nail. (The cut should also reach two fingerbreadths *above* the epicondyle to leave room for resection.)

[1] S. Guild and B. Stookey, *Surgery, Gynecology and Obstetrics*, 1919, **28,** 612.

TWO EXPOSURES IN THE HAND

A MEDIAL APPROACH TO
MID-PALMAR SPACE AND ULNAR BURSA [1]

Adams McConnell—the first by many years, this side of the Atlantic, to give Kanavel's work a practical appreciation—described in 1913 a method of draining the mid-palmar space (*Medical Press and Circular*, 1913, **95**, 328).   His dorsal incision of the web between the fingers, remote alike from vessels, nerves and palmar skin, has not been bettered.[2]   It is a part, however, of its charm that surgery leaves room for new alternatives. The one I shall describe gives access to the space and ulnar bursa. Advantage will be taken of a loop-hole in the *edge* of the hand to gain entry to the palm.   The skin incision, like McConnell's, leaves no palmar scar, and gives dependent drainage both of space and bursa when the hand lies semi-prone, in its most comfortable attitude.

ANATOMY

The floor of the palm is formed by alternate bones and interosseous muscles covered with a loose carpet of fascia—a carpet separated from the ulnar bursa by mid-palmar space.   The bursa wraps the superficial and deep flexor tendons of middle, ring, and little fingers and almost fills the space.[3]

The way in.—Opponens of the little finger, the deepest hypothenar muscle, lies on the ulnar side of palmar floor concealed by the short flexor and the large bulge of abductor.   It is fastened proximally to the hook of unciform and to the transverse carpal ligament ;   distally, to the distal three-quarters of the fifth

---

[1] *The Lancet*, 1939, **1**, 16.

[2] There is, I know, a prejudice abroad which holds that specialists, like cobblers, should stick to their last.   And so, in case it were believed by any that the hand of *one* employment " hath the daintier touch," the fact is worth attention that this neurosurgeon was amongst the first (if not the first) to integrate Cushing's technique outside America ; certainly first (as Dandy notes) to use ventriculography in Europe.   But never any man's disciple—a grade most fit to rank beside the legendary *second* class of the nipponic Order of Chastity.

[3] *Mid-palmar space.*—A healthy, undissected man has no mid-palmar space—if " space " means " interval " ;   nor has he any popliteal space :   *both* are convenient myths (though most anatomists long looked coldly at Kanavel's).   There is, however, in the hand between the palmar floor and ulnar bursa a fissile plane—an ' *espace décollable* ' that easily distends and shows a special shape when it becomes unstuck by pus or by injection.

metacarpal shaft, on the ulnar side of the volar face (Fig. 78). Between these terminal attachments there is a small ' free ' portion of opponens belly, and this when isolated by a touch becomes the palmar boundary of a loop-hole that is framed behind by fifth metacarpal base and the joint it makes with unciform—the hamate of B.N.A. (Fig. 78). An instrument thrust through this loop-hole

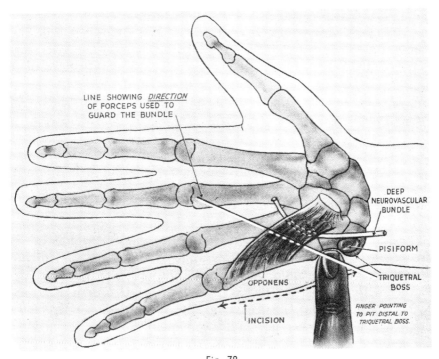

Fig. 78

The landmarks

1. The triquetral boss from which the knife will cut along the edge of the fifth metacarpal.
2. The pit marked by the finger distal to the boss. Opposite the pit we find the loop-hole to mid-palmar space. A forceps *aimed* along the sloping line goes through the loop-hole *for a fingerbreadth* to form a tangent that will guard the curving ulnar bundle.

meets and overcomes a check; then it goes on and either penetrates mid-palmar space, or is a menace to the deep branch of the ulnar nerve or to the ulnar bursa.

The hypothenar fascia.—The check is caused by the most radial portion of a fascia that sheathes the hypothenar muscles and loops them loosely, like a sling, to the shaft of fifth metacarpal. The toughness of the membrane and its erratic spread to neighbouring interosseous bellies vary in different persons.

The *deep branch of ulnar nerve* with its satellite artery and veins must be carefully avoided. The branch leaves the main trunk opposite the pisiform and sinks gradually into the palm between the two superficial muscles of the hypothenar group— abductor and short flexor of the little finger. It enters the field of operation as it grazes the ulnar side of the hamate (or unciform) hook and is there bridged or embraced by opponens fibres. Just distal to the hook the nerve and vessels fortunately bend thumb-wards, almost at right angles, and, fortunately again, the bend lies a good fingerbreadth radial to the loop-hole's mouth. Whatever instruments we turn toward the space will thus avoid the nerve if pointed distally—for choice, towards the *head* of third metacarpal (Fig. 78).

THE OPERATION

The site allows a long, benignly placed, incision, and this will give advantage for inspection combined with thorough drainage of a part where pus is liable to pocket. Blind use therefore of the loop-hole as a means of access should be condemned ; it is a mere lucky breach that must be *widened* for surgical attack.

Position.—With the patient recumbent under general anæs-thesia, either pronate and turn his upper limb till the *back* of the thumb rests on the table, or bring the half-pronated forearm into contact with the biceps. The first position has the merit of ulnar-flexing the hand and thus relaxing skin and muscle so that bony landmarks are easy to feel. At the moment, however, of making the incision the wrist should be propped straight to unwrinkle the skin.

Two ways of finding the pit which is the surface guide.—(1) Run a thumbnail down the ulnar border of the patient's *wrist* ; a thumb's breadth dorsal to the pisiform the nail will override a boss—the cuneiform or os triquetrum—and sink at once into a pit just distal to the boss. In this depression (which dips towards the loop-hole) the nail will touch the hard base of the fifth metacarpal immediately behind the hypothenar mass. (2) The thumb, slid proximally *up* the subcutaneous edge of fifth metacarpal, is checked by the triquetral boss exactly opposite the pit (Fig. 78).

The incision.—This begins on the triquetral boss and goes— through skin only—down the whole length of metacarpal edge ; skin and fat are reflected just sufficiently to show the bone and let us see the fascia that ensheathes the bulging belly of abductor—

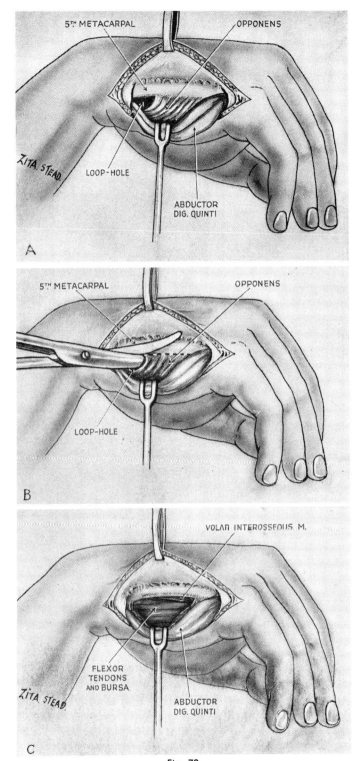

Fig. 79

The loop-hole and the exposure.—To find the loop-hole, A, slit the fascia binding abductor belly to the ulnar edge of fifth metacarpal. Retract the belly palmwards. Open a deeper fascia that lies just palmar to the metacarpal base. Deep to the fascia a touch of blunt dissection will dislodge the short 'free' portion of opponens towards the palm and so define the loop-hole. B. Widen the loop-hole by severing opponens. Open the fascia deep to the muscle. C. Retraction draws the severed opponens palmwards, with the abductor. The ulnar bursa lies with its back to mid-palmar space.

a muscle recognised by its mobility before and during operation.
Pick up this fascia close to the ulnar edge of metacarpal; open
it lengthwise without injuring abductor or the *dorsal* branch
of ulnar nerve, which runs along the sheath; liberate and retract
the muscle palmwards. Then pick up and divide a thin fascia
just in front of the metacarpal base.

It is now easy to define the loop-hole (Fig. 79, A) by raising the
free portion of opponens from bone with the blunt nose of Mayo
scissors; withdraw and open the scissors; pass one blade through
the loop-hole and cut opponens close to metacarpal shaft, dividing
all but distal fibres (Fig. 79, B); open the screen of fascia beyond.
The ulnar bursa then appears—through the wide gap between
hypothenar mass and palmar floor—bulging into the mid-palmar
space (Fig. 79, c). Widen the gap still further by flexing the hand,
especially its little finger. The deep neurovascular bundle can be
protected during this operation with a closed forceps introduced
along the palmar floor in the direction shown in Fig. 78—a safeguard which I owe to Wing-Commander R. Shackman, my former
colleague.

The final scar escapes the rubs of ordinary use.

MEDIAL APPROACH TO THE DEEP TERMINAL
BRANCH OF THE ULNAR NERVE

Exposures made through palmar skin can sometimes be exceed-
ingly refractory; and, if we use that route to deal with the deep
ulnar branch, we split the palm from wrist to finger leaving the
scar ill-placed.[1]

Instead we can adapt for this exposure the medial approach
to the mid-palmar region (p. 116), prolonging the incision four
fingerbreadths into the forearm (Fig. 81, A), disarticulating the
pisiform, and—for the widest view—dividing the opponens.

THE OPERATION

After incising skin and fascia look for the ulnar trunk beside
and radial to the tendon of flexor carpi ulnaris; then trace it down
to where it ends—just radial to pisiform—in deep and superficial
branches. The *deep* branch lies next pisiform, and after trivial
contact with its fellow nerve dips through the hypothenar mass.

---

[1] See Fig. 10 in a paper by C. A. Elsberg and A. H. Woods: *Archives of Neurology and
Psychiatry*, 1919, **2**, 658.

We know already how to find the distal part of the deep branch in the palm, opposite opponens loop-hole (p. 117) ; in order, therefore, to expose the nerve in continuity from the medial side we must displace the interrupting block of pisiform.

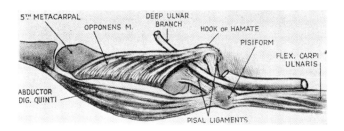

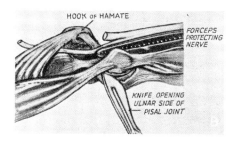

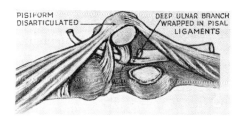

Fig. 80

Exposure of the deep terminal branch of ulnar nerve (anatomy)

Diagrams which show that when the pisiform is raised within its band (like a patella), and turned in such a way that the articular facet looks to the ulnar side, the pisal ligaments wrap round the nerve. A. The undisturbed lay-out seen from its ulnar aspect. B and C are ulnar views : B. The pisal joint is opened while we guard the nerve with intervening forceps ; C. The pisiform is raised and turned to let the ligaments be cut in safety close to the facet.

Mobilising the pisiform.—The tendon of flexor carpi ulnaris inserts on this bone, and abductor digiti quinti springs from it ; the pisiform, therefore, detached from the wrist, remains (like a patella) in the band formed by these muscles. The bone is also moored by two ligaments which pass distally, and they are reinforced

with fibres from the tendon of flexor carpi ulnaris (Fig. 80) ; the
weaker goes to the base of fifth metacarpal ; the other—a stout
cord (crossed by the deep ulnar branch) goes to the hook of hamate.
When therefore we lift the pisiform from its articulation (guarding
the nerve with a metal tool while we divide the capsule of the joint)
we see only the *start* of the deep branch ; the rest of its proximal
portion is wrapped in ligaments (Fig. 80). These can be safely
cut if the mobile bone (still in its band of muscle) is turned through
a right angle so that the oval articular facet looks to the ulnar
side ; then we divide the ligaments against the pisiform.

The deep branch may now be traced through fibres of abductor
and opponens digiti quinti, and seen to great advantage (Fig. 81, B).
But, if we need a wider access, dividing the opponens near the
edge of metacarpal will let us reach two extra fingerbreadths of
this short nerve (Figs. 79, B and 81, c).[1]

THE INNOCENT EFFECT OF PISAL DISARTICULATION

My readers should be warned. A piece of pure anatomy—most
properly consigned in other pages of the book to footnotes—lies
right ahead, and those who steadily pursue the by-pass of the text
must now skip over an intrusion. But some that disarticulate the
pisiform may wonder why they have not spoilt the ' flexor retinaculum ' (a recent alias of transverse carpal ligament). For in the
current text-books which favour that nomenclature the proximal
and ulnar corner of the retinaculum is fixed (they say) to pisiform.
Detachment therefore of the pisiform should free the corner and
impair restraint. It, happily, does nothing of the kind.

To think it might is to suppose that an important piece of band

---

[1] I have recently seen a lad whose superficial and deep branches of a left ulnar nerve had
been completely divided at the wrist. Six months after the accident he was operated
on by Mr J. C. Sugars, using the method here described. After continuing a forearm
incision into the hand by making it curve closely round the heel of the hypothenar
eminence, detachment of the pisiform gave clear access for suture and was followed by
no bowstringing of flexor tendons. Recovery of function has so far been remarkable.

Fig. 81

Exposure of the deep ulnar branch (the operation)

A. Mobility test to find abductor digiti quinti ; incisions for the skin and fascia follow its
dorsal edge and then go up the forearm—ulnar to flexor carpi tendon.
B. The disarticulated pisiform, detached from pisal ligaments, stays in its compound band.
Obscuring fibres of opponens are cleared away to bare the nerve. For wider access
mobilise opponens with Mayo scissors ; cut through the muscle close beside the edge of
fifth metacarpal (B and C).

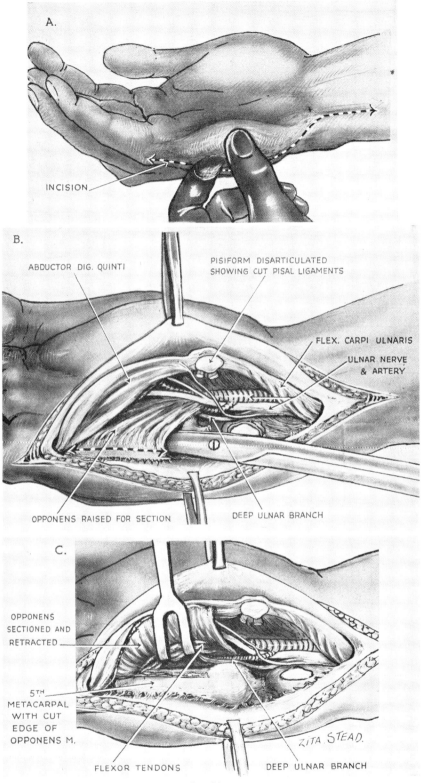

A.

INCISION

B.

ABDUCTOR DIG. QUINTI

PISIFORM DISARTICULATED
SHOWING CUT PISAL LIGAMENTS

FLEX. CARPI ULNARIS

ULNAR NERVE
& ARTERY

OPPONENS RAISED FOR SECTION

DEEP ULNAR BRANCH

C.

OPPONENS
SECTIONED AND
RETRACTED

5TH
METACARPAL
WITH CUT
EDGE OF
OPPONENS M.

FLEXOR TENDONS

DEEP ULNAR BRANCH

ZITA STEAD.

Fig. 81

concerned in curbing tendons would be attached for *that* upon a mobile and unstable bone—an almost blasphemous conception.

Like every legend, this account of pisiform attachment is the distortion of a fact. There *is* a retinaculum whose proximal and ulnar corner is firmly fixed—not in a futile way to pisiform, but to the stable cuneiform (the os triquetrum of the Basle nomenclature). Then comes that old appurtenance of fairy-tale, the cloak of darkness : the cardinal attachment to the cuneiform is hidden underneath extrinsic fibres from the pisal coat. These fibres spread in part from the insertion of flexor carpi ulnaris, and partly (on a deeper plane) from an oblique band that also coats the pisiform— a portion of the so-called *radio*carpal ligament. But far from working as a retinaculum this band (which springs, despite its name, from ulnar styloid) *relaxes* when the wrist is palmar flexed. The retinaculum of course does not ; and it is just in virtue of its ulnar corner, fixed as it is to cuneiform, that flexor tendons are restrained from tearing pisiform away from carpus.

Current descriptions of this quondam transverse carpal ligament (once the anterior annular) call for revision. First, it is wrong, I think, to give the structure *as a whole* the name of flexor retinaculum ; it does not all by any means deserve it. Something also might be done to better the nomenclature which lumps as " radiocarpal " a ligamentous band whose proximal extremity springs only from the *ulna*—a band that may be found to play a part in wrenching off the styloid process in a Colles fracture.

The golden age of ligaments is gone. So has the silver age (with John Bland-Sutton) ; and rust begins to gather.

SECTION II

ACCESS AT THE SECOND LEFT COSTAL ARCH

SINCE 1922 I have used this arch in the following sequence of exposures :—

    I. Resection of a *posterior segment* gave access to

        A. The stellate ganglion (1922).

        B. The first stage of the left subclavian artery (1923).

(By removal of a transverse process in *A* and *B* the operation became a costotransversectomy.)

    II. Resection of an *anterior segment* gave access to

        A. Pulmonary emboli (1940).

        B. Upper thoracic ganglia, sympathetic and spinal, plus relevant nerve roots. (This last with T. P. Garry in 1949.)

Exposure of the stellate ganglion from behind achieved a certain currency when Adson adopted it at the Mayo Clinic (*Proceedings of Staff Meetings*, 1928, **3**, 266), where I had the privilege of seeing him use it. The sole important modification of the method came later with the transverse muscle-splitting incision through trapezius, devised by J. C. White. Description, therefore, of the stellate exposure—the first, Professor Leriche tells me, designed to reach the ganglion from the back—would be redundant. The other three I shall describe ; they, like certain features they present, have gained no current recognition.

A METHOD OF LIGATING THE FIRST STAGE OF THE LEFT SUBCLAVIAN ARTERY FROM BEHIND [1]

While investigating a posterior approach to the stellate ganglion, I came on a simple method of exposing and tying the first stage of the left subclavian artery.

After demonstrating this method on several occasions in the School of Anatomy of the Royal College of Surgeons in Ireland,

[1] *British Journal of Surgery*, 1923, **10**, 367.

I found that another posterior approach had been used by Sherrill in 1910 and published by him in 1911.[1]

Only twenty-one cases of ligature of the left subclavian artery in its first stage were on record when my paper appeared in 1923, and of these, seven had been performed since Sherrill's operation, which was then the solitary other instance of a posterior approach to this forbidding vessel. But in February 1925 I received a letter from the late W. A. Hailes of Melbourne, which is still a cherished memory, for it described success with the method I had published, giving me my first experience of what in bishops' parlance might be termed *translation* from dissecting room direct to theatre.

The aneurysm in Hailes' patient had the size of a cricket ball, and the ligature was placed about $\frac{9}{4}$ in. above the aortic arch. In his letter Hailes expressed the belief that the case would have been inoperable from in front " even with resection of the clavicle and sternum." [2]

This belief of Hailes reflected the sinister repute of anterior access to the first stage of the *left* subclavian artery. Thus, in spite of Halsted's successful case in 1892, and others since, ligation of the first stage—right or left—got no mention in the 1934 edition of Carson's text-book, nor was it dealt with in Thorek's *Modern Surgical Technique* (1938). A place was therefore clear for the simple means on which I chanced in a quite unescapable " marriage of observation upon accident."

During an approach to the left stellate ganglion of a hunch-backed cadaver, after a costotransversectomy at the level of the second left rib followed by depression of the pleural dome, the first stage of the left subclavian artery stood out in the field. Further depression of the pleura exposed the artery from its point of origin at the aortic arch to the first rib, and definition of all its branches except the thyrocervical trunk was easy. These structures were rendered surprisingly superficial by the kyphotic deformity of the back. Examination of normal subjects showed that in them the left subclavian artery and its branches are farther from the dorsal surface of the trunk. The first stage of the artery,

---

[1] Sherrill raised a flap of skin and muscle and removed about 3 in. of the second, third, and fourth ribs. After pushing aside the pleura, the artery was exposed at the level of the fourth dorsal vertebra as it left the aorta. *Transactions of the Southern Surgical and Gynecological Association*, 1911, **23**. Quoted by W. S. Halsted in *Johns Hopkins Hospital Reports*, **21**, fasc. 1.

[2] The case was later published by R. J. Wright-Smith, then Medical Registrar in Melbourne Hospital (*Medical Journal of Australia*, 21st May 1927, p. 754).

however, is just as easily tied in spite of the depth at which it lies, for once the lung and pleura have been depressed, the artery, except for a delicate sheath, lies naked in the thoracic cavity, and is immediately accessible. There is no barrier of vein or nerve ; the vessel is directly under the finger. With a suitable needle it is easy to pass a ligature round the artery, and at my request this was done by students who had never previously tied any vessel in the body. Before describing the steps of the operation, certain anatomical points must be dealt with.

ANATOMY

The muscular planes.—The part of the second left rib which is removed lies between the scapula and the vertebral spines : it is

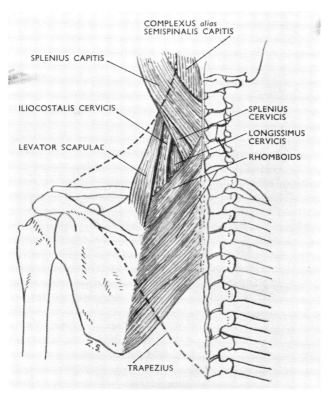

Fig. 82
Showing the muscles that lie deep to the trapezius, which is indicated by the dotted line.

concealed by muscles which anchor the scapula to the vertebræ. The trapezius is spread over the rhomboids, which cover the upper serratus posterior. Division of these muscles allows the surgeon to widen the space between the scapula and the spine, and it is essential that the transverse width of the wound should be as great as possible. Deep to the muscles of the shoulder girdle, the splenius spreads upwards from the dorsal spines; and lateral to the splenius are the cervical extensions of the sacrospinalis (Fig. 82).

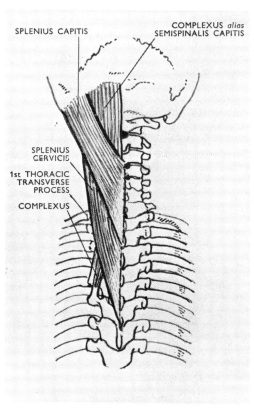

SPLENIUS CAPITIS

COMPLEXUS *alias* SEMISPINALIS CAPITIS

SPLENIUS CERVICIS

1st THORACIC TRANSVERSE PROCESS

COMPLEXUS

Fig. 83

The first thoracic transverse process is the first which projects beyond the edge of splenius. It forms a deep landmark for identifying the second rib.

The second rib.—The second rib must be accurately identified. It is not difficult to mistake it for the first, and thus in error to remove the third rib. The second rib and transverse process viewed from behind lie dorsal to the first, and the body of the first rib runs steeply down and forwards from the costotransverse articulation; it is difficult to palpate. When, however, the trapezius and the other muscles passing to the scapula have been divided and retracted, the first rib can be felt from behind by hooking the finger deeply down along the neck.

The *first* dorsal transverse process is a good landmark (Fig. 83): it lies at the level of the seventh cervical spine, three fingerbreadths from the middle line. It is the first transverse process to project beyond the edge of the splenius. *Here its tip is felt but is not seen*, being covered by two cervical extensions of sacrospinalis (iliocostalis cervicis and longissimus cervicis). Reckoning from this landmark, the surgeon finds the second transverse process and the second rib.[1]

---

[1] For additional security, the second rib should be localised by radiography before operation, and the radiologist should be asked to examine the thoracic inlet for accessory cervical or rudimentary thoracic ribs which might confuse the surgeon approaching them from behind.

The left subclavian artery.—The anterior relations of this artery in its first stage make an impressive list. Deep to the muscular planes consisting of the sternomastoid, sternohyoid, and sterno-thyroid, lie the left innominate, internal jugular, and vertebral veins, together with the vagus and phrenic nerves, the carotid artery, and branches of the cervical sympathetic. In the posterior

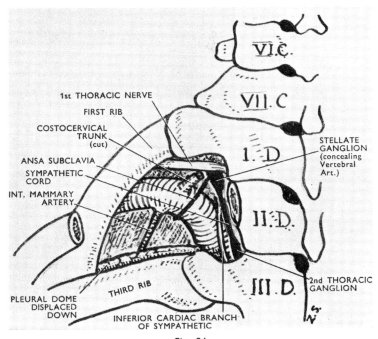

Fig. 84

The relations of the first stage of the left subclavian artery seen from behind after removal of the second thoracic process and part of the second rib. The œsophagus, and the thoracic duct which stripes its left side, are not shown in the figure : they are nearer the middle line. To see the origin of the subclavian artery from the aortic arch and to tie the *proximal* part of the artery stand behind the head of the table.

approach, however, when the pleural dome has been depressed, only one small structure intervenes between the surgeon and the artery—the ansa subclavia of Vieussens. This tough but slender loop crosses the back of the subclavian as the vessel arches after giving off its vertebral branch (Fig. 84). The depth of the proximal part of the artery from the dorsal surface is about 3 in. ; that is to say, if the index finger could be thrust through the skin it would just touch the artery. By making a large flap as described below, the thickness of the skin and subcutaneous tissue is eliminated from the field, and suitable division of the muscles to the shoulder girdle allows the surgeon to work *from the plane of the thoracic wall.* The ' working depth ' of the artery is thus reduced to 2 in., which is the actual depth of the artery from the upper border of the manubrium in front. The ' working depth,' therefore, is the same whether the approach is from the front or back.

The left vagus.—The presence of the left vagus need not be feared. The relations of the nerve depicted in most text-books of anatomy are those which it assumes after it has been freed by dissection. It then falls away from the common carotid, and lies close in front of the first stage of the subclavian. If this were its

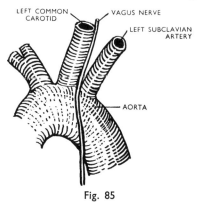

Fig. 85

The aortic arch viewed from the left side, showing left vagus related to the left common carotid and left subclavian arteries like the oblique stroke of the letter N. The vagus is safe from inclusion when the left subclavian artery is tied from behind.

true position, it would be in danger when the artery was tied from behind. Actually the nerve is, as Charpy [1] states, a satellite of the common carotid, and passes downwards and inwards close along this artery, coming gradually forwards as it descends : it thus lies beside, rather than behind, the left carotid at the root of the neck, and is on a plane anterior to the left subclavian (Fig. 85). About a finger-breadth above the aortic arch the direction of the vagus changes ; the nerve passes out, down, and back, to cross the root of the left subclavian artery, so that this part of the vagus lies between the vertical carotid and subclavian origins of the left side like the oblique stroke of the letter N.

Further, there is a barrier between the vagus and the subclavian which protects the nerve from inclusion when the artery is tied by the posterior route. This barrier consists of a layer of areolar tissue which contains : (1) The middle and sometimes the superior cardiac branch of the cervical sympathetic ; (2) descending œsophageal and tracheal branches of the inferior thyroid artery ; (3) an occasional thymic tributary of the vertebral vein. These structures not only make it difficult to expose the subclavian from in front, but obscure the origin of the vertebral artery, which tends to lie at a relatively low level on the left side.

The left vertebral artery.—This vessel during development is often absorbed into the aortic arch, and seen from in front may be mistaken for the subclavian, since it then arises from the arch

---

[1] Poirier and Charpy, *Traité d'Anatomie*, 2nd edn., vol. ii, pt. 1, p. 426.

to the left of the left common carotid. This error will not be made in ligation from behind.

The thoracic duct and the inferior cardiac nerve.—The thoracic duct will not be injured from the back; it stripes the left side of the œsophagus in the superior mediastinum, and only leaves it to pass in front of the root of the vertebral artery. In an anterior attack the duct, though not in contact with the first stage of the subclavian, may be injured as it arches outwards over the vertebral origin.

The inferior cardiac branch of the sympathetic also lies medial to the artery. With the most ordinary care it is easily avoided (Fig. 84).

THE OPERATION

A good headlight should be used, but in the cadaver I have repeatedly tied the artery without artificial illumination. The

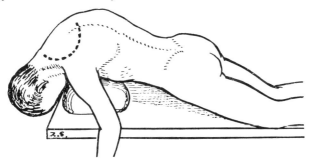

Fig. 86

Showing the position securing a maximum abduction of the scapula. The original incision is shown. (It might, of course, be replaced by White's transverse muscle-split of trapezius, which should be stopped a thumbwidth medial to the scapula to avoid the accessory and cervical innervation.)

patient lies prone, with the left shoulder clear of the table and the left upper limb hanging vertical (Fig. 86). Make the upper dorsal region as kyphotic as possible. This gives the space between the scapula and the vertebral column its maximal width.

1. Find the seventh cervical spine. Mark : (*a*) A point four fingerbreadths above it and one fingerbreadth to the *right* of the middle line ; (*b*) a similar point six fingerbreadths below the seventh spine ; (*c*) a point over the middle of the spine of the left scapula. Join these three points by the incision shown in Fig. 86, which is carried down to the sheath of the trapezius muscle. Raise the flap of skin and subcutaneous tissue thus outlined and turn it over to the *right* of the middle line.

2. With a vertical cut one fingerbreadth to the left of the vertebral spines, divide the origins of (*a*) the trapezius, (*b*) the rhomboids, and (*c*) the serratus posterior superior. Do this first at the middle of the wound where the silvery tendon of the serratus indicates the depth reached. Extend this incision throughout the entire length of the wound. Retract the divided muscles outwards. The pointed caudal end of the fleshy splenius is now exposed.

3. At the level of the seventh cervical spine, and three finger-breadths from the middle line, find the tip of the first left dorsal transverse process, remembering that it is the first which projects beyond the edge of the splenius. Find the second left rib.

4. Clear the transverse process of the second dorsal vertebra as far as the lamina. Clear at least 3 in. of the second rib. Divide the transverse process at its root and remove it. Divide the rib as far as the wound will permit from the costotransverse articulation.

5. Raise the proximal cut end of the rib. With a finger push the pleura away from its head and neck. Rotate the rib segment and divide its attachments. The sympathetic cord is now seen close to the vertebral body, lying on the pleura like a tape.

6. Very gently push the pleural dome downwards and out-wards from the vertebræ. A small strand will now be found holding the pleura to the neck of the first rib. This strand is a branch of the superior intercostal artery. Divide and tie it. The pleural dome can then be freely depressed, and the left subclavian is felt by the finger passed vertically and at a tangent to the vertebral body. *The removal of the transverse process, together with the costal neck, permits of this direct approach.* A broad malleable retractor keeps the lung and pleura out of the field. It should be polished so as to reflect light into the cavity. The artery is isolated under direct vision by blunt dissection, and its sheath is opened in the usual manner, using a long dissecting forceps. The ansa subclavia should be avoided.

7. The surgeon stands facing the head of the table. An aneurysm needle with a slot eye (or, better, the cup-and-ball needle described on p. 133) is passed with the *left* hand from within outwards : introduction of the right forefinger into the wound facilitates this manœuvre. The eye is threaded with a ligature, or with a guiding thread to which a broad definitive ligature can be attached. Ample space is afforded for securing the knot.

The internal mammary and costocervical trunks can be tied

at their origins. The vertebral artery is obscured by the cervico-dorsal ganglion of the sympathetic, but can be safely ligatured by opening the subclavian sheath close to the vertebral origin and passing an aneurysm needle round the parent trunk so that its point appears in the angle between the subclavian and the vertebral artery. The thoracic duct may thus be avoided. The thyrocervical trunk is difficult to secure by the posterior route.

A CUP-AND-BALL ANEURYSM NEEDLE FOR DEEP LIGATIONS [1]

While investigating the posterior approach to the first part of the left subclavian artery, which is described in the preceding pages, I asked the students in the dissecting-room of the Royal College of Surgeons, Ireland, to test the description and simplicity of the method. Using ordinary aneurysm needles, they tied the vessel correctly, but it was plain that a better tool would have made the task yet more simple. When the needle was threaded and then passed, the ligature lay back along the shaft, and was difficult to catch in the deep wound, while if the needle were passed unthreaded, it was not easy to expose and thread the terminal eye.

On experiment I found that an ordinary dental stopping instrument (Fig. 87, A) passed easily under the artery, and it occurred to me that if the smooth ball-tip of the instrument were detached and pierced like a bead, and if the stem were hollow, with a mouth wide enough to seat the ball, the ball could then be strung on a thread going through the stem. The thread, pulled taut, fixed the ball firmly to the cupped end of the stem, and the implement passed like an ordinary aneurysm needle under the vessel. It then remained merely to pick up the ball beyond the artery and thus retrieve the thread, which was done very simply under the guidance of vision, or of *touch*, by means of a fine hairpin bent into the shape shown in Fig. 88.

Keeping the thread taut, the ball was first made to enter the wide part of the loop, and was then caught at the constricted end ; the thread was relaxed and the ball withdrawn.

I had another and smaller model of this needle made for ligating the middle meningeal artery as a preliminary to operation

[1] Shown at the Section of Surgery, Royal Academy of Medicine in Ireland, April 27, 1923. Reprinted from the *Irish Journal of Medical Science*, October 1924.

on the gasserian ganglion (Fig. 87, c). With ordinary technique the aperture in the temporal fossa has a diameter of about 3 cm., while the distance of the artery from the surface of the zygoma is some 5 cm. Thus here, too, a deep vessel is tied through a small unyielding gap. Mr (now Regius Professor) A. A. McConnell found that with my instrument ligation of the artery at the foramen spinosum became extremely simple—but that, of course, was before plugging the foramen had replaced ligation.

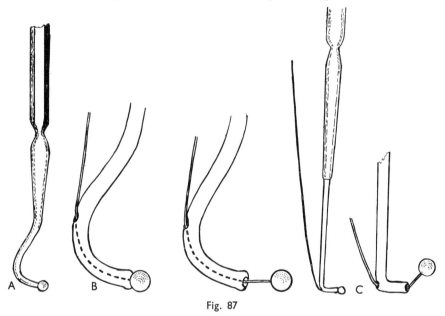

Fig. 87

When the ball is being strung on the thread, instead of knotting one end to secure the ball and passing the other through the hollow needle, it is better to slide the ball half-way along the thread and then to pass the *two* ends through the tubular stem.

The first of these cup-and-ball needles was made for me in 1921 by the late Edwin Haines of Dublin, a most skilled artificer who had long worked on astronomical instruments and, in World War I, on submarine equipment. It is to him that my needles owe the distinction of being perhaps the first surgical tools that were modelled in duralumin. They were afterwards made by Messrs Down Bros., London, in stainless steel.

There is nothing new. Long after describing the cup-and-ball needle I read, in a selection from the works of Abraham Colles published by the New Sydenham Society in 1881 (p. 342), that during the first ligation of the subclavian artery it became impracticable to retrieve the ligature although the aneurysm needle had been successfully passed round the vessel. An assistant suggested that Colles should make a knot on one *end* of the ligature, sufficiently large to prevent it from slipping through the needle's eye, so that when needle and knot had passed together under the vessel, the knot might be picked up on the far side. Unfortunately the eye of the needle was so long that it allowed the knot to slip back when the needle was pushed forward. Yet,

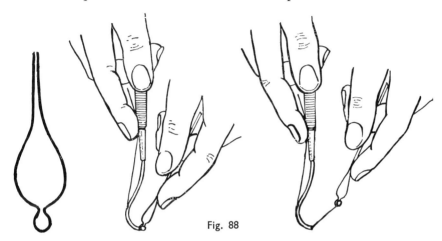

Fig. 88

despite the fact that the cup-and-ball principle was already foreshadowed in 1811, I feel privileged in following (though unawares and over a century later) a suggestion born at the crisis of an operation by Colles.[1]

A TECHNIQUE FOR REMOVING PULMONARY EMBOLI

Excepting for an obsolete paragraph on restoring the heart beat, this article is reprinted by kind permission of the *Lancet*

---

[1] A memoir by the editor of this New Sydenham Society volume records two unfamiliar tales regarding him. One of them, with perhaps a grain of truth in a halo of myth, tells how a flood of the River Nore, near his Kilkenny School, swept away the side of a house and took with it a treatise of anatomy which Colles found later in a field, " and soon preferred to his Horace or Lucian." The other, from a letter in his own hand, adds an unlooked-for gleam to the quiet portrait in the Dublin College. In April 1796 he writes from Scotland : " I must begin by telling you that I am much improved in point of personal appearance and accomplishments ; for having this day cast aside my winter clothes and put on my summer dress, my landlady could not be restrained even by the dictates of female modesty, from telling me to wear hair-powder. I need scarcely tell you that, strong as my pride is, it could not persuade me to go to the expense of six guineas a year."

much as it stood (*Lancet*, 1940, **1**, 349). I have three reasons for including it here :—

First, the method (which discards classic instruments) was welcomed as simple and bloodless by René Leriche, who for many years has occupied a place in surgery one thinks of as the growing point (*Les Embolies Pulmonaires*, 1947, pp. 52, 53, Paris : Masson et Cie).

Secondly, the exposure is extensile in that its early stage affords an extrapleural access to upper thoracic ganglia, both sympathetic and sensory (p. 147).

Thirdly, pre-operative practice of its technique can provide surgical teams with the finest test I know of smooth unhurried speed.[1]

It has, of course, long been obvious that many lives might be saved by the organisation of hospitals in respect of emboli ; O'Shaughnessy found that those unorganised were lucky if they could claim a single success. But in these islands how many have ever installed the warning bells that twenty years ago were rung in Sweden ? If bells rang here, how many competently practised ' residents ' would they alert ? How often would these find their patients or their instruments prepared ? Success, at best, will be infrequent ; yet now, when hearts are trumps in surgery, " live and let *die* " is a poor motto for ' residents ' with decent sporting instincts. But instinct without guidance would be disastrous, and guidance in this matter is lamentably overdue.

In eight months (1939-40) I performed pulmonary embolectomy on three patients, and, though none was saved, a procedure has taken shape from these attempts which serves at least to meet some of my own difficulties.

FIRST OPERATION

The first operation, except for one detail, followed tradition. Four inches of second left rib and cartilage were resected through a T-shaped incision ; and, after the medial edge of the pleural sac had been displaced outwards by gauze dissection, an opening was made in the pericardium. The special hooked sound then looped a rubber tube through the tunnel of the transverse sinus behind the aorta and pulmonary artery. With both vessels thus controlled, I opened the blue and bulging pulmonary trunk and

---

[1] In 1939-40 I was exceptionally privileged in housemen : Barber, from Toronto; Billimoria, from India (via Barts); Dunlop of Melbourne ; Harty, from Dublin *en route* for Cambridge ; Yeates, from Sydney.

drew out a long clot like a tapeworm folded lengthwise, using the bulky forceps supplied for this purpose. The lips of the opening in the artery were held with small hæmostats. Cardiac movement ceased as the patient reached the theatre, only returning after fifteen minutes—a tardy response to the combination of two restorative measures, injection of the left auricle with adrenaline and compression of the heart at systolic intervals between a hand inside the chest and one passed under the diaphragm by laparotomy. Meanwhile artificial respiration with carbon dioxide and oxygen was maintained by the anæsthetist. A pulse presently beat at the wrist and was felt for an hour ; for this hour, too, the dulled eyes became living and bright ; then the patient died—apparently a second time.

It is worth note that, once the clot was out, crossing the hæmostats on the lips of the pulmonary opening checked bleeding from this source and gave leisure to close the vessel. No use, therefore, was made of the special clamp designed in the original technique to seal the opening between removals of clot and during final suture.

Slight delays in passing the hooked sound through the transverse sinus and fastening on its rubber tube led me to relinquish their use.

There are two sources of delay : (1) Even with practice it is not always easy to deliver the end of the retrieving sound and make fast the rubber tube ; the end will sometimes hide behind the sternal edge or engage pericardium. (2) In haste one may screw the bayonet catch of the tube into the sound while—wrongly—holding the rubber tube itself ; the catch snaps out when the tube untwists. This has happened to at least three other surgeons (Nyström, 1930). The vessels, too, have been wounded by the sound or injured by the tube ; even the right auricle has been opened. Lake (1927) used his finger for hooking up the vessels when no sound was available.

It was just as easy to pass a finger through the sinus in cadavers and then hook up and handle aorta and pulmonary artery. Thus I came to question the need of occluding both these main trunks, for I could hold at pleasure the pulmonary with finger and thumb and free the aorta. But tradition blinds ; and forceful use of the transverse sinus—with fingers now instead of tube—still seemed the way to gain control of the pulmonary trunk.

It is well, however, to know how to *find* the transverse sinus, in order to tell pulmonary trunk from aorta, and especially to steady the trunk. More than once the wrong vessel has been opened, for the aorta may be pulled in front of the pulmonary by the tube or, because of sclerosis, be mistaken for pulmonary filled with clot ; the aorta can even be hooked up separately by anyone really determined. But books still fail to guide the tyro. I have found each of the following methods useful in locating the sinus : (1) The right index finger, slid vertically inside the pericardium opposite the second rib and kept in contact with the lining of the left wall of the sac, crosses over the left auricular appendix and goes straight into the sinus ; (2) outward retraction of the left wall of the pericardium brings to view the blunt, free tip of the appendix ; a finger enters the sinus a little behind and medial to this landmark. The pulmonary artery is the trunk next the left end of the sinus.

SECOND OPERATION

My second operation was performed shortly after the first. This time the patient's heart was beating when the chest was opened, but it stopped at once when I passed a finger into the sinus and hooked up the two great vessels. I immediately let slip the aorta and kept hold of the pulmonary trunk. Emboli had already reached its smaller branches ; and, though most were removed in the way described presently, the outlook for the patient—even from the standpoint of pulmonary embolectomy— could only be desperate. This time I discarded the special clot-forceps that seemed so large in the previous case and used an aspirator instead. Attached to it was a cannula curved to the shape of a favourite dissecting scissors, which happened, when introduced from the main trunk in cadavers, to enter, like sword into sheath, branches arising from the right and left pulmonary arteries.

I had found, through the courtesy of the late T. H. Belt, that with this cannula the aspirator, in dead lungs, removed emboli from small branches and in my second case was able to extract, as I have said, most of the peripheral clot. But the real virtue of the aspirator—at least as yet—is not in these peripheral extractions ; at present it seems impossible to save a patient who has been gradually overcome by clots that reach remoter branches. Advantage lies in the cannula entering a small and easily controlled incision in the main trunk and then cleaving at once by suction to adjacent clot, which may either stick in its mouth and thus be drawn out or else pass on through the lumen. Nyström (1930) has long used aspiration for removing pulmonary emboli and cites Trendelenburg as using it many years before him in animal experiments.

An unexpected source of delay in this case was the peculiar depth and density of the propericardial tissue—rich, perhaps, in thymic remains—which appeared on retracting the pleura. After dividing this tissue I lost time through mistaking the smooth face of pericardium for the exposed wall of a great vessel. I had till then not learnt to rely on the likeness of pericardial wall to thin dural membrane as sure guidance for opening the sac.

THIRD OPERATION

The third patient—like the second—was alive in the early part of the operation, though obviously dying. The heart stopped immediately after the pericardium was incised.

Professor B. O. Pribram (a refugee in 1940, but formerly Professor of Surgery in Berlin) told me that he too, on opening the pericardium, had seen the heart stop and require massage to restore its beat. Others have stopped it, as I did in my second case, by hooking up aorta and pulmonary artery. It would be well to know how these stimuli act, and meanwhile, perhaps, to atropinise the patient thoroughly before operation.

This time I did not hook up or disturb the aorta; it was, however, easy to grasp and control the pulmonary artery separately between finger and thumb while I made a short opening in its wall. The lips of this opening were caught with delicate hæmostats, and the cannula after a moment's check found the way in (Fig. 89, A, B, and C). There were no clots in the main trunk, but several were sucked from right and left branches and quickly reached the flask of the aspirator. I thought afterwards how useful a manual control would have been with which I could interrupt aspiration myself and then redirect the cannula while circulation continued round it.

It is by no means difficult to stop hæmorrhage from the pulmonary artery where pressure averages a fifth of that of systemic trunks and through sympathetic influence may rise during systole to perhaps 50 to 60 mm. Hg. Mr R. Shackman and I have found by experiment on fresh post-mortem material that the crossing of two hæmostats placed on the lips of the small opening by which the cannula enters prevents leakage (Fig. 89, B and C), even if pressure within the vessel is equal to the

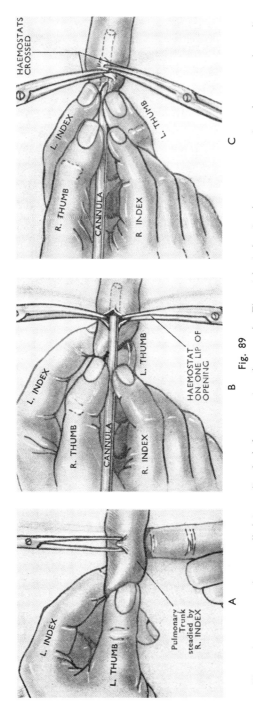

HAEMOSTATS CROSSED

L. INDEX

L. THUMB

R. THUMB

CANNULA

R. INDEX

C

R. THUMB

CANNULA

R. INDEX

L. INDEX

L. THUMB

HAEMOSTAT ON ONE LIP OF OPENING

B   Fig. 89

L. INDEX

L. THUMB

Pulmonary Trunk steadied by R. INDEX

A

A. The pulmonary trunk controlled immediately before opening the vessel. The right index in the transverse sinus locates and steadies the trunk, while the first assistant picks up a fold of its front wall with a fine-toothed forceps. The surgeon withdraws his right index from the sinus and uses his right hand to open the artery. Then, and not till then, he occludes the lumen between left thumb and index. If the artery wall is friable the finger of a second assistant should replace the surgeon's in the sinus to relieve strain by supporting the vessel. The aorta is not disturbed nor is the pulmonary trunk hooked up.

B. The pulmonary trunk is opened and the cannula passed. The lumen of the trunk is still momentarily occluded by the surgeon's left thumb and index. He has opened the vessel by cutting through the fold (A). The first assistant has caught each lip of the opening with a Dunhill hæmostat.

C. Prevention of leakage. The momentary occlusion of the trunk's lumen has ceased. The first assistant has crossed the hæmostats to prevent leakage. The surgeon, after releasing the lumen, is now using his left thumb and index to fix and further seal the opening by pressing its lips against the cannula.

maximum found in normal life. At the low pressures, therefore, that go with pulmonary embolus risk of hæmorrhage is small indeed. None the less, however, in operating on our patient we took care to reinforce closure by pressing the lips of the opening with finger and thumb against the wall of the cannula (Fig. 89, c).

A DRAFT OF TECHNIQUE

The following provisional scheme, based on my three operations, will serve for epitome.

1. **Skin preparation.**—As soon as operation is even considered,

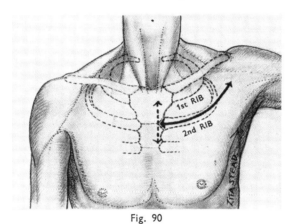

Fig. 90
The incision
Its sternal limb allows the wide exposure of thoracic skeleton from which alone the 'working-depth' is reckoned.

prepare the whole front of the chest and upper part of the abdomen.

2. **Local anæsthesia.**—If likelihood of operation increases, infiltrate a triangle whose base on the left edge of the sternum measures a liberal span from the sternoclavicular joint, and whose apex lies a span out along the second left rib. The epigastrium, too, should be injected in view of cardiac massage. (My second and third operations were performed under local anæsthesia.)

3. **Incision** is T-shaped (Fig. 90); it cuts down on 7 in. of sternal border and on 7 in. of second rib and cartilage. (Beginners —for fear of opening pleura—should by no means follow the expert who cuts between ribs.) The flaps of skin and pectoral muscle are then turned back from the costal plane widely enough to let the operator proceed unhampered from this new surface and so

reduce the working depth of the wound. It is prudent to open the epigastrium at this stage.

4. **Resecting the second left rib and cartilage.**—After superficial

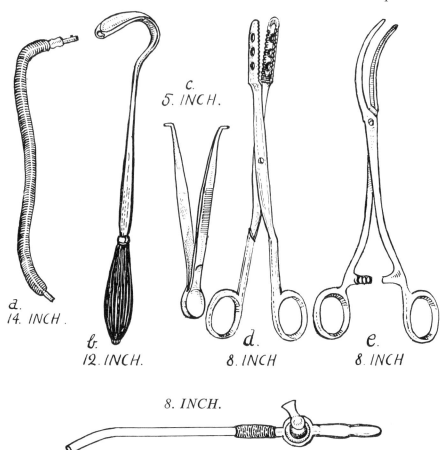

Fig. 91

Above—**Five discarded instruments, originally used for pulmonary embolectomy**

a. The rubber tourniquet for controlling the ascending aorta and pulmonary trunk.

b. The sound for withdrawing the tourniquet through the transverse pericardial sinus.

c. The forceps for keeping the opening in the pulmonary trunk patent during introduction of

d. the massive forceps for removing the embolus ;

e. Forceps for controlling the opening in the pulmonary trunk during suture.

Below—The polythene 8 in. cannula, with stop-cock, for aspirating clot in the technique described here.

division, above and below, of intercostal muscles, begin with the cartilage, near the sternum. In this place a streak of fat clothes the internal mammary vessels, which lie deep to the cartilage, and with them keeps the pleura far enough off to give a safe plane of cleavage to any common raspatory that is slightly curved on the flat near its edge. Divide the sternal end of the cartilage and use it for drawing the rib gently away from the pleura while the curved raspatory helps a finger to finish the extraperiosteal separation. Resect at least 6 in. of rib-plus-cartilage—a wide removal which gives the great advantage of *oblique* access.

5. **Exposure of the pericardium.**—With the pulp of the finger draw the edge of the left pleural sac outwards. To do this without

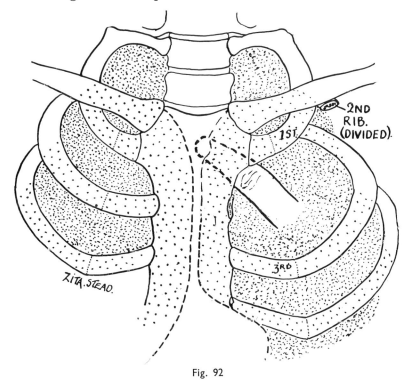

Fig. 92

opening the pleura choose a spot at the lower border of the first costal cartilage and work a finger in gently under the mammary vessels, then under the manubrium. Aim the finger so as to reach the middle point of the manubrium, and, when that point is reached, but not till then, flex the finger and begin to mobilise and retract the pleural edge ; for there the left sac leaves its fellow and goes to its own apex (Fig. 92). This is only another use of the old trick of tracing planes of cleavage from the place where structures part, and after learning to apply it here I never opened the pleura once in all the material put so generously at my disposal by Professor J. H. Dible ; nor was it opened in any of my three patients.[1]   A very little care leaves the internal mammary vessels unharmed and close to the sternum.   The gap left by the wide resection of rib allows the apex of the lung to be mobilised and then flattened in a posterior direction within the sac of the pleura, a flattening which liberates the side of the pericardial cone and so gives better access to the pulmonary trunk, which slopes backwards.   Withdrawing the pleura reveals a variable thickness of propericardial fat, which is sometimes pink and feebly vascular ;   pick this up in forceps and divulse it boldly with blunt-nosed scissors down to the smooth, unmistakable face of pericardium.

6. **Opening the pericardium.**—Catch this membrane near the sternal edge with a fine-toothed forceps ;   open it longitudinally for at least 3 in. with the same scissors and expose the conus arteriosus of the right ventricle in company with the pulmonary trunk and ascending aorta.

7. **Catching and opening the pulmonary trunk.**—Slide the tip of the right index into the transverse sinus (see the description of the first operation) and locate and steady, but *do not hook up*, the pulmonary trunk (Fig. 89, A).   The assistant, standing on the right of the patient, then catches the middle part of the trunk with a fine-toothed forceps held in his left hand, making a small transverse fold in its anterior wall (Fig. 89, A).   The surgeon withdraws his right finger from the sinus and occludes the stem of the pulmonary trunk between left thumb and index close to the heart. To prevent the forceps from tearing a friable trunk the surgeon's finger must be replaced in the sinus by that of a *second* assistant, who thus relieves strain by supporting the vessel.   Scissors in the surgeon's right hand now cut longitudinally into the artery through the small transverse fold held by the first assistant.   The opening in the vessel should be just large enough for the cannula. The scissors are then put down and the cannula is picked up. The first assistant, using his right hand, meanwhile grasps in turn each lip of the opening with a delicate hæmostat, taking care to keep his original hold of the vessel with the toothed forceps till the second hæmostat is on (Fig. 89, A and B).   (I used Dunhill's goitre hæmostats for this purpose and found them excellent.)   It is worth noting that some pericardia contain oily fluid, which makes the pulmonary trunk slippery ;   it might thus be well for the surgeon to wear cotton gloves over rubber ones.

---

[1] Behind the sternal *body*, on the other hand, the two pleural sacs are sometimes in wide apposition ;   separation there is done at great disadvantage.

8. **Passage of the cannula, hæmostasis, and removal of clot.**— The surgeon, still occluding the lumen, passes the cannula through the opening. The first assistant then forestalls hæmorrhage by gently crossing the hæmostats over the cannula (Fig. 89, c). This control of the opening is the cue for the surgeon to release his grasp of the lumen ; he now uses his *left* thumb and index and presses instead the wall of the vessel against the cannula to fix the opening and keep it shut when the cannula moves from branch to branch (Fig. 89, c). A tap controls suction (Fig. 91). Small clots go clean through the cannula ; the large stick in the nozzle and can then be drawn out. By this method, therefore—with fingers and aspirator in place of tourniquet and clot-forceps—the lumen of the pulmonary trunk is only closed during the very few seconds required for opening the wall and passing the cannula in. Aspiration is stopped while the cannula moves from branch to branch, so that blood may circulate past it. (The directions of the main branches of the artery—the left almost perpendicular to the table, the right nearly horizontal—must be remembered.) *There is at no time interference with the aorta ;* indeed, the hooking up of this trunk seems in retrospect an unnecessary act of violence.

9. **Closing the incised trunk.**—After removing the cannula, keep the hæmostats crossed at the lips of the opening and close the trunk with mattress sutures. Then close the pericardium and chest wall.

I would stress here the need of training oneself and others for embolectomy on fresh unhardened cadavers ; formalin stiffens and withdraws parts otherwise supple and easily reached, while stale material tends to exaggerate difficulties due to friability. I have had recently to demonstrate the operation on preserved cadavers ; in all but one of them the heart and great vessels had withdrawn to the right and backwards. Even in that awkward abnormal situation it was easy to gain separate control of the pulmonary trunk—not indeed as usual with left thumb and index but between the two index fingers of an assistant standing on the right side of the subject. Approach in a difficult case of this sort, or in any case, is greatly helped by tilting the chest with a pillow under the left scapula. The surgeon will then appreciate in full the value of oblique access given by a really wide resection of the second costal arch.

SUMMARY

Attention is called to certain points in the operation for removing pulmonary clot.

Flaps are reflected widely enough to reduce 'working' depth by making a new surface at the level of the ribs. The epigastrium is opened early for possible cardiac massage. Wide resection of the second left rib gives oblique access to the pulmonary trunk, for through the large gap the lung apex can be mobilised and flattened backwards within its pleural sac. These parts are seen best when a pillow is put under the left scapula of the patient. The likeness to thin dura of pericardial wall helps the surgeon to find it through any thickness of propericardial fat.

Two methods of finding the transverse sinus are described. No sound or tourniquet is passed through it ; *the sinus is used merely in locating and steadying the pulmonary trunk.* The aorta is left undisturbed. The pulmonary trunk is separately controlled with the fingers ; it is *not* hooked up. An aspirating cannula, properly curved, is used instead of forceps for removing clot. The cannula requires only a short opening in the pulmonary trunk, and, when it enters the lumen, hæmostasis can be secured at once. The time during which fingers occlude the lumen of the trunk is thus reduced to the few seconds spent in making the opening and passing in the cannula. Bleeding from the pulmonary trunk after the introduction of the cannula is prevented by crossing the two hæmostats which have caught the lips of the opening in its wall ; this opening is further sealed by pressing it against the cannula. A tap stops aspiration so that circulation may proceed while the cannula is redirected from branch to branch.

REFERENCES

Lake, N. C. (1927). *British Medical Journal,* **2,** 1180.
Leriche, R. (1947). *Les Embolies Pulmonaires,* pp. 52, 53. Paris : Masson.
Nyström, G. (1930). *Annals of Surgery,* **92,** 498.
O'Shaughnessy, L., and Sauerbruch, F. (1937). *Thoracic Surgery.* London : Arnold.

ANTERIOR EXTRAPLEURAL ACCESS TO UPPER THORACIC GANGLIA, SYMPATHETIC AND SPINAL [1]

Years ago, during a former appointment at the Royal College of Surgeons in Ireland, one of us came upon a dorsal route—procured by costotransversectomy—for dealing with the upper part of the thoracic sympathetic chain (1922). Before that date, in Continental surgery, and later here (though not in the United States, where Adson gave the Dublin method currency in 1928), emphasis lay most on a cervical path for entering the chest by way of the thoracic inlet. From 1934, however, the dorsal route—adapted then for sectioning preganglionic fibres—acquired new prestige.

A choice of means uncramps the mould of surgical procedure, and so we venture to describe a third approach.

In 1942 a Service class held at the British Postgraduate Medical School was shown how a cannula could aspirate a pulmonary embolus without the added use of clamp, or tourniquet, or anything but fingers, scissors, and mosquito forceps. And, afterwards an officer, who hurried out and left no name, drew our attention to a windfall we had missed—the reach of sympathetic chain accessible on drawing down the pleural dome through the large gap produced by wide removal of a second rib and cartilage.

Division of this second cartilage beside the sternum is easily performed without incising pleura : the sac is buffered off the cartilage by internal mammary vessels which run within a streak of fat, and often by a portion of the sternocostal muscle. So, when the knife has freed both borders of the cartilage, a little-finger tip and then a curved director find room to pass beneath it and protect the pleural sac.

The lifted cartilage provides a handle for gently raising up the rib from the undamaged, close-adherent pleura, and safely clearing it far into the axilla ; there the rib is either cut away or, better, cracked across for subsequent replacement.

The way of entry next the sternum thus obtained will let us separate the pleural sacs ; for these are parted best—like other structures—from levels where they naturally trend apart. The

[1] T. P. Garry and A. K. Henry, *Irish Journal of Medical Science*, October 1949, p. 757.

index finger, therefore, sliding in until its *nail* lies close behind the
midpoint of manubrium (Fig. 93) will, when the finger tip is
flexed, engage the separation of the pleural domes (Henry, 1940).
A little movement sideways soon makes room for entry of the
middle finger ; and presently the whole hand slipping in can peel
the dome intact from the thoracic inlet.   The dome, with the
included apex of the lung, is drawn easily towards the diaphragm,
and so leaves bare (excepting for a lining of translucent fascia)

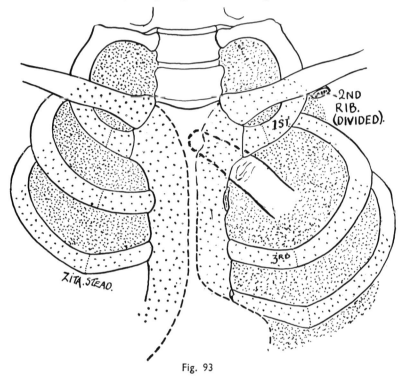

Fig. 93

the inner face of the thoracic cage.   The sympathetic chain
is often obvious at once ; its upper ganglia—all but the stellate,
which lies across the costal *neck*—lie on the heads of corresponding
ribs, and can be dealt with as desired, from stellate down to
fourth thoracic.   Behind the chain lie intercostal nerves and
vessels.

The present-day objective.—Resection of some inches of the
third and second of these nerves with rami grey and white,
including, too, the hinder primary divisions, and, finally, a subarachnoid section of their *roots*, both sensory and motor—these
steps to-day afford a favoured means for burking the regrowth

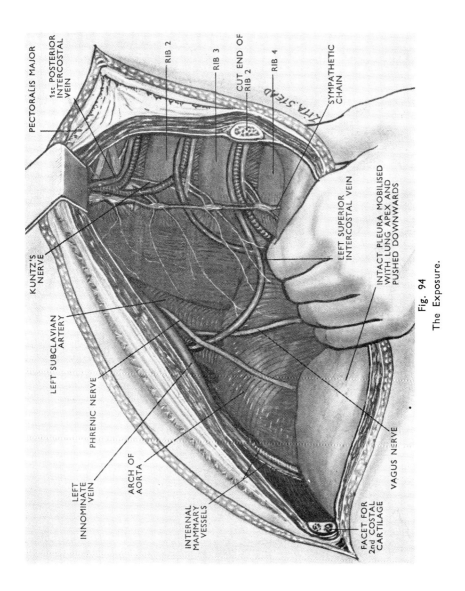

Fig. 94

The Exposure.

of upper-limb *pre*ganglionic fibres that govern sweating and constrict the vessels (White and Smithwick, 1942).[1]

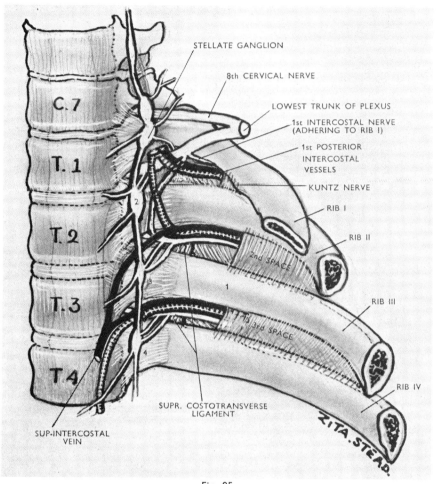

Fig. 95

Diagram of parts seen in the transthoracic extrapleural approach to upper thoracic ganglia. Kuntz's nerve has its common relation to the anterior primary ramus of Th. 1, joining the ramus close to where the first intercostal nerve separates. (M. Stranc.)

We find it easier to trace and clear and resect nerves Th. 2 and Th. 3 (together with the chain) through the anterior route than through the dorsal path obtained by costotransversectomy : the prospect from in front is very wide indeed. The intervertebral foramina are readily accessible between the heads of ribs, though

[1] These authors' own account of their technique with costotransversectomy suggests they would be glad if it were possible to drop the part concerned with root resection. This, from behind, can sometimes be most difficult, though easy from in front.

each is covered and concealed. Except in the obese, the trunks of intercostal veins and arteries (which pass behind the chain) are plainly visible (Figs. 94 and 95).

ANATOMICAL CONSIDERATIONS

Finding the second rib in the chest.—It is, unfortunately, easy, as was stressed in the former Dublin method, to miscount ribs when working from the back ; the natural kyphosis of the upper dorsal vertebræ brings first and second ribs confusingly together. The same is true when working from within the chest—a fact which matters in determining the number of a sympathetic ganglion or of an intercostal space beside the spine. We find it can be curiously baffling to try to follow back the second rib from where it has been cut in the axilla : the finger slips unwittingly along the third.

Within the chest the sharp front edge of the first rib (though out of sight) is clearly felt two fingerbreadths lateral to the vertebral bodies, and is, of course, the spot from which to find the second. Pass in the hand, therefore, palm up, left on left side, right on right, with the index touching the vertebral bodies. The middle finger goes through the thoracic inlet, and is made to bulge the tissues of the neck above the clavicle, a sign that it certainly lies above the first rib. Then travelling down and back into the chest the middle finger nail slides over the sharp edge of the first rib, and—after moving only through the thickness of the finger tip —strikes the second rib, below and behind the first. It is easy to pass an instrument along the palm and mark the second rib for recognition by means of dye or a clip.

Foraminal coverings.—A handbreadth from the bodies of the vertebræ each intercostal nerve is screened by tense translucent fascia, and, followed centrally, is lost to view (together with the vessels) ; for fat accumulates between the costal heads behind the fascia, and there occludes and hides each intervertebral foramen.

Considered from the surgeon's point of view, this cellophane or onion-skin-like membrane forms a single barrier, but one of us (T. P. G.) has found the ' skin ' is really double, consisting of two demonstrable coats : (1) An inner fascia called till lately *endothoracic*, which, though the name has dropped from books, continues still to line the chest after we strip the wall of pleura.

This layer where it lies on the ribs is loosely joined, but normally not fused, with periosteum. (2) The second ' skin,' which partly coats the outer surface of the first, invests the flattened *endocostal* bellies (sternocostalis alias triangularis sterni, subcostales, inter-costales intimi) ; and fusing where it touches periosteum, spreads in and out *between* each pair of ribs, across the intervals that part these scattered groups of muscle. This outer patchy ' skin ' might well be called the *intracostal* fascia.

Ligaments.—Two sets of these are relevant. The first, the superior costotransverse, is formed of thumbwide bands that lie a thumbwidth lateral to vertebral bodies : one in each intercostal space unites the nuchal crest belonging to the lower rib with the preceding transverse process next above (Fig. 95). Each slopes just lateral to and partly screens the stout posterior primary ramus ; it also lies *behind* the anterior ramus, which is, of course, the intercostal nerve. The ligament affords a useful base for scissors to divide the hinder ramus (p. 158).

The second ligament, remarked by one of us (T. P. G.), is small, inconstant, and, so far as we can find, unnamed. It matters, for, when present, it lies in front of, and blocks our access to, the very short thoracic trunk formed by the union of motor and sensory nerve roots (p. 158). We shall therefore liberate the obvious trunk and use it plus its anterior ramus as a handle for getting control of the far less obvious roots.

The second and third thoracic nerve roots.—The roots of Th. 2 and Th. 3, if measured from their highest levels of attachment to the cord, begin about two fingerbreadths or, more exactly, 33 and 38 mm. above the points where they escape from inter-vertebral foramina (Soulié). These segments of the cord leave no more room in the canal they occupy than that which lies around a little fingertip encircled by a dorsal vertebra, and in that tiny space the roots are almost vertical to any transverse section of the cord. Then, suddenly, on leaving the canal at a foramen, the roots turn through a full right angle (Fig. 96). Both facts are useful to the surgeon. For, firstly, since these roots converge downward, towards the point of exit, their sensory and motor parts—which on the cord are separated only by about 5 mm.—come close enough together to be cut ' in one ' as they emerge from each foramen. And, secondly, the sudden bend as they emerge protects the cord from minor operative pulls whose brunt will fall instead on the foramen's mouth.

A recent windfall (1956), photographed as Fig. 97, bears out our draft of 1949 (Fig. 96). This draft was put forward in lieu of ocular proof of the supposed true lie of upper dorsal roots. We had inferred this layout from tables of nerve-root length (due separately to Soulié and to Hovelacque), considered with our measurements of cord and dural-sheath diameters.

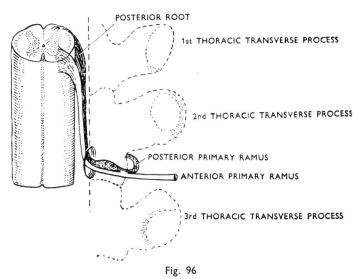

POSTERIOR ROOT

1st THORACIC TRANSVERSE PROCESS

2nd THORACIC TRANSVERSE PROCESS

POSTERIOR PRIMARY RAMUS

ANTERIOR PRIMARY RAMUS

3rd THORACIC TRANSVERSE PROCESS

Fig. 96

The second thoracic segment

This draft of the lie of roots of Th. 2 was inferred (1949) : (*a*) from their average intradural length at this level—33 mm. or two fingerbreadths ; (*b*) from estimates of cord and dural-sheath diameters. (Compare the actual specimen in the next figure.)

Note how the spinal ganglion at upper thoracic levels is *not* framed by the foramen but lies outside on a sill formed by articular processes where T. P. Garry's ' jolt ' test detects it in the dead *and* in the living subject (Professor P. Fitzgerald).

Comparing that draft (Fig. 96) with the actual specimen, one sees in both the surprising—almost vertical—drop of an upper dorsal root, so very like the more familiar lumbosacral declivities.

In the draft figure (Fig. 96) the intradural root length was made to equal Soulié's mean of 33 mm.—an average length of two fingerbreadths. In the actual specimen photographed in Fig. 97, the root length of Th. 2 was considerably longer (44 mm. on the right side ; 46·5 mm. on the left side), which proves our inference to be an understatement.

Two months later, however, another specimen was found with Th. 2 root lengths of 35 mm. (right) and 37 mm. (left), which gave a close agreement of inference and fact.

Thus it would seem that the splayed-out courses of upper

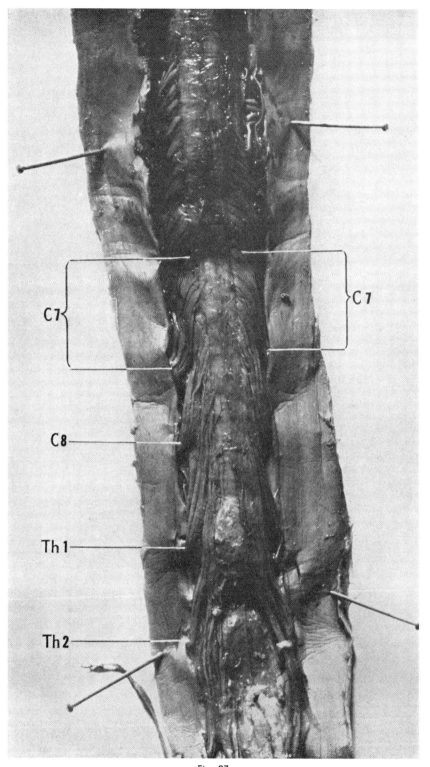

Fig. 97

Photograph of a hardened spinal cord with opened membranes (slightly enlarged)

Despite the widely gaping dura a rare chance has let thoracic roots stay put. They thus go steeply and unsplayed to reach their dural openings, just as though they still were crowded in the narrows between cord and close-encircling sheath.

dorsal roots shown in the text-books are nothing more than artefacts—" errors of retraction," essential for presenting nerve-root pictures (Fig. 98).

Our draft, however, failed in one respect : it did not demonstrate that individual rootlets cling to the cord through half their length as they stream down and mould themselves to its circumference.

This *moulding* is clearest in the photograph at the seventh cervical segment where (unlike their thin thoracic fellows, from Th. 2 to Th. 12) rootlets suggest the back of a child's head with hanks of hair smeared down to right and left and parted widely (Fig. 97).

The position of thoracic spinal ganglia.—The text-books (Buchanan, Cunningham, Gray, Piersol) state that these ganglia lie *in* the intervertebral foramina. From this agreement one would think that if the intervertebral foramen were, as the Latin word implies, a hole, or like, perhaps, an open window, it then should frame the ganglion. In point of fact the ganglion appears to lie *outside* the window—on the sill. Each sill is formed by joined articular processes, protruding right and left so that they show beyond the bodies of each pair of vertebræ ; and looking from above directly down on a recumbent spine one does not see the intervertebral foramina ; one sees the sills that bear the ganglia (Fig. 96).

A barrister, however, might contend that ' intervertebral foramen ' may apply not only to the obvious and rounded hole between two vertebræ but also to an orifice, elliptical in shape, whose longer axis and whose plane slope back and outward from the bodies. The inner pole of this ellipse would then be figured by the front edge of the hole ; the outer, by the outer edge of the combined articular facets. And so, by thus imagining a funnel sliced obliquely, he could contrive to bring the sill within the bounds of the foramen. The barrister might, therefore, argue that a ganglion—like an evasive member of the Commonwealth— can be both ' in ' and at the same time ' out.' Anatomists, we hope, will leave that kind of shift to older callings, and either rule that these upper intervertebral foramina are simply holes (resembling their congeners elsewhere), or that they constitute a special order of foramen—the silled or liminate.

Meanwhile what matters to a surgeon is the fact that ganglia of the thoracic nerves do *not* lie in a hole, but clean outside it on a dorsal sill—so far outside, indeed, that we shall show they can

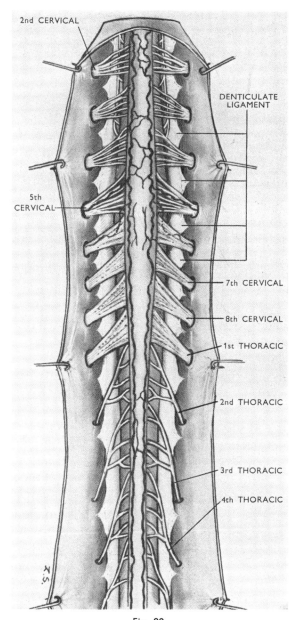

Fig. 98

The upper spinal nerve roots (after Hovelacque)

The wide abduction of the roots in this figure is required to demonstrate three of the different types of rootlet distinguished by Hovelacque—upper cervical, lower cervical, thoracic.

Current illustrations in other hands are misleading and often fail in four respects : (1) they do not distinguish variety in upper spinal roots ; (2) they greatly shorten their intradural length ; (3) they change an almost vertical trend below C7 to a frank outward slope ; (4) they fail to mould the rootlets to the cord.

be lifted forward (with their roots intact) and *felt* by pressing them against a rib head.

In case experience should clinch the usefulness of spinal-root division, there follows a technique for its performance from the *front*.

SECTION FROM IN FRONT OF SENSORY AND MOTOR ROOTS

A special instrument.—Apart from means of lighting up the field, the only special tool that helps in the performance of the operation is a very long-handled pair of Bozeman's gynæcological scissors, which one of us (T. P. G.) discovered rusting in a junk shop on the Dublin quays. These scissors (Fig. 99) have two

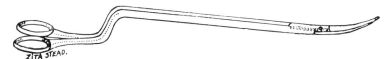

Fig. 99

Bozeman's 10-in. scissors, invaluable for dividing anterior and posterior nerve roots.

useful curves : their 10 in. shaft is (like a rifle) cranked near the grip ; the nose is oppositely bent (and slightly twisted) on the flat. So, when the user sights along the shaft, he has unbroken view of what he wants to cut.

The sympathetic chain.—The chain where we divide it lies in front of intercostal nerves and vessels ; therefore divide it first. Cut it below the third thoracic ganglion, counting the first as portion of the stellate. Displace the upper segment of the chain towards the patient's head, dividing rami communicantes and medial branches. This gives access to the site of intervertebral foramina. (The surgeon deals with the divided chain as he prefers —resecting it below the stellate, encasing it in silk, displacing it to dorsal muscle, or blocking it with alcohol injected neat or laced with phenol.)

Rami, roots, and ganglia of Th. 2 and Th. 3.—Divide each anterior ramus alias intercostal nerve 2 in. lateral to bodies of the vertebræ, and take it as a guide. Lift the cut central end and trace it medially. (Use clips and then divide the vessels where they screen the lifted nerve.) A thumbwidth from the vertebræ the nerve is tethered by its dorsal ramus which lies beside the inner edge of the superior costotransverse ligament, and travels with a dorsal vein and artery. The ramus and the vessels should be therefore ' clipped ' *en masse* before we cut them.

Dividing the dorsal tether.—Its section is accomplished by passing the tip of the Bozeman scissors in along the intercostal space, letting its convex aspect slide on the front of the superior costotransverse ligament. (When cutting through this tether take special care the scissors' tip does not rise forward off the ligament and cut by accident the nerve *trunk* with the ramus.) Clip the tether as far back as possible. There will seldom be room enough for two clips between which to cut, so do not hesitate to cut the bundle in *front* of a single clip : bleeding from *central* ends of the divided vessels—if not already checked by clips put on the screen of major intercostal veins and arteries—at once becomes accessible by severing the dorsal tether. Should the clip fail to close the dorsal vessels, division of the costotransverse ligament gives access to the bleeding point, which will retract towards the dorsal muscles. The *second* ligament, in front of the thoracic trunk—if present—must be cut (p. 152). The trunk thus liberated leads us to the spinal nerve roots.

Finding the spinal ganglion and dividing the nerve roots.—The closed tip of the scissors can now locate this ganglion, which is both firm and inconspicuous : the metal sliding out across the ganglion jolts on to bone, as if it had crossed a knot (T. P. G.). The bone may be the foramen's sill or the rib head, depending on the direction given to the handle formed by the liberated trunk and the divided intercostal nerve. And once it has been felt its shape will be descried.

Next, with the ganglion located on the dorsal root, divide the root just central to the ganglion, turning the scissors' tip conveniently to cut through motor roots as well. The presence of recurrent vessels at each intervertebral foramen makes it advisable to catch the roots with clips before dividing them.

Division of the roots necessitates, of course, an opening of the subarachnoid space, so spinal fluid leaks ; but Smithwick finds that this gives no occasion for concern.

The method we describe already claims the signal privilege of having been used in Dublin by Mr (now Professor) P. Fitzgerald, at St Vincent's Hospital, in June 1948.

Two anatomical points are worth emphasis :—

1. The accessibility of the upper thoracic spinal ganglia which are more laterally placed than text-books suggest and can thus be felt by Garry's ' jolt ' test.

2. The intradural lie and length of upper spinal roots are quite unlike their current portraits.

REFERENCES

Adson, A. W. (1928). *Proceedings of the Staff Meetings of the Mayo Clinic*, **3**, 266.

Adson, A. W., and Brown, C. E. (1929). *Surgery, Gynecology and Obstetrics*, **48**, 577.

Henry, A. K. (1922). *Transactions of Royal Academy of Medicine in Ireland*, reported in *Lancet*, **2**, 1385.

—— (1927). *Exposures of Long Bones and other Surgical Methods*. Bristol : Wright.

—— (1940). *Lancet*, **1**, 349.

Hovelacque, A. (1927). *Anatomie des Nerfs*. Paris : Masson.

Smithwick, R. H., Freeman, N. E., and White, J. C. (1934). *Archives of Surgery*, **29**, 759.

Soulié, A. (1904), in Poirier and Charpy's *Traité d'Anatomie Humaine*, vol. 3, fasc. 3, p. 821. Paris : Masson.

White, J. C., and Smithwick, R. H. (1942). *The Autonomic Nervous System*, 2nd edn. London : Kimpton.

SECTION III

THE HYPOGASTRIC ROUTE

THE MIDLINE EXTRAPERITONEAL HYPOGASTRIC ROUTE

This route allows us to reach and deal with various objectives such as the following :—

> The pelvic stage of both ureters in relation to stone and stricture.
> Femoral hernia, single or bilateral.
> The blood supply of the prostate and of other pelvic organs.
> The bladder pedicles in relation to cystectomy.
> Obturator-nerve trunks (for bilateral resection in adductor spasm).
> Hip-joint nerves in a complete exposure from in front.

I shall not deal with bilateral exposure of the pelvic stage of the ureter : stone and, in Egypt, stricture due to schistosomiasis have made this a matter of routine.[1]

Use of the midline route for femoral hernia is sufficiently established. Retropubic prostatectomy has its own literature, and the simple bilateral *pelvic* resection of obturator-nerve trunks for adductor spasm needs nothing but mention in the paragraphs on complete exposure of hip-joint nerves (p. 171).

I shall deal with only two objectives, each in relation to one of the following procedures :—

> 1. Prelusive vascular control in extraperitoneal prosta-tectomy.
> 2. Complete exposure of hip-joint nerves by anterior access.

But though the midline route itself, aside from a particular objective, has seen long service, some of its features still need notice.

---

[1] I have described these strictures and their treamtent in the section ‘ Schistosomaisis,’ *British Surgical Practice*, vol. vii, 1950.

INCISION : ' RETZIUS ' : CLOSURE

Skin incision and rectus separation.—Owing to the slight overlap (unpredictable as to side) that occurs below the navel at the medial borders of the recti, and owing also to the fact that only *there* is linea alba actually linear, clean separation of the recti is often missed ; incidentally, too, midline incision in this part usually opens both rectus sheaths. Separation, however, is easy to effect, since the recti—as at a traffic roundabout—pass the navel on opposite sides. If, then, we prolong the top of our midline incision to skirt the navel (Fig. 100), we can there expose

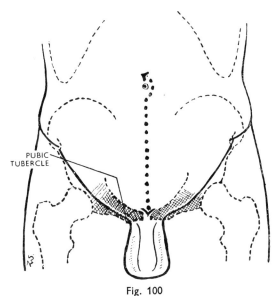

PUBIC
TUBERCLE

Fig. 100

For a clean and complete access to ' Retzius ' the midline incision meets the pubic symphysis and goes to skirt the navel.

the wide umbilical parting of the muscles, and follow down their cleavage to the symphysis. And, if we require maximal exposure of the lateral pelvic limbs of ' Retzius,' rectus separation *should* reach that level—leaving the joint unscotched.

The space of Retzius.—The midline hypogastric route allows us to open and explore the pelvic part of the potential space of Retzius. (The *abdominal* part goes up towards the navel between the two obliterated umbilical arteries.) The large pelvic component is frequently and wrongly called ' retropubic ' or ' prevesical '—naming the whole space from the smallest part. Its full extent spreads far from the 2 in. width of pubic bodies and the sharp bows of the empty bladder, going obliquely back a further handbreadth on either side. Here it separates the inferolateral vesical surfaces from structures that are either lightly held or firmly fixed to the side walls of the true pelvis.

The ground plan of the opened *pelvic* portion of the space is, therefore, like a massive U whose thick loop lies behind the symphysis, while the somewhat splayed-out limbs spread backwards and embrace the sides of the bladder. These limbs end posteriorly, to right and left, at a frontally disposed septum. This important structure carries the ureter from the pelvic wall to the bladder in company with relevant vessels. In the male it includes those vessels that supply the organs sandwiched by the two layers of rectovesical fascia—the vesicles and vasa. Each of these two isolable septa forms, to right or left, a bladder *pedicle*, and thus becomes a major key to radical cystectomy. (Through the courtesy of Mr T. J. D. Lane, I had the privilege of demonstrating the potential value of these two pedicles in regard to that operation before a distinguished group of visiting British urologists at the Meath Hospital, Dublin, in October 1947.)

The surgeon opening the space of Retzius by stripping up pelvic peritoneum exploits and magnifies the change produced by a filling bladder. For this reason, in the absence of previous infection, the peritoneum lifts easily and, if gently handled, without hæmorrhage.

Stripping pelvic peritoneum.—This, I find, is done best by beginning anterolaterally, towards the *side* of the bladder rather than straight in front.

Adherent structures.—In the male four things related to the pelvic part of ' Retzius ' adhere normally to *raised* peritoneum in some at least of their extent : (1) the urachus ; (2) the obliterated umbilical artery in its distal, or front, portion ; (3) the vas as it lies between the internal ring and the back of the empty bladder ; (4) the upper and major length of the pelvic stage of the ureter.

Two of these structures will be seen or felt as cords crossing the opened space : (*a*) the proximal and pervious part of the umbilical artery—free of peritoneum—slopes up and inward either from the end of the undivided internal iliac trunk, or from the beginning of its anterior division, to reach the side of the bladder ; (*b*) the vas deferens—stuck tightly to peritoneum—goes to reach the *back* of the bladder at a higher level than the umbilical artery.

As peritoneal stripping proceeds, the vas comes to lie at the forward and concave edge of a peritoneal fold that forms a shelf above the posterior limb of ' Retzius.'

Rectus-sheath closure.—When separation has been carried *right* down to the pelvic symphysis, a precautionary stitch is advisable ; otherwise a hernia may show at the upper edge of the joint in a matter of weeks. For that reason I have found it well to place a single mattress suture in the divided aponeurosis at this level, bringing the two deep faces of sheath flatly together like the palms of hands. The rest of the aponeurotic layer can be closed with a ' running mattress,' leaving a low ridge of sound union palpable through skin.

JUXTASYMPHYSEAL HERNIA AFTER MIDLINE INCISION

A neglected detail of anatomy perhaps explains the need for placing the single mattress suture immediately above the symphysis. The linea, a fingerbreadth below the navel, becomes a strip whose thin edges look front and back ; its width (because of slight rectus overlap) lies in a plane a trifle off the sagittal. Towards their pubic ends the two thin *edges* of linea (anterior and posterior) widen out, most often like river deltas (Fig. 101), though sometimes the hinder edge may thicken and bifurcate. These anterior and posterior widenings are known as the *feet* of linea.

The two feet of linea alba.—The *anterior* (and lesser) widening, or foot, shows a featureless triangular surface whose base gains attachment to the anterior and upper border of the symphysis and pubic crests. It lies concealed behind the *superficial* suspensory genital ligament (the fundiform or sling) that is attached to linea and joins on either side with Scarpa's fascia. (The *deep* suspensory ligament springs from the symphysis and linea.)

The widening of the *posterior* edge of linea goes to the corresponding upper border of symphysis and pubic crests. It is unsuitably called the adminiculum or *prop* of linea alba. (Paturet's ' posterior foot,' in spite of tradition, is a better term, which pairs well with its anterior fellow.) This hinder foot, or ' adminicular ' widening, is sometimes simple and imperforate like the forefoot ; more often it either forks before reaching the symphysis, or else is pierced at the centre of its triangular face. These openings, whether forked or perforate, transmit a *cul-de-sac* of thinned out transversalis fascia that goes a thumbwidth forward between the lower parts of the two recti and ends behind the blank triangular face of the forefoot. The sac is filled with

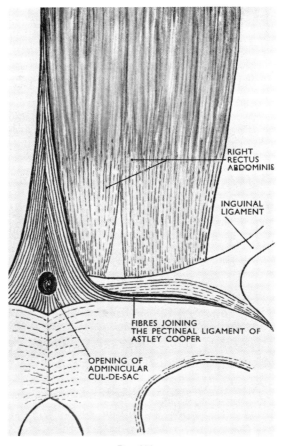

Fig. 101

The so-called prop (the *adminiculum*) of linea alba, seen from behind. The variety shown here has an opening that leads into a fascial *cul-de-sac*, filled normally with fat—a combination which, if unregarded, may favour juxta-symphyseal hernia after a low midline section of the rectus sheath. (The adminicular opening is sometimes arched. It may be absent.)

extraperitoneal fat supplied by a twig from the pubic branch of the inferior epigastric artery.

Thus, when the anterior end of the *cul-de-sac* is unmasked or split by a midline incision that reaches the symphysis and cuts through the fibrous barrier provided by the forefoot of linea plus portions of the two suspensory ligaments, a path may open for the sort of hernia which calls for a deterrent juxtasymphyseal ' mattress.'

I have seen three of these post-operative protrusions immediately above the symphysis, small at first but soon expanding.

PRELUSIVE VASCULAR LIGATION IN PROSTATECTOMY [1]

The wide access we obtain to the pelvic part of the space of Retzius by the midline route (p. 161) suggests a means of controlling blood supply as a first step in extraperitoneal prostatectomy.

Control of blood supply at *source*, which is the rule in thyroid resection, is not a recognised procedure in dealing with the prostate. Yet in open prostatic surgery the loss of blood will often fall on persons unsuited by their age for ordinary deprivations.

The blood supply of the prostate comes through branches that spring directly or indirectly from the internal iliac artery, but we cannot count much on diminishing the arterial inflow to the prostate (or indeed to any other pelvic organ) by tying that main trunk : its anastomoses with offsets that stem at pelvic level from the external iliac, and in the thigh from profunda femoris, are far too free.

We are thus led to seek for vessels that reach the gland directly, and in particular the vessels *named* prostatic. They, in presence of moderate glandular enlargement, may have calibres equal to the average bore of radial arteries—a fact which on ordinary grounds would seem to call for their ligation as a first step in open prostatectomy. I say ' seem ' advisedly, because countless successful operations have been performed without thought for any bleeding excepting that from ultimate prostatic twigs.

It would none the less be interesting to know in what proportion of these fortunate patients there has been significant bleeding after operation, and, more recently, to learn how many have received post-operative blood transfusion.

Supposing then that we should wish to limit the blood supply of the prostate before operation as we do that of the thyroid, we must first review the visceral branching of the internal iliac artery in relation to the space of Retzius.

[1] The work embodied here was completed in 1952. It was published in the *Irish Journal of Medical Science*, August 1954.

VISCERAL BRANCHES OF THE INTERNAL ILIAC ARTERY

The origins of these branches vary so much that Poirier (*Traité d'Anatomie Humaine*, 1902, vol. ii, fasc. 2, p. 786)

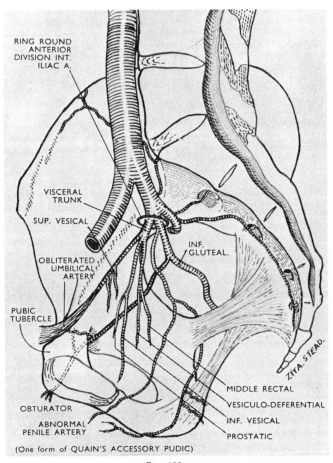

Fig. 102

High 'terminal' forking of the anterior division of the internal iliac into pudendal and inferior gluteal (*alias* sciatic) arteries.

abandons the attempt to give average accounts of how they spring from parent stems. Thus, to quote extreme cases, they may arise (1) like tentacles, as a single bunch from the anterior limb of the internal iliac trunk—as if their several stems were absorbed at one place into it (Fig. 102) ; or (2) they may spring separately along its length (Fig. 103). Between these extremes of concentration and dispersion there is a rich variety of pattern.

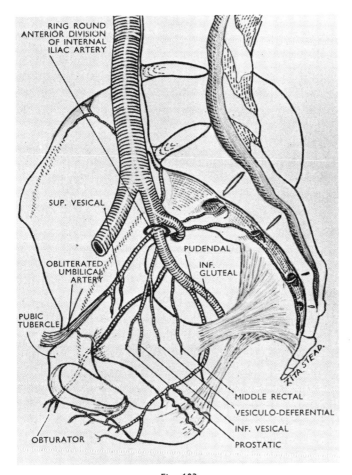

Fig. 103

Low 'terminal' forking of the anterior division of the internal iliac into pudendal and inferior gluteal (*alias* sciatic) arteries.

Poirier therefore begins his account by refusing to classify *origins* of visceral branches, and describes them instead according to their goals. He does this, for the male, as follows :—

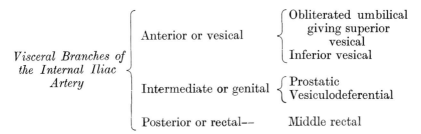

Visceral Branches of the Internal Iliac Artery	Anterior or vesical	Obliterated umbilical giving superior vesical Inferior vesical
	Intermediate or genital	Prostatic Vesiculodeferential
	Posterior or rectal—	Middle rectal

Our first object is to identify these arteries so that we can tie relevant vessels at points immediately prior to their distribution. It is also important to leave sufficient blood supply for the bladder and prostatic bed, and to avoid damaging the penile inflow.

These requisites call for a rapid survey of internal iliac branchings, whose pattern on the two sides of the pelvis is often asymmetrical and sometimes widely different. There is, too, a further complication.

Intrapelvic penile arteries.—Poirier's table has the merit of showing the common distributive order of visceral branches from before back, but interloping arteries may break in. These are most often penile arteries that have an intrapelvic course—an arrangement so frequent that Vesalius gave it as orthodox.[1] The vessels may come from the obturator or the inferior gluteal (the old sciatic) artery ; but far more commonly the whole main stem of internal pudendal is as it were diverted from the ischiorectal fossa to course *above* levator ani and reach the penis through the space of Retzius (Figs. 102 and 104).

In virtue of their goal all intrapelvic penile arteries before emerging from the pubic arch will closely *precede* prostatic branches. It is well, therefore, to keep lively watch for this Vesalian breach with orthodoxy lest we tie the wrong artery.

A survey on both sides of the pelvis will also prevent unwise ligation of common stems. Thus, if an inferior vesical artery gives rise to the prostatic and to the vesiculodeferential vessels, its closure may compromise the blood supply to the prostatic bed or to the bladder. So, if we are to have the chance of testing effects of transient occlusion, the patterns of *origin* as well as those of distribution must be producible for prompt assessment.

These considerations stress the need for some physical means that will literally and quickly find and *bring out* the relevant pattern of internal iliac branching. The want is met by the obliterated umbilical artery which—used as a leash—can be made to serve both as clue and as tractor (Fig. 104).

The arterial leash.—The umbilical artery is a constant feature; it varies little, aside from the extent of its patency and the number of its vesical branches. It springs from the extreme end of the internal iliac *trunk*. Fortunately for our purpose, this origin gives the leash attachment to the precise spot where traction best brings out the pattern of visceral branching. The leash then crosses the hinder part of the space of Retzius, going obliquely up, forward,

---

[1] Poirier (loc. cit., p. 808) quotes Krause to this effect.

and in to, the side of the bladder, where it clings to the vesical wall, lying just below the flat upper face of the empty viscus. Leaving the front of the bladder it again crosses ' Retzius,' this

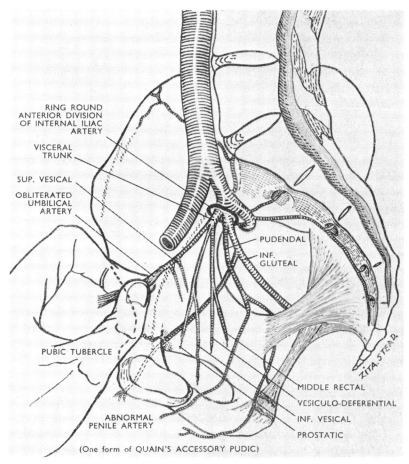

RING ROUND
ANTERIOR DIVISION
OF INTERNAL ILIAC
ARTERY

VISCERAL
TRUNK

SUP. VESICAL

OBLITERATED
UMBILICAL
ARTERY

PUDENDAL

INF.
GLUTEAL

PUBIC TUBERCLE

ZITA. STEAD.

MIDDLE RECTAL

VESICULO-DEFERENTIAL

INF. VESICAL

PROSTATIC

ABNORMAL
PENILE ARTERY

(One form of QUAIN'S ACCESSORY PUDIC)

Fig. 104

**The obliterated end of the umbilical artery freed from the pubis
and used as a tractor**

This yields an ideal windfall ; from it sprang the axial vessel which became the parent stem of every artery that serves the limb—and half its girdle. Traction made thereon elicits in particular the *visceral* pattern of pelvic branching on the ipsilateral side.

time through its prevesical part, and reaches the pelvic wall in the region of the pubic tubercle ; from there it slopes up to the navel.

As a rule the vessel loses its lumen while it lies on the side of the bladder, and before the lumen shuts it gives off one, two, three, or rarely four superior vesical arteries ; it may, however, be patent up to the navel.

Most commonly we find the vessel first as a whitish band flattened by contact with the pubis and raised with the peritoneum, to which it sticks. If we separate this band towards the pelvis, we are supplied with the tough handle of a leash whose deep end is attached to the source of visceral arteries. With it—if used discreetly—we can draw their whole ipsilateral pattern sufficiently away from the pelvic wall to let us recognise and test constituent vessels from stem to distribution.[1] This can be done because the pattern is elastic and is *thinly* pasted to the pelvic wall by a translucent areolar covering from which we have already detached the thick sheet of parietal peritoneum.

Two precautions are essential : gentleness first, for the pull will pass from the fibrous handle of the leash to the softer patent portion, and thence by way of the anterior limb of the internal iliac trunk to the pattern of branches ; secondly, the pull should be made in the antero-mesial direction in order to reduce strain on the often delicate superior vesical twigs that leave the unobliterated reach of the artery.

THE ARTERIAL SUPPLY OF THE PROSTATE

The prostatic artery comes from the anterior limb of the internal iliac trunk, though seldom directly. It shares more often a common stem with the inferior vesical, or with the middle rectal and vesiculodeferential arteries. It may even spring from the patent part of the obliterated umbilical, being then merely an enlargement of one of the fine anastomotic twigs which normally link the two vessels. These fine twigs are liable to rupture when we open the space of Retzius, and their value in maintaining a residual supply to the prostatic bed must be uncertain. (The risk of confusing prostatic and intrapelvic penile arteries has already been stressed.)

The vesiculodeferential artery generally arises in common with the prostatic and middle rectal. It passes between the two stout layers of rectovesical fascia which enclose and sandwich the seminal vesicles together with the ends of the ureters and the ends of vasa deferentia. After branching widely to supply the front of the vesicle, the artery sends branches to the base (or postero-inferior aspect) of the bladder, and so to the prostatic bed. The deferential artery is given off above the branching,

---

[1] It is likely that the small non-damaging clamps used for *temporary* vascular occlusion will serve in testing residual vascularity in the prostatic bed.

and its fine descending twig goes with the vas to the prostate. (An ascending recurrent twig follows the vas to reach the epididymis and anastomose with the testicular artery—a link which is broken by vasectomy.)

SUMMARY

These paragraphs suggest that in prelude to certain prosta-tectomies (1) the whole pelvic part of the space of Retzius be opened up ; (2) that the obliterated umbilical artery be used on either side as a tractor leash which will bring out the variable pattern of visceral pelvic arteries for recognition, assessment, and possible ligation.

My own work of necessity was done on bodies prepared for the dissecting room and my thanks are therefore due to my colleague Mr W. A. L. MacGowan, F.R.C.S.I., who has confirmed the innocuous and satisfactory effect of adequate traction on the obliterated umbilical artery at post-mortem in *fresh* cadavers of very different age and obesity : in each the pattern of visceral branching was plainly elicited. It has been a pleasure to have the help of so accurate and critical an observer.

COMPLETE ACCESS TO HIP-JOINT NERVES FROM IN FRONT [1]

Current procedures on arthritic hips include resection of nerves that bring painful stimuli from the joint, and if the surgeon deals first with anterior nerves and then with posterior, his patient will be turned from a supine to a prone position.

With that change from recumbency to ' face down ' goes a threefold nuisance, viz., the need for incisions front and back ; renewal of sheets and towels ; the chance of shock.

The object of this paper is to show that *all* nerves to the hip joint can be reached, exposed, and resected *from in front* in the recumbent patient, with a maximum regard to anatomy and a negligible sacrifice of muscle innervation.

THE TWO METHODS

(*A*) If the surgeon has no scruple about denervating the main mass of the adductor group, he will take the simple course of dividing the obturator *trunk* on the side wall of the pelvis after

[1] T. P. Garry and A. K. Henry, *Irish Journal of Medical Science*, April 1953, p. 177.

he has displaced the peritoneum. In that event an abdominal extraperitoneal approach suffices, and the incision (excepting for a small extension at the navel) is mesial and hypogastric. But use of (A) prevents resection of certain contributions from the femoral nerves.

(*B*) If, on the other hand, he should think it well to hesitate

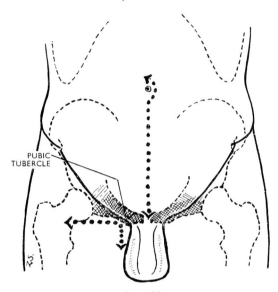

PUBIC
TUBERCLE

Fig. 105

The two incisions

The **abdominal incision** is the same as that used by one of us for extraperitoneal access to the lowest part of both ureters. (The extension at the navel allows *clean* separation of the recti, since that is where they separate (p. 161).)

The **thigh incision** (*a*) lets us liberate parts of the obturator nerve below the obturator tunnel and thus makes possible our 'pull-through' technique ; (*b*) gives access to extra-abdominal recurrent contributions from the femoral nerve to the front of the hip joint (Figs. 106 and 107).

before he gravely jeopardises muscles of adduction—known abroad as 'muscles of chastity' though taking part as well in usual, uncanonised activities—then, in the case of such demur, the surgeon will add a *thigh* incision (Fig. 107).

This extra cut allows him to spare the branches of the obturator nerve that supply the bulk of the adductor mass while he resects those obturator twigs that serve the hip joint.

The thigh incision, too, gives access to certain *femoral* branches that carry articular nerves.

Whether he chooses (A) or (B) the surgeon stands on the side of the patient remote from the seat of operation.

METHOD B.—Let us suppose Method B is used. The obturator nerve, after peeling off peritoneum, is found at once on the side wall of the pelvis, lying directly above the companion artery and

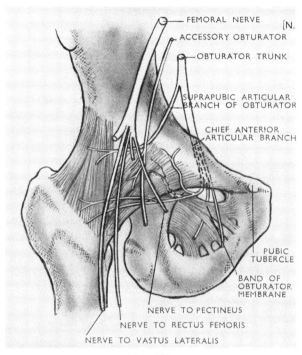

Fig. 106

Anterior nerve to the hip joint (after Paturet)

Note the unlabelled dotted twig, deep to pubofemoral ligament. This twig forms part of a neurovascular bundle that makes a constant but undescribed groove at the ' exit ' of the obturator tunnel (see text). This ' exit ' is often masked by a well-developed pubofemoral ligament, which then requires division for access to anterior offsets.

vein. Mobilise the nerve as far up as possible, then loosen it and its divisions at and through the $\frac{1}{2}$ in. length of obturator tunnel, in which the nervous structures keep their superior relation to artery and vein. This mobilisation lets us note whether—as in 12 per cent. of subjects—the nerve lying on the pelvic wall gives off a suprapubic articular branch (Fig. 106, after Paturet) *before* entering the obturator tunnel—a branch which, of course, we cut.

The thigh incision.—Next, passing to the thigh, find first the pubic tubercle. At this level make a hockey-stick incision with a short limb descending for 2 in. from the tubercle down the thigh, and a long *transverse* limb measuring a wide handbreadth outwards from the tubercle (Fig. 105). From this tubercle the plane of cleavage between pectineus and adductor longus slants down and out. Open the plane and part these muscles widely, but, if pectineus is thick and resistant, sever the medial half of the belly from its J-shaped linear attachment to the pectineal face of pubis and turn the muscle outwards. With either means, pectineus buffers the femoral vein whose upper end lies in the groove between pectineus and psoas.

The superficial opening, or ' exit,' of the obturator tunnel can then be reached from the thigh, but the upper portion of the ' exit ' is still masked by an overhang of the part of the pubo-femoral ligament that goes medially to join the pubic tubercle (Fig. 106) and sometimes, too, by an associated piece of obturator externus muscle.

The *anterior division* of the obturator nerve is found at once as it passes down from the tunnel's ' exit ' over the outer face of the outer obturator to supply the *front* of adductor brevis. The upper course of the *posterior division* varies ; it may run in front of, through, or deep to obturator externus : and when it lies deep to the muscle, it may also go deep to a strong outlying band of obturator membrane—which the French call by, what is to us, the misleading name of ' subpubic ligament '—a band which may be strengthened by an offshoot of fibres from the pubofemoral (Fig. 106).

The obturator nerve and the ' pull-through ' method.—Our object is to mobilise a whole segment of the obturator nerve together with its branches—a segment that lies above, in, and below the obturator tunnel—so that we can get a to-and-fro ' pull-through ' movement of the nerve constituents. The obturator branches now appear and can be classed very simply as *thick* and *thin*. The thick we spare ; they go to adductor muscles. The thin, which include anterior articular branches to the hip, are indiscriminately cut. This, of course, means that branches going to obturator externus and perhaps to pectineus are sacrificed. The sacrifice is minimal. Downward traction on the two obturator divisions—which now begin to slide through the obturator tunnel—drags on the small articular twigs, so that they are seen to run *proximally* from the parent trunks. One of these is very constant ; it turns backwards from the parent stem and helps, with offsets from the obturator vessels, to make a definite but undescribed groove on the hinder lip of the obturator ' exit ' within a fingerbreadth of its arched top. The nerve then passes through the acetabular notch bridged by the transverse ligament. There is a certain risk of missing twigs, like this one, that arise just within the tunnel's ' exit,' when they are masked by an overhang of pubofemoral ligament (Fig. 106). For that reason it is well to divide the overhang in order to see these offsets springing from main divisions.

The accessory obturator nerve.—This nerve, described first by Schmidt in 1774, occurs (on the average of findings by six different authors) in 17 per cent. of subjects. It will be looked for above the pelvic brim, descending vertically in front of and often touching the obturator trunk, which should be stroked gently with a ball-ended dental burnisher to avoid missing an adherent but easily separable accessory obturator. Lower down it becomes more difficult to reach, for it may lie deep to the external iliac vein and run within the psoas sheath before going under Poupart's ligament to supply pectineus, hip joint, skin, and femoral artery.

The chief and most constant anterior articular branch to the hip springs from the back of the obturator trunk (Fig. 106), or from the posterior division of the trunk, just before or just after the trunk enters the obturator canal—a variation that lends value to the ' pull-through ' technique which delivers the branch for section when the trunk is drawn up towards the pelvic cavity. The *back* of the trunk or the back of its posterior division will then be stroked with the burnisher, and any *thin* branch that the ball-end separates off will be resected in due conformance with our classification of ' thick ' branches to be saved and ' thin ' to be cut.

Femoral branches to the joint.—Twigs to the hip joint stem from three branches of the femoral trunk :—

(1) *From the branch to pectineus* which goes behind the femoral sheath. It has its origin, however, within the abdomen and leaves the parent trunk *above* and very close to Poupart's ligament. (Soulié, in Poirier and Charpy's *Anatomie*, describes *two* nerves to pectineus—one from the femoral trunk ; one from its so-called internal musculocutaneous division (see footnote, p. 231).)

The branch or branches slope inwards from the trunk and, therefore, can be hooked by drawing the dental burnisher *up* along the medial edge of the femoral nerve, after that nerve has been clearly defined.

(2) and (3) *From branches to rectus femoris and from branches to vastus lateralis.*

These are small recurrent *upper* branches to the muscles. They reach the lateral part of the anterior face of the hip joint, and may either form a plexus on the joint or unite before they reach it or spring from a common stem. They are the first lateral offsets that leave the femoral nerve in the *thigh*.

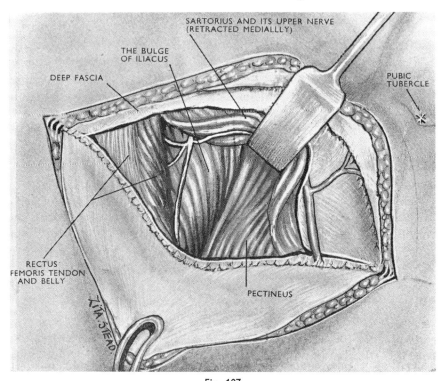

Fig. 107
The transverse part of the thigh incision opened up
Two proximal branches of the femoral nerves are seen passing deep to rectus femoris. In this subject they sprang from a common stem : one branch supplied rectus, the other vastus lateralis ; each ended in recurrent twigs to the front of hip joint.

These branches are easily found through the transverse part of the thigh incision. Mark a point level with the pubic tubercle and distal by one handbreadth to the anterior superior spine of ilium. At this point displace sartorius medially ; separate rectus femoris from vastus lateralis. Then you will see the forward bulge of iliacus belly (*lateral* to its attachment to psoas tendon). The nerve, or nerves, to rectus femoris and vastus lateralis pass obliquely down and out on the steep slope of this forward bulge. Still farther out they turn up towards the joint (Fig. 107).

It is difficult to isolate the tiny articular twigs that spring from these recurrent branches ; and since the branches themselves are small, and since they form only a minor fraction of the large nerve supply to rectus femoris and vastus lateralis, they may be resected without anxiety.

POSTERIOR NERVES TO THE HIP JOINT

Approached from in front, after reflecting pelvic peritoneum, these nerves, despite their depth, are easier to deal with than the anterior nerves we have just reviewed : their stems are found in close and definite relation to a single bony point—the spine of ischium ; they spring from the *front* of the sciatic trunk ; they can be felt and picked up blindfold after dividing a single layer of fascia.

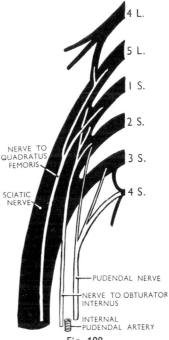

Fig. 108

The pelvic part of right sciatic trunk

A front view showing the order in which branches leave its anterior face. The quadratus branch is the most lateral.

In general, *one* nerve (Fig. 108)— that shared by the quadratus femoris and gemellus inferior—gives a branch to the back of the hip joint. The articular twig, however, may be double, and in 12 per cent. of subjects it is supplemented by a further twig that comes *direct* from the sciatic trunk and may itself be double (Paturet).

The nerve to quadratus and Garry's manœuvre.—Stand on the side of the patient *remote* from the seat of operation. Separate the peritoneum from the side wall of the true pelvis until you can feel the curved anterior edge of the greater sciatic notch. At the caudal end of the notch locate the spine of ischium. A strong but loose sheet of fascia occludes the bight of the notch. *Open the fascia a fingerbreadth headwise to the spine of ischium.* Make an inch-long opening. For the patient's *right* side use the longest finger of your *left* hand, turning its palm towards the patient's head. Use a right finger for the patient's left side. Pass the finger

through the opening you have made in the fascia ; the soft
resistance that you feel is the sciatic trunk.

With the finger press the trunk gently backwards towards the
table. Flex the finger tip towards the spine of ischium. The

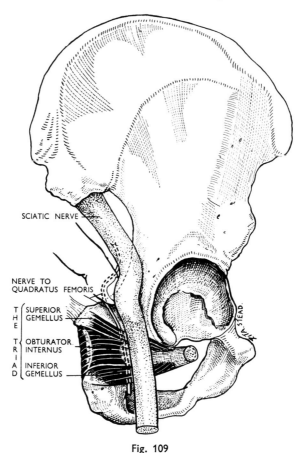

Fig. 109

Quadratus nerve and sciatic trunk

The diagram shows how a muscle triad (*a*) parts the nerve
from its parent trunk ; (*b*) straps the nerve to the bone.
The free trunk, therefore, moves back when a finger thrusts
against it from in front, but the nerve stays forward and is
felt *in situ.*

firm, thin cord now felt crossing the pulp of the finger is the nerve
to quadratus femoris, and any other similar cord found at this
level (a fingerbreadth headwise to the spine of ischium) is either
a twin nerve to quadratus or the occasional direct articular branch
from the sciatic trunk.

Anatomical relations (Fig. 109) make this simple manœuvre

feasible. Just below the level of our fascial opening the *back* of the nerve to quadratus (with its articular twigs) is crossed by a transverse muscle triad—gemelli plus obturator-internus tendon ; the triad straps the nerve to the back of ischium. The sciatic trunk, on the other hand, from which the nerve to quadratus springs, lies free *behind* the triad and, at the level of our opening, is backed by the loose belly of piriformis. For that reason a finger pushing through the opening thrusts the yielding, unfettered trunk dorsally towards the table, while the nerve to quadratus— caught between triad and bone—stays ventrally and feels like tight string. (This interpretation, like the manœuvre, is Garry's— each of them a *tour de maître*.)

We would add that caudal to the site of the quadratus nerve three structures hug the spine of ischium. From without inwards, these are :—

(1) The nerve common to obturator internus and gemellus superior ; (2) the pudendal vascular bundle ; (3) the pudendal nerve (Fig. 108). We need disturb none of them, though if we cut the thin nerve shared by obturator internus and gemellus superior it would scarcely matter.

Before attempting these procedures, the surgeon will waste no time if he consults Gimbernat's favourite text-book of anatomy— the cadaver.

Soon after this paper appeared the operation we described was carried out at the Richmond Hospital, Dublin, through the initiative of my former colleague, Mr W. A. L. MacGowan, by Mr C. Gleadhill, then Assistant in the Department of Neurosurgery. The patient, a man over 70, was bedridden with marked osteoarthritic changes in both hip joints. A month after a bilateral resection of hip joint nerves he walked to his church and back, a total distance of about a half mile.

EXPOSURES IN THE LOWER LIMB

VESSELS AND NERVES IN THE BUTTOCK

I PUT this first. Of all exposures in the lower limb a method for the buttock was, I found, the principal concern of an experienced majority.

We have been taught to look for the gluteal vessels by splitting gluteus maximus, perhaps because its well-marked grain is almost irresistible. But if we split the grain, we play into the hands of entities that tend to give a narrow, bloody field. The parts are thick ; skin felts with fat, and fat with fascia covering thick gluteal muscle. Then, too, the vessels sprawl on the deep face of maximus, much as they sprawl on the placenta, spreading their arteries (as Bell remarks) " with sudden and crooked angles " ; so they diverge and run *across* the grain ; and here those cursed things of surgery, the veins, are large. These handicaps of mere anatomy grow uglier with wounds : the part becomes " a clotting mass adrip with blood."

In this exposure, therefore, we must spare and see—two things which can be done well only when we lift the lid-like shape of maximus as we might lift the lid nailed on a packing-case. Thus we can either raise the muscle by setting free a pair of sides that meet, and prising up the corner (like Fiolle and Delmas) ; or else (with Stookey)[1] we can set *two* corners free and turn the whole lid back. The plans themselves are simple, but neglect of detail leads to sorry execution.

ANATOMY

The gluteal lid (Fig. 110).—The cover formed by maximus is like a parallelogram whose *shorter sides*—the femoral and pelvic— are almost longitudinal, the one aligning roughly with the femur, the other fixed from ilium to coccyx.

The *longer sides*—cephalic and caudal—are oblique, like the

---

[1] B. Stookey, *Journal of the American Medical Association*, 1920, **74,** 1380. (In the exposure described below, Stookey's ' question-mark ' has been shifted *forward* to exploit the Fiolle and Delmas drum-head.)

grain of maximus ; the lower side descends across the gluteal fold

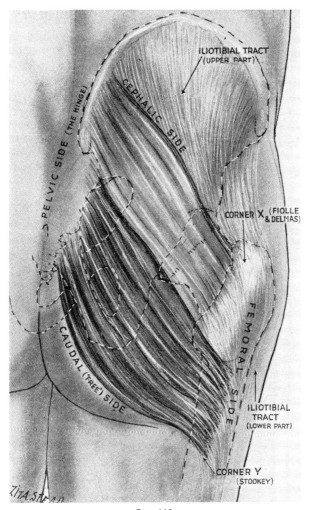

Fig. 110

The gluteal lid or parallelogram

Note its four sides—two long (cephalic and caudal), and two
short (femoral and pelvic). *All* the superficial fibres plus the
upper half of deep fibres are attached distally to iliotibial tract
(see Fig. 111). The lower (deeply shaded) half of the *deep*
fibres are fixed to femur. X is the corner to free in order to
prise up the lid in the partial exposure of Fiolle and Delmas.
Y is the second corner which must be freed with X to let us
raise the lid and hinge it back for the complete exposure, after
Stookey.

and is (as Boyer notes) the ' free ' side of the muscle—united to
surrounding parts by *loose* connective tissue.

Of these four sides two which meet in front—the short femoral,

the long cephalic—need close consideration.   All the fibres of
gluteus maximus have their
distal attachments at the
short, *femoral side* of the
muscle.   These attachments
are of two kinds, fascial and
bony.   The superficial fibres
join the part of iliotibial tract
which slides on great trochanter ; so, too, does the
upper half of deeper fibres ;
the lower half, however, im-
plants itself on bone, marking
the back of femur and forming there the distal point of
the gluteal parallelogram.

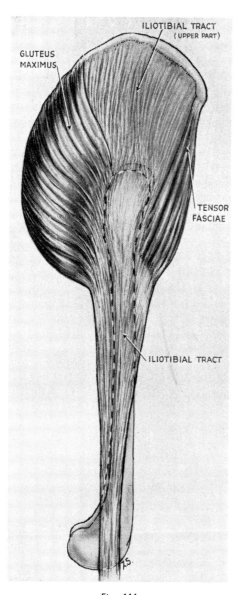

Fig. 111

The ' pelvic deltoid '

The fibrous middle part (formed by iliotibial
tract) covers gluteus medius and is stuck to it
in front. Behind, near great trochanter where
medius slopes inward, the tract covers the muscle
like a drum-head (see Fig. 114 A).

The long *cephalic side* that
joins with the short femoral is
bound, in muscle-sheath relation, to a special piece of
tract—the proximal expanse
which hides gluteus medius,
and occupies the gap between
the maximus and tensor
muscle.   Indeed, we may
regard these three (the tensor,
tract and maximus) as figuring
a pelvic deltoid (Fig. 111)
whose middle part consists
of fibrous tissue—a useful
myth in practice but one
condemned by strict mor-
phology.

If we set free these two
adjoining sides—cephalic and
femoral—dividing their attachments to the tract, we
liberate a corner of gluteal
lid which we can now prise
up. But if we need the widest
possible exposure (to reach
in comfort, say, the great sciatic) we must unfix a second corner—

the distal piece of maximus that joins the femur. Then every side is free except the pelvic ; for (as we know from Boyer) the caudal edge is virtually unattached. And so, with three sides free, we raise the lid.

THE OPERATIONS OF PARTIAL AND COMPLETE EXPOSURE

Position.—The patient lies face down. Take advantage of this position to mark out the points through which the knife will pass : (1) the posterior superior spine of ilium ; (2) a point on the crest a handbreadth in front of this ; (3) most difficult of all to find, a point midway between the front edge and the back edge of great trochanter. (Be sure you find the front *edge* under the covering wad of tensor belly) ; (4) a similar point on the femoral shaft level with gluteal fold ; (5) a point on the back of thigh midway between ischial tuberosity and the back of great trochanter, just below the gluteal fold (Fig. 112).

The skin incision.—Since it is difficult to know beforehand if our exposure must be full or partial, I shall describe the full incision— a question-mark on the right side, its mirror image on the left (Fig. 211)—and indicate the portion that gives room for *circumscribed* approach.

The ' question-mark ' needs rigorous attention ; a lapse will hamper us persistently.[1] Begin first at the posterior superior spine of ilium ; carry the knife a handbreadth along the iliac crest. Then cut obliquely down the outer face of hip to reach the top of great trochanter. The knife proceeding distally bisects the outer face of the trochanter and travels down the shaft till level with the gluteal fold ; *that* is enough for circumscribed exposure. But, for full access turn the knife in transversely at this level ; stop at the midline of the thigh, half-way, that is, between the great trochanter and the tuberosity of ischium. Then cut vertically down the thigh as far as you propose to liberate the great sciatic nerve. The ' question-mark ' should reach but not divide deep fascia.

The posterior cutaneous nerve of the thigh.—The *trunk* of this large nerve (once named the small sciatic) lies in the midline of the thigh just under the deep fascia ; *and there it stays*, sending out perforating twigs and coming to the surface only in the calf

---

[1] It is, for example, remarkably (and ruinously) easy to follow the hinder edge of great trochanter instead of bisecting its outer face—

> " *I told them once, I told them twice :*
> *They would not listen to advice.*"

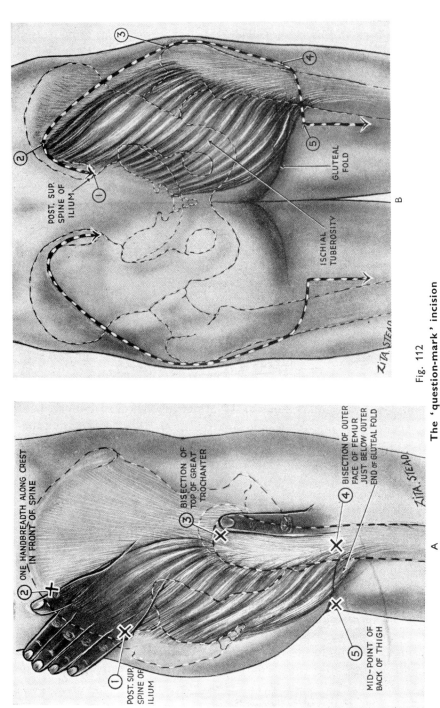

POST. SUP
SPINE OF ILIUM
①

②

③

④

⑤

GLUTEAL
FOLD

ISCHIAL
TUBEROSITY

B

ZITA STEAD

Fig. 112

The 'question-mark' incision

A. Note the five points which map its course. The 'difficult' point (3) is a fingerbreadth behind the front edge of great trochanter. For the partial exposure of Fiolle and Delmas, incision stops at point 4. B shows the full 'question-mark' on the right; its mirror image on the left.

② ONE HANDBREADTH ALONG CREST
IN FRONT OF SPINE

③ BISECTION OF
TOP OF GREAT
TROCHANTER

④ BISECTION OF OUTER
FACE OF FEMUR
JUST BELOW OUTER
END OF GLUTEAL FOLD

① POST. SUP.
SPINE OF
ILIUM

⑤ MID-POINT OF
BACK OF THIGH

ZITA STEAD

A

(Fig. 113). This nerve will be imperilled by a full exposure ; it clings, ensheathed in fat, to the deep face of maximus, close to the long ' free ' caudal edge. So, when the edge is raised, the nerve is cut unless we make a point of finding it *as a first step*, using the *stem* of the ' question-mark ' — a method which I owe to Major C. W. Clark of the Canadian Army. His plan works well, for nerve and stem are mesially placed. The nerve, remember, lies beneath deep fascia (and just beneath) ; so we can find it much more easily than if it lay in superficial fat. Open deep fascia therefore longitudinally and trace the trunk up to the edge of the gluteal lid. When presently we raise the lid and hinge it back, the nerve is easily detached—together with its perineal branch, the *ci-devant* pudendal nerve of Sœmmerring.

Liberation of the adjoining femoral and cephalic sides.—We next set free the shorter, *femoral* side of maximus by cutting down on bone and splitting lengthwise the piece of iliotibial tract that slides on shaft and great trochanter. Our cut accordingly bisects the outer surface of the femur and divides the main (and fascial) insertion of the maximus (Figs. 112, A and 113).

We then proceed to free the long, *cephalic* side of maximus, which, as we know already, is fastened by a sheet of iliotibial tract ; and this we must divide. A detail of arrangement makes it well to place the cut correctly.

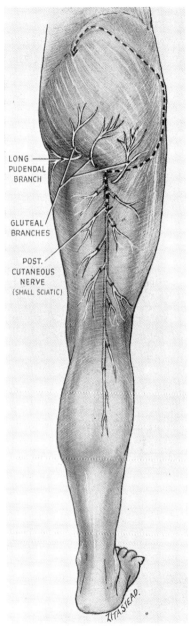

LONG PUDENDAL BRANCH

GLUTEAL BRANCHES

POST. CUTANEOUS NERVE (SMALL SCIATIC)

Fig. 113

The posterior cutaneous nerve of the thigh (the small sciatic)

Note its long course under deep fascia. Find it through the *stem* of the ' question-mark,' and thus, with C. W. Clark, protect the nerve (which sticks to the deep face of maximus) *before* you mobilise the caudal edge of gluteal lid.

The useful drum-head.—This sheet of tract (the fibrous portion of the pelvic ' deltoid ') covers the several parts of gluteus medius with different degrees of contiguity. In front, the tract and muscle stick together ; behind, the two are separate. So, when medius is lax, it leaves the hinder piece of tract stretched like a drum-head over it. The opening of this drum-head through a small extension upwards of the cut already made along the femur will let us put a finger in the shallow cavity and use a thumb to grasp the rubbery

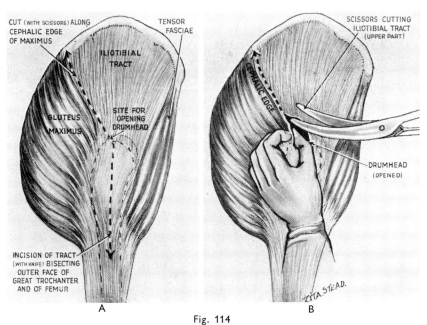

Fig. 114

Line for dividing iliotibial tract

A. The *knife* bisects the outer face of great trochanter and of femur ; it opens the drum-head at the top of the bisection. B. Finger and thumb locate the rubbery cephalic edge of maximus, and *scissors* cut the tract along beside it. Knife and scissors thus detach the *first* corner of the lid (X in Fig. 110) by setting free its femoral and cephalic sides.

transition that marks the meeting-place of maximus and tract. Use scissors to divide the tract along this sloping edge (Fig. 114).

And now with two sides free we raise one corner of the lid and look for structures underneath. That is the method of Fiolle and Delmas. But for fuller view we must set free a second corner.

The second corner of the lid.—We have already found the ' free,' or caudal, edge of maximus along with the posterior cutaneous nerve (once called the small sciatic). Raise both together from the hamstrings. Hook a finger round and then cut through the

thick insertion of maximus to femur ; the muscle there is sometimes vascular and should be pressed between assistant fingers on
the medial side of the dividing knife (Fig. 115). Before we turn

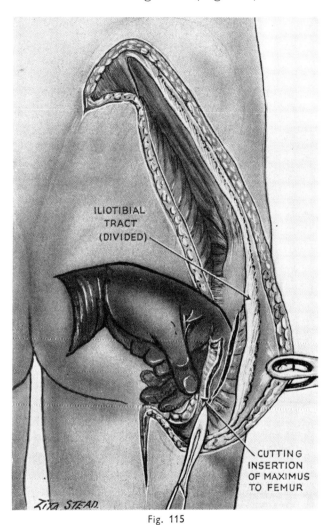

ILIOTIBIAL
TRACT
(DIVIDED)

CUTTING
INSERTION
OF MAXIMUS
TO FEMUR

Fig. 115
Freeing the second corner (Y in Fig. 110)
This is done by dividing the fleshy attachment of maximus to femur.
Fingers control the proximal extremity which is often vascular.

the muscle over we must see that the posterior cutaneous nerve is
finally detached and safe. The whole gluteal lid can then be hinged
back on its pelvic fastening, but very gently ; for though the great
arterial and venous stems that branch into the lid are favourably
placed—close to the pelvic hinge—the veins are always weak, and,
in the old, the arteries are brittle.

STRUCTURES UNDER THE GLUTEAL LID

The key and the trap.—There is a key muscle for this region; each main nerve and vessel leaves the pelvis at one or other edge of pyriformis; and as a rule we find this 'key' immediately. Sometimes, however, a deep fold in gluteus medius marks off a

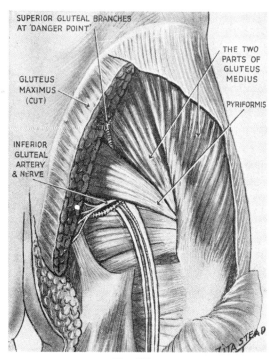

neighbouring piece of belly close beside the 'key' (Fig. 116); then a small effort will separate the hinder part of medius into a disconcerting replica of pyriformis. I have twice seen confusion follow this detachment. (The transverse plane grazing the top of great trochanter is at the caudal edge of pyriformis—a muscle sometimes fused above with medius and minimus.)

Fig. 116

Pitfalls under the gluteal lid

(This figure is anatomical and is not part of the exposure.)

Note the posterior part of gluteus medius which is sometimes separated off and mistaken for pyriformis, causing complete disorientation. Note also the 'danger spot' where a branch of superior gluteal artery, accompanied by *veins*, spreads into maximus. It lies three fingerbreadths in front of the posterior superior spine of ilium and three fingerbreadths below the crest.

The muscles.— Seven *transverse* muscular parts cross the wound from above down: the hinder piece of gluteus medius, pyriformis, gemellus superior, the tendon of obturator internus, gemellus inferior, quadratus femoris, adductor magnus. The *vertical* muscles seen under the lid are proximal parts of the hamstrings (Fig. 117). A narrow tongue, more deeply placed, and lateral to where the fleshy fibres of maximus insert on femur, is vastus lateralis.

Structures related to the borders of pyriformis.—At its *upper edge* are the superior gluteal vessels and nerve. The nerve runs forward with offsets of the vessels, and is concealed at once by

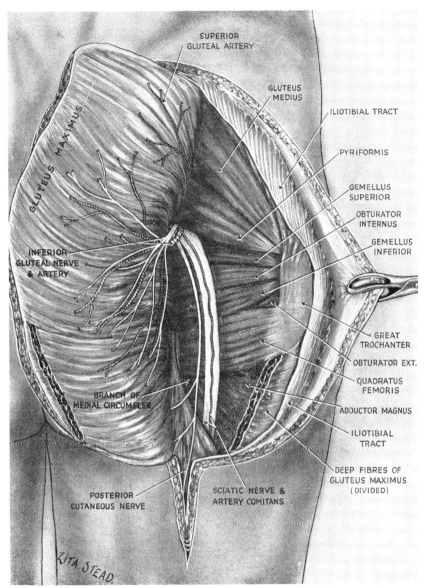

Fig. 117

The gluteal lid hinged back

The exposure is completed except in respect of the subgluteal arc formed by pudendal bundle (see the next figure—Fig. 118). Biceps is left in place to stress the fact that on its way to fibula the sloping belly crosses the sciatic. Therefore in following the nerve prolong the stem of 'question-mark' and mobilise the biceps : raise the belly like a bucket-handle and trace the nerve deep to it. (Only the *infra*bicipital part of sciatic lies between inner and outer hamstrings.)

gluteus medius. The artery and *large* companion veins continue into maximus and constitute a veritable danger spot—three finger-breadths in front of the posterior superior spine of ilium and three below the crest—a point to keep in mind when hinging back the lid.

At the *lower edge of pyriformis* the most superficial structure to emerge is the inferior gluteal nerve whose trunk breaks up at once in branches of supply to maximus and screens the lower gluteal vessels. These last send offsets down beside the structure next in depth—the small sciatic or posterior cutaneous nerve, already seen and spared (p. 183). It lay (before we had displaced it) along the posteromedial edge of the " huge great sciatic nerve "—the one oasis of description Gogarty could find in ' Cunningham ' [1] (Figs. 116 and 117).

Still deeper is the nerve to quadratus femoris—deep to the gemelli group and reaching the *deep* face of its own muscle. Its course is covered by a finger laid beside and lateral to the ischial tuberosity.

The internal pudendal bundle.—This, too, emerges at the lower edge of pyriformis, curving between the great and small sciatic notch, and lying deep and slightly medial to the lower gluteal screen of nerves and vessels—a source of hæmorrhage to think of once gluteals are controlled, and one whereon we might be called to pounce ; which we can do as follows.

FINDING THE SITE OF THE PUDENDAL BUNDLE.—Use the left hand for the right side, and *vice versa*. Abduct the thumb *widely*. Slide the forefinger up across the sciatic trunk and then along the back of the ischial tuberosity. Keep the palmar surface of the finger flat against the bone and let the distal phalanx pass deep to pyriformis, into the great sciatic notch. The finger will advance until the web of the outstretched thumb is stopped against the great trochanter (Fig. 118). Then the tip of the finger, slightly flexed, will press on the arc of the pudendal bundle ; this as a rule sticks fast to its background and will not let itself be hooked without a little blunt dissection.[2]

Thus, after hinging back the gluteal lid, a single rapid movement finds the bundle and allows precise insertion of a tampon

---

[1] Failure to realise that the long head of biceps slopes across the back of sciatic may cause confusion—especially if we attempt to trace the nerve through insufficient stems of ' question-marks ' (see Fig. 117, and legend).

[2] The bundle, one should know, consists of three parts : pudendal vessels flanked by two nerves. The vessels lie more or less on the tip of the ischial spine ; the internal pudendal nerve is on the inner side of the vessels; the small nerve to obturator internus (which also gives a twig to gemellus superior) lies on their outer side.

(Mikulicz for choice). This may stop the bleeding, or, at least, will stanch it and give time to reach and tie the parent trunk by means of laparotomy. The pudendal artery can then be found

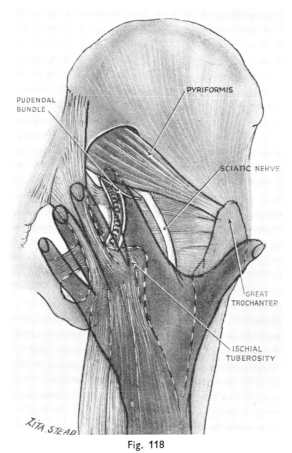

Fig. 118

Finding the pudendal bundle

Using the left hand for the right side and vice versa, the index slides on the tendon-covered back of ischial tuberosity, lengthwise, till the hand is stopped by great trochanter making contact with the web of the outstretched thumb. The tip of index passes *deep* to pyriformis into the great sciatic notch and comes to rest on the pudendal bundle.

extraperitoneally, in the space of Retzius, by means of light traction on the obliterated umbilical artery (p. 168).

Repair.—We must most carefully reconstitute the field of operation—especially the proximal expanse of iliotibial tract. Smooth function here depends on normal interplay of all three portions of the pelvic ' deltoid '—of tensor, tract and maximus. A hernial defect (with bulging of gluteus medius) may lead to snapping-hip, or to recurring, noiseless subluxation of tract on great trochanter. In either case the consequent imbalance makes and unmakes a postural deformity which certain temperaments are haunted by, and some (however innocent) exploit.[1]

THE ROLE OF GLUTEUS MAXIMUS IN CERTAIN MOVEMENTS

I have been urged (and even begged!) by some to omit the pages relevant to this heading; others, again, write *stet* to them.

A voice, now vanished, has decided me : these pages caught at least the fancy of the late Frederick Wood Jones—who vouched in no way for their accuracy. So far as they go they are, I know, true ; but I am also sure that the observations they record were made, by force of circumstance, on too few subjects ; they thus suggest the " always " that never happens in anatomy.

I am convinced, however, that certain critics—for two reasons, or even three—rejected them without sufficient pause : they may have been misled, as I have been myself, by palpating a taut hamstring in mistake for gluteus maximus ; others have touched the neighbouring upper part of vastus lateralis. Between the Scylla and Charybdis of that lively pair, fingers are easily persuaded to a wrong decision on the *in*activities of maximus.

Another source of error stems from the fact that most of the human guinea-pigs at my disposal in the last war were " of the greyhound breed " : their bellies, however fair, were never round, in Shakespeare's sense—an autonomic state whose lasting upkeep seems to demand a ' guy rope ' contraction of the maximi.

A third and less excusable mistake is to forget that even if we bend a *finger* against enough resistance, almost every scrap of striped body muscle—from neckline to sphincter—contracts ; though few can claim to be protagonist.

Other generations, aside perhaps from Leonardo's, knew little of the workings of the large, mysterious bulk of maximus ; they called it " abductor," etc., etc. I remember my own surprise when a recumbent subject under test was able to raise his pelvis

---

[1] Two examples : (1) Gluteus medius hernia (after Ober's operation of fascial division for backache) which caused undue preoccupation with shifting aspects of a great trochanter. (2) A rather simple individual with snapping hip, who drew a useful pension for " recurring *dislocation* " of the joint. A loud click synchronised with three-inch shortening of the limb—apparent, but extremely lucrative.

from the floor *without* contracting either maximus. We are, indeed, still groping.

The following is my grope. It was, I feel, worth making—if only to distract a chief Anatomist of one's time.

A sitting man cannot raise himself if the part of his body which is in front of his centre of gravity does not weigh more than that which is behind his centre of gravity without the use of his arms.

The sinew which guides the leg, and which is connected with the patella of the knee, feels it a greater labour to carry the man upwards in proportion as the knee is more bent; and the muscle which acts upon the angle made by the thigh where it joins the body has less difficulty and has less weight to lift because it has not the additional weight of the thigh itself. And besides it has the stronger muscles, being those which form the buttock.[1]   LEONARDO DA VINCI.

If when you grasp a muscle you can shift it easily from side to side, you may be sure the muscle is relaxed sufficiently to make it—at the moment of your test—unfit to work as a prime mover. That state of idle relaxation is the state of maximus in most of the activities which text-books claim for it [2] (though fingers must be careful not to take for its contraction the *neighbouring* activity of hamstrings).

---

[1] These are in no way final and decisive statements : each is a *note*—" the shadow of a thought in process of formation."

[2] A pair of these accounts (with comments in parenthesis) appear below. They may, I think, be handled as unfeelingly as fossilised remains : the uncoordinated " actions " of a single muscle are parentless survivals, out of date since the Renaissance.

From Gray's Anatomy, 1942, 28*th Edn., p.* 634.—" When the Gluteus maximus takes its fixed point from the pelvis, it extends the thigh and brings it into line with the trunk." [*The muscle is lax during the movement.*] " Taking its fixed point below, it supports the pelvis and the trunk upon the head of the femur, and, so far as the hip-joint is concerned, the maintenance of the erect attitude is ensured by the balanced tone of the Gluteus maximus and the other extensors of the joint, on the one hand, and of the flexors of the joint on the other hand." [*The maximus is absolutely lax in static natural erect positions, but if we spring to full ' attention,' and (in our zeal) incline to thrust the pelvis forward, it thrusts the pelvis forward* (see footnote p. 195),—*a fault that has no part in keeping us erect.*] " Its most powerful action is to raise the trunk after stooping by drawing the pelvis backward." [*The maximus is lax throughout the movement.*] " It is a tensor of the fascia lata, and through the iliotibial tract it steadies the femur on the tibia during standing when the extensor muscles are relaxed." [*See the last comment but one, above.*]

From Cunningham's Text-Book of Anatomy, 1943, 8*th Edn., p.* 508.—" The gluteus maximus is mainly an extensor of the thigh and has a powerful action in straightening the lower limb, as in climbing or running." [*Does this imply : when acting from its origin ? For presently we find the phrase :* " Acting from its insertion "—*as if to signify antithesis. If the antithesis is meant, the words suggest a retropulsion during climbing, just as they did when used in 1922 (5th Edn., p. 417).*] " Its lower fibres also adduct the thigh and rotate it laterally." [*The fibres meanwhile are relaxed.*] " Acting from its insertion the muscle is a powerful extensor of the trunk when the body is being raised from the sitting

The muscle, for example, is relaxed if we extend the hip ; in standing still ; in rising from the exercise of touching toes with straightened knees ; in leaning back when seated. Tradition has enjoined on maximus the task of moving *back* the femur and the pelvis. These movements in reverse are fortunately absent, else we should never climb the stairs, or leave a seat by voluntary act : gluteus maximus would guarantee that we were damned (like Sisyphus) to lasting retropulsion.

The muscle works quite otherwise. Taking a fixed and distal point in front, at the insertion of the ilio*tibial* tract upon the *front* of the tibia, its action (leaving seats or mounting stairs) helps to effect the raising of the pelvis and the femur *forward*, strapping each to each in such a way as to combine great solidarity with requisite mobility.[1]

The task indeed seems herculean, befitting well the bulk of maximus. But looking closer at the muscle we find the *length* of fibre far too short for the achievement : it measures roughly half the length of the required range of movement, and even maximal contraction could only bring the trunk through less than a quarter of the path it actually travels to surmount the foot.

I think it therefore possible that maximus may work instead like a *supporting* giant—a kind of Atlas—bearing the body's weight with fleshy hands while quadriceps, relieved of strain, procures the movement up and forwards of a mass maintained at every stage in levitation.

What happens when, unaided by our arms, we rise to full height from a chair ? Before we leave the seat the trunk tilts slightly towards the knees—a movement due, I think, to iliopsoas, not to rectus femoris. The feet are usually drawn back, and thus reduce the distance which the trunk must go to reach a stable

---

or stooping position ; " [*But these are movements made in* opposite *directions : the trunk moves forward from the sitting posture ; backward from the stooping posture.*]

Perhaps, since 1498, sufficient time has passed to let our text-books try the plan of Leonardo and link the muscles with descriptions of our common *acts*. Their total is, he notes, eighteen—a figure whose correction would do nothing to reduce his genius or evince a trace of it in others.

[1] The *femur* is slung forward as a whole by maximus in virtue of the junction which the lateral intermuscular septum makes with the part of iliotibial tract that constitutes the tendon of maximus. The septum at its inner edge is fixed to linea aspera ; its outer edge, as we shall see below (p. 218 and Fig. 136, B), joins with the hinder border of the tract. And so, by way of tract and septum, maximus secures a purchase on the shaft throughout its length.

The ' strap ' effect is due to *tightening* of the tract whose pressure on the great trochanter forces the backward-sloping neck to drive and hold the head of femur up against the *front* of acetabulum.

equilibrium. Then both the maximi contract, and—like a pair of hands passed from in front to curve behind the pelvis— begin to lift the trunk and thigh (this last through the iliotibial tract and lateral septum, see p. 218) together forward on the legs. In front the quadriceps conducts the movement. And then surprisingly, while hip and knee are still in flexion, first maximi, then recti, cease to act and leave the *final* straightening of the limb to semitendinosus.[1]

This action of a hamstring may seem strange, because we learn (by rote) to call the hamstrings "*flexors* of the knee." And so they are—provided that the foot is off the ground and quadriceps is lax. But the semitendinosus differs from its fellow hamstrings : it is attached in front of—not behind—the ' centre ' for the move- ment of the knee ; its lower tendon curves like fingers round the lever of the tibial shaft. So, when the foot is standing firm, and while the ankle acts as fulcrum, then a contraction of the muscle will pull the top of the tibia *back* and bring the knee to full extension. And you will find that if the trunk is vertical (and therefore does not need the aid of other hamstrings to check a forward plunge), semitendinosus, alone of all the local bellies you can feel, is genuinely taut throughout the movement. It is, in fact, a service-pattern ' muscle of attention '.

A model made in plasticine of the half pelvis seems to throw further light. Let it be flat at first, on the Mercator principle ; string it with thread attached like maximus from ilium to coccyx and thence continued into ' iliotibial tract '. Pivot the slab upon its ' acetabulum ' ; pull the loop forwards, letting your hand sink slowly as it pulls. Almost at once the ' semi-pelvis ' tilts. Now mould the plasticine which stands for ilium in close accordance with the bone : make it look backward at its hinder part, and

---

[1] The sudden laxity of maximus is fortunate perhaps if we consider how the *hyperactive* muscle lifts the pelvis nearly to the summit of the arch of opisthotonus produced by strychnine or by tetanus, in gross exaggeration of the movement which a patient makes to let the nurse remove a bed-pan. In this routine event the quadriceps is not protagonist, and maximus, behaving now as a *protrusor of the pelvis*, must put forth all its strength— a thing it rarely does, leaving to other muscles acts it might perform, and working when it must ; and then with notable economies of effort.

  That is a common character of muscle. A palmar flexion of my wrist against the force of gravity, and made with fingers loose, tightens the tendon of my flexor carpi radialis, which stands out like a ridge. Then, if I close my grip, the radialis ridge goes limp and fades, throwing the work instead upon a broader ridge of finger flexors. A loosening of the grip restores the *status quo* : the radialis juts ; the finger tendons fade. And while the order of this devolution fluctuates in wrists which (unlike mine) possess a long-palmaris tendon, the principle remains. No wonder, therefore, that we sometimes note a will to do the minimum and ' pass the buck ' ; these traits—united with the most unhuman *readiness*—are in the grain of all our striped activity.

splay it out ; stagger the ' coccyx ' inward from the ' ischium '. Pulling once more you find that a large fraction of the force which made the model nod when it was flat is now absorbed in twisting it : the downward pull instead of causing an immediate nutation begins to turn the slab in such a way that if the plasticine were living bone the pubis would be forced towards its fellow at the symphysis, and ilium would try to wrench itself away from sacrum.

Here—in connection with nutation—our plasticine perhaps illuminates the problem of the deeper caudal piece of maximus affixed to the gluteal mark : the fibres ought, one feels, to pull the upper part of femur *back*. Yet, if we force the thigh to full extension on the trunk, and then as far as it will go behind the buttock, though hamstrings harden, maximus is limp. And, when we rise from chairs, the upper part of femur travels *forward*. (The only backward-moving portion is the lower end—drawn backwards as we saw (p. 195), by semitendinosus when maximus had *ceased* to act.) Possibly these caudal fibres help in countering the forward inclination of the pelvis produced by rectus femoris and upper parts of maximus.

With plasticine (as in the art of surgery) experience may be fallacious ; but, as one handles it, a feeling grows that maximus could play a Titan's part—moulding the shape of pelvis, and re-doubling special portions of the bone predestined to *withstand* the stress of moulding—a dual part that might be found to mark for anthropologists, the hillman, say, from certain dwellers on the plain. And, if the skull shape alters rapidly with new environment (as Ridgeway thought in 1908, and Boas tried to prove in 1912),[1] may not the shape of pelvis too ? Or could a faster change, in favour this time of obstetrics, be got by early training of the muscle ?

It seems, perhaps, that Aristophanes was right when (in the *Clouds*) he let his students of astronomy look skyward with their rumps : gluteal muscles bring a host of problems into focus.

The care of convalescent maximi.—A brace of simple rules emerge from these conceptions. The patient, while recumbent,

---

[1] Sir W. Ridgeway, 1908, *Presidential Address to the Section of Anthropology*, British Association for the Advancement of Science ; Franz Boas, 1912, *Changes in Bodily Form of Descendants of Immigrants*, Washington D.C. 61st Congress, 2nd Session, State Documents 64, Document No. 208.

must be *lifted* on to bed-pans in order to prevent the all-out effort of the maximus that goes with a protrusion of the pelvis (see footnote, p. 195). Then, when he leaves the bed, we *lift* him to his feet and keep him on the level. There he may walk (gently and making short steps) with maximi as limp as battle-dress—a gait that we must teach *before* the patients rise. (In normal gait the fibres of the maximus stretch while the moving limb swings past its fellow, till, as we ground the heel, they harden suddenly—a little on the flat, but more and more with rise of gradient. Contracting thus they help the pelvis on to overtake the foot.)

So, in his *early* convalescence, the patient need not use the damaged maximus ; and if, as well, we lower him to sit or lie and do not let him stoop, he will not strain its fibre.

THE FRONT OF FEMUR

This (like its brachial homologue) is covered by a half-sleeve of muscle ; and whether we explore the back of humerus or front of femur our practice is identical : we look first for a *seam*, then open it to find a deep head coating bone and crossed obliquely by a neurovascular bundle. Accordingly, to reach the shaft in either case we rip the seam, loop the bundle, and split the deep head.

I shall return to these points later.

APPROACH TO THE FEMORAL SHAFT
FROM IN FRONT

Exposure of the femur from the outer side was once the fashion : it called for no reflection—the surgeon cut directly down on bone. The inconvenient, unsightly and bloody wound seemed to suggest a price exacted for security, together with a certain disregard of structure. The knife thus used transects the slanting fibres of vastus lateralis, a goal of all four perforating arteries and of the branch descending from the outer circumflex. The patient, too, must lie upon his side, or else the surgeon works at disadvantage.

The method found below [1] respects anatomy, is relatively bloodless, and gives a wide exposure : over twelve inches of the *shaft*—

[1] *British Journal of Surgery*, 1924, **12**, 84.

from small trochanter to the lower end—are easily accessible. We look in comfort on the front and sides of femur ; and while the patient still lies flat, we can secure a safe, dependent drainage.

Let us now take up the points of the first paragraph.

The *half-sleeve* consists of the quadriceps, enclosed in fascia ; its seam (which shapes the course of our incision) lies between vastus lateralis and rectus femoris—a pair of heads that part towards their origins and form a V-shaped entrance to the sleeve. This entrance will be found a handbreadth distal to the great trochanter, in line, of course, with the incision which runs from anterior superior spine down to the outer angle of patella (Figs. 119 and 120). For further guidance grasp the long and relatively mobile rectus head below the ' spine,' and move the muscle crosswise ; the outer margin of the mobile zone will mark the seam (compare p. 115).

The upper part of Fig. 119 shows that we must separate two other bellies—sartorius and tensor fasciæ—a very simple act for those who take the care to mark out incisions precisely. Then when the seam is ripped two structures must be kept in mind before exposing bone—suprapatellar pouch and neurovascular bundle.

The neurovascular bundle.—Coating the femur, when we rip the sleeve, we see a silvery fish-like belly—the deep, investing belly of crureus (or vastus intermedius in B.N.A.). A bundle slopes across its face consisting of the nerve (or nerves) to vastus lateralis plus outer branches (with companion veins) of lateral circumflex artery. This bundle can be found—in providential fat—a handbreadth distal to the great trochanter ; and when it has been mobilised and looped up like a bucket-handle, *then* we can split the muscle deep to it and reach the shaft (Fig. 120).

The *suprapatellar pouch* spreads, when the limb is straight, three fingerbreadths above patella. Pouch and bundle are described below in further detail.

THE OPERATION

Position.—With the patient flat on his back, extend the knee on the side of operation ; then raise the heel well off the table, relaxing rectus femoris.

Incision.—Divide the skin (and afterwards deep fascia) from anterior superior iliac spine to the outer angle of patella (Fig. 119, B). It is important to make this cut in such a way that we can open fascia *between* the tensor muscle and sartorius.

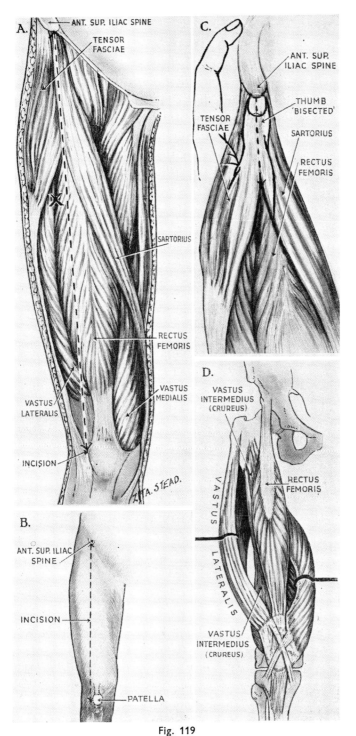

Fig. 119

The quadriceps sleeve in relation to the anterior incision

The cut goes from anterior superior spine to the outer angle of patella—close to the seam between rectus femoris and outer vastus (A and B). Find the entrance, X, to the sleeve one handbreadth below the top of great trochanter (or *two* handbreadths below anterior superior spine). From there the seam rips easily. The common mistake is to make the cut too far out. Avoid this by catching the thumb-nail squarely under the *notch* of the 'spine' (C). The knife 'bisects' the thumb and parts sartorius from tensor fasciæ. D (*after* Poirier) shows the segments of the sleeve, and how part of vastus intermedius (crureus) lies *behind* the distal half of vastus lateralis, though these last two are often fused.

Begin exactly at the centre of the very shallow notch immediately below the ' spine.'

It is impossible to find it by approaching from above ; feel therefore from below. The thumb does this best, catching the notch with its nail. A cut can then be made as if to split the thumb

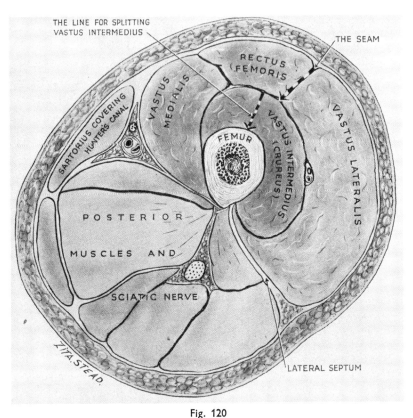

Fig. 120

The quadriceps sleeve in cross-section

Note the position of the seam, which must be ripped, and the line for splitting vastus intermedius—the deep, investing head which coats the femur.

in half (Fig. 119, c). The common error is to choose too lateral a point ; the knife strays into muscle and butchery begins.

Planes of cleavage.—The finger finds the V-like interval between rectus femoris and vastus lateralis, a handbreadth distal to the great trochanter ; and passing down between the bellies meets with minor vessels, which are caught and cut. More distally the finger will be checked where the vastus fibres join the rectus margin ; then we use a knife.

The trilaminar tendon of quadriceps.—A working knowledge here will let us rip the sleeve still farther down and thus obtain a maximal exposure.

The stout component from the rectus femoris lies in a groove provided by the distal parts of medial and lateral vasti (Fig. 121). Adjacent portions of these vasti, flush with rectus tendon, fasten on its borders and send their deeper fibres of insertion round behind to make a common sheet which cradles it. This interwoven sheet (the second lamina) lies on the third and deepest—formed, of course, by tendon from the vastus intermedius (the part of quadriceps once called crureus).

So, if we wish to mobilise the distal portion of the rectus and

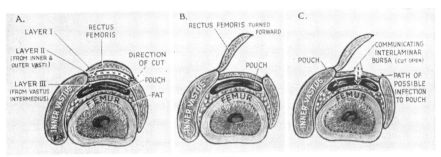

Fig. 121

Delamination and rotation of quadriceps tendon to secure further distal exposure of shaft

A. Divide the edge of rectus tendon from vastus lateralis ; then, with the knife laid flat, detach the *back* of rectus tendon down to patella. This will let you twist the tendon (B)—and, with it, all the rectus—farther forward, exposing more of vastus intermedius *belly*. (In order to avoid the pouch, the splitting of intermedius belly (Fig. 122, A) is checked four fingerbreadths above patella—a point which lies, of course, above the level shown in these pictures.) Note the fat between pouch and bone, which (with the extra access got by delamination) lets us separate the pouch intact and reach the distal limit of the shaft. C. Shows the theoretical risk of delamination in presence of sepsis—if any interlaminar bursa should happen to communicate with suprapatellar pouch.

bare the shaft still farther down, we separate at first the *edge* of rectus tendon from the vastus lateralis ; then, with the knife blade in the frontal plane, we cleave its hinder surface from the vastus sheet and so delaminate the tendon of the quadriceps (Fig. 121, B). After this cleavage we can twist the outer edge of rectus *as a whole* much farther forward and so get extra room to see and split the fish-like, bone-investing belly of the vastus intermedius.

The frontal cut to cleave the laminæ of quadriceps should not be made in presence of infection : bursæ are found at times between the layers, and might (if they were sliced, and chanced as well to join with the synovial pouch) bring sepsis to the knee (Fig. 121, c).

The neurovascular bundle.—Now that the sleeve is ripped the slanting bundle shows, a handbreadth distal to the top of great

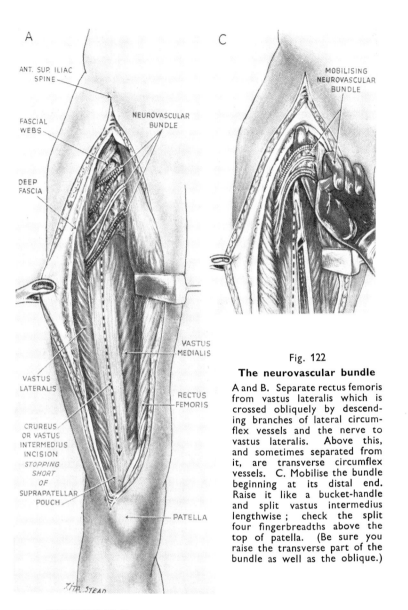

A

ANT. SUP. ILIAC SPINE

FASCIAL WEBS

DEEP FASCIA

VASTUS LATERALIS

CRUREUS OR VASTUS INTERMEDIUS INCISION *STOPPING SHORT OF* SUPRAPATELLAR POUCH

NEUROVASCULAR BUNDLE

VASTUS MEDIALIS

RECTUS FEMORIS

PATELLA

C

MOBILISING NEUROVASCULAR BUNDLE

Fig. 122

The neurovascular bundle

A and B. Separate rectus femoris from vastus lateralis which is crossed obliquely by descending branches of lateral circumflex vessels and the nerve to vastus lateralis. Above this, and sometimes separated from it, are transverse circumflex vessels. C. Mobilise the bundle beginning at its distal end. Raise it like a bucket-handle and split vastus intermedius lengthwise; check the split four fingerbreadths above the top of patella. (Be sure you raise the transverse part of the bundle as well as the oblique.)

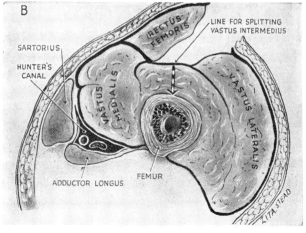

B

SARTORIUS

HUNTER'S CANAL

RECTUS FEMORIS

LINE FOR SPLITTING VASTUS INTERMEDIUS

VASTUS MEDIALIS

VASTUS LATERALIS

ADDUCTOR LONGUS

FEMUR

trochanter. The nerves and vessels reach the outer vastus and sink into it. Often they spread out fanwise (as in Fig. 122, A) or else divide into quadrants, two or three in number. A thin transparent fascia binds them (with surrounding streaks of fat) to vastus intermedius. The presence of this fat makes mobilising easy. Division of the binding film along the lowest streak will often let us raise the bundle as a whole upon the finger— like a bucket-handle. An upper transverse part is sometimes missed through carelessness; and sometimes quadrants widely separate may need a further opening of the film (Fig. 122, A).

Under this arching 'handle' cut to bone by splitting through the length of vastus intermedius. Watch for sharp bleeding from a vein divided in the upper fibres.

The suprapatellar pouch. —Avoid a penetration of this pouch which spreads three fingerbreadths above the top of patella and therefore check the split through vastus intermedius a trifle higher up (Fig. 122, A).

If we delaminate the tendon of the quadriceps, we can—in case of need— detach the pouch from bone.

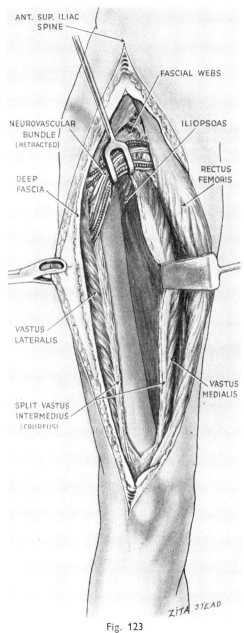

Fig. 123

Anterior exposure of femur

Detach the split vastus intermedius and expose as much of the shaft as you wish.

A broadly bladed osteotome, close against the shaft and moving distally, will take advantage of the lucky weft of fat that lies between the bone and pouch—a thing to practise first upon cadavers, for round the uninfected knee we should not make too bold with cobwebs.[1] Displace the flaccid pouch towards the joint and so get access to the lower end of shaft.

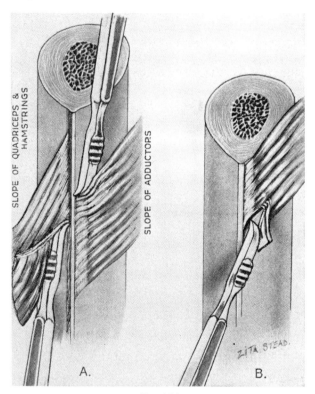

Fig. 124

Stripping the femoral shaft of muscle

A. Work the rugine into the acute or stripping angle which muscular attachments make with bone, *i.e.*, *up* the shaft for all the muscles excepting adductors. Note how the rugine tears into muscle when used in the wrong direction (B) against the obtuse angle.

Retraction of the halves of intermedius will presently reveal a foot or more of shaft—a wide span plus a handbreadth (Fig. 123). But first it must be cleared of muscle.

Stripping the femoral shaft.—The slope of muscle varies : vasti and the short head of biceps travel down *from* the femur ; adductors, *to* the femur. We strip them off most cleanly by working the rugine against the *lesser* angle which the fibres make at their

---

[1] Attempts at separating pouch from *quadriceps* will nearly always tear the pouch.

attachments—the stripping angle of the muscle. Used in the opposite direction the instrument will tend to leave the shaft and tear the fibres—especially at linea aspera where rugged edge and toughly planted tendon contribute (with the effort they evoke) to sharp and sudden deviations (Fig. 124, B).

Beginning at the inner side detach from linea aspera the origin of vastus medialis, which forms the medial intermuscular septum (Poirier) by working *up* the bone ; then separate adductors in the opposite direction.

On the outer side of shaft the rugine works in one way only—

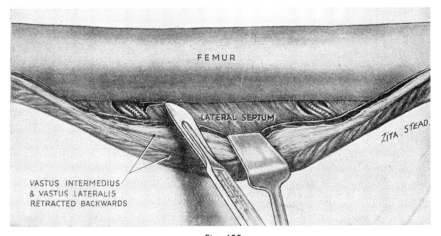

Fig. 125
Stripping the shaft of lateral septum

(The sleeve is open and the femur stripped of quadriceps.)   Sit, looking level with the bone. Press back the vastus lateralis and outer moiety of intermedius.   Find the perforating bundles coming through the septal archways.   The pressure on the muscle draws the vessels back sufficiently to let a *knife* divide the septum from the linea.

upwards : at first against the vasti origins ; and presently—behind the septum—against the shorter head of biceps.

The *lateral intermuscular septum*, irregular in grain and giving passage to the perforating vessels, requires special treatment. Sit looking level with the wound and *see* the vessels coming through their roomy archways. Retraction of the vasti will draw these vessels back sufficiently to let you *cut* the septum close to bone and leave them safe (Fig. 125). (A surgeon, Maurice Pearson, in South Africa—*British Medical Journal*, 1930, **1**, 910—has paid this femoral approach the compliment of making it a ' one-man job.' He has devised retractors (Fig. 126), weighted at the ends, which lever up the shaft and press the muscles back.)

Drainage.—Counter-openings, too, are made with perfect safety

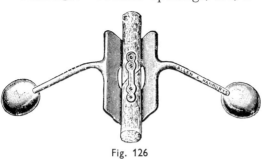

Fig. 126

Maurice Pearson's retractors

These are self-retaining ; they lift the shaft, press back the muscles, and take the place of an assistant.

(The block for this figure has been kindly lent by Messrs Allen & Hanburys.)

by cutting down upon a forceps passed between the outer part of vastus intermedius and the bone. The outer face of lateral septum shuts the forceps off from the sciatic nerve (Fig. 127) and guides it back to skin behind the field of operation. For with the limb recumbent the

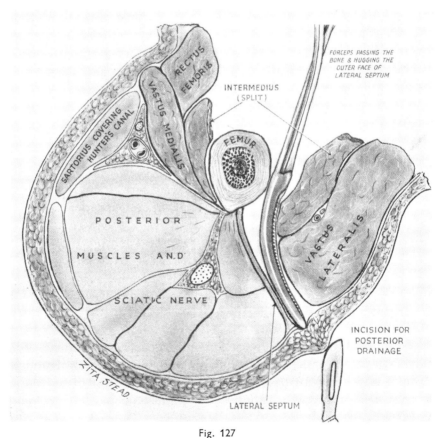

Fig. 127

Posterior drainage after anterior exposure of femoral shaft

When you have ripped the seam and split vastus intermedius, slide a forceps past the outer side of shaft, and make it hug the outer face of septum till the skin is bulged behind. Note how the septum buffers the sciatic nerve.

septum is approximately vertical—a statement true of every portion that we use in making *this* exposure. The reason seems to be as follows. Close to the knee for a few fingerbreadths the septum keeps a frontal plane and faces fore and aft ; that is because the mass of quadriceps in front of it is almost equal to the biceps mass behind. But farther up the thigh the quadriceps preponderates so quickly as to turn the septum back into a plane that faces right and left. I stress the point to meet suggestions that exposure of the femur from in front is incompatible with proper drainage.

Extension of Anterior Femoral Exposure to the Knee Joint.—The distal part of this approach is easily continued with the wide benign exposure devised by Timbrell Fisher for the knee joint.[1] He brings his own incision down along the inner edge of the patella. Let us, instead, continue ours along the *outer* edge (keeping, like Fisher, clear of tibial tubercle so that the scar will not be knelt on). This outer cut lies parallel to the main cutaneous nerves and is remote from the medial, transversely placed saphenous branch whose injury gives trouble after meniscectomy. Bring the cut a fingerbreadth below the level of the tubercle (Fig. 128). Reflect the skin medially and expose the *inner* edge of patella ; expose also the inner edge of quadriceps tendon to the height of four

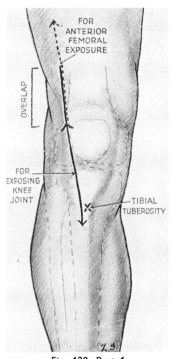

Fig. 128, Part 1

Incision including knee joint with anterior femoral exposure

The black line shows the incision for separate exposure of the joint. The knife avoids the tibial tuberosity.

fingerbreadths. Then split the fibrous covering of the patella along the middle line ; reflect the cover inwards just beyond the margin of the bone; cut along that inner edge into the joint. Continue this cut upwards (avoiding inner vastus) through the *tendon* of quadriceps sufficiently to let us dislocate the patella (strung between ligament and tendon) so that its articular face rests on the outer side of outer femoral condyle. Flex the knee to a right angle and make the joint yawn. I have used Fisher's fine, original exposure to pick

[1] *The Lancet*, 1923, **1**, 945.

shot-gun pellets from the back of a condylar recess, and also—with the trivial change described above—for excising knees through straight incisions (p. 7).

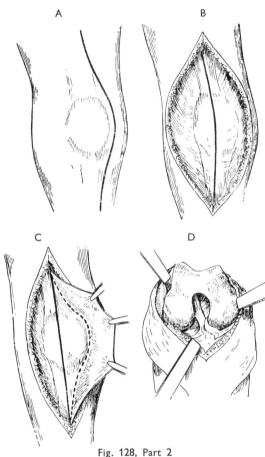

Fig. 128, Part 2

These four drawings, copied by kind permission of Mr A. G. Timbrell Fisher and of *The Lancet*, show that author's original wide exposure of the knee joint through a medial skin incision, A. The procedures figured in B, C and D—reflection inwards of the prepatellar fascia (B), medial arthrotomy (C), and lateral luxation of patella, with flexion of the joint (D)—can all be performed through the *lateral* incision continuing anterior femoral exposure (Fig. 128, Part 1).

Repair will (if we wish) seal the cavity with three staggered rows of suture. Drainage can be got in the face-down position—the only way (without resection of a condyle) of using gravity to empty pools in either blind posterior pouch. But drainage damns the knee joint to adhesions; and where the joint and not the life is threatened, as happens often in the early case of knee infection, I have secured quick healing and good function by injecting 10-15 c.cm. of mercurochrome (1 per cent. in water) after thorough aspiration of pus, repeating the procedure three or four times with two-day intervals. Mercurochrome, I found, was harmless to the joint, and was bacteriostatic in that dosage. (This was before the advent of more recent drugs about whose action on and in synoviæ I have no personal experience.)

THE UPPER PART OF THE ANTERIOR FEMORAL APPROACH

Let us consider certain details of a region shared by this exposure of the femur and by Smith-Petersen's exposure of the hip.

The fascial webs.—After we part the muscles and move towards the femoral neck, two, three, or four superimposed and separate layers of fascia, remarkable in strength and shape, cross the path of the knife. These layers occupy the space between the origins of the rectus femoris and tensor fasciæ muscles, uniting the *deep* aspects of their sheaths (Fig. 129). Each—like the web between two ' Victory ' fingers—is furnished with a clear-cut margin, concave distally. *One* of the webs (but which, it is impossible to prophesy) has on its deeper face and near its edge an artery the size of radial —the ascending branch of the lateral circumflex ; so it is well before we cut the webs to clamp their margins till we find the vessel.

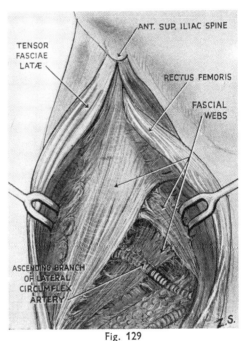

Fig. 129

The fascial webs

These cover the front of hip joint and join the deep aspects of the sheaths of rectus femoris and tensor muscles. Note the relation of web and artery.

These webs deserve a study which I found no time to give them. A glimpse of a figure in Paturet's *Traité d'Anatomie Humaine* (1951), Vol. II, p. 599, a fascinating book, which I owe to the gift of Sir Gordon Gordon-Taylor, led me to suspect a link between my so-called webs and Paturet's ' recurrent ' (or third) head of rectus femoris. I have no sure warrant for that surmise, nor (in a very limited search) have I had the fortune to find a convincing third head. I leave Fig. 130 as a guide for more thorough explorations.

The double bonnet.—These web-like structures screen the joint in front. When they are cut a finger-tip pressed firmly on the capsule can just squeeze in above its upper face and force a path between the capsule and a hood which covers it—a double hood or bonnet formed by gluteus medius and minimus, whose deeper part (the minimus) is moulded down in streamline on the joint. So, to expose the deep articular machinery, we raise the bonnet (Fig. 131).

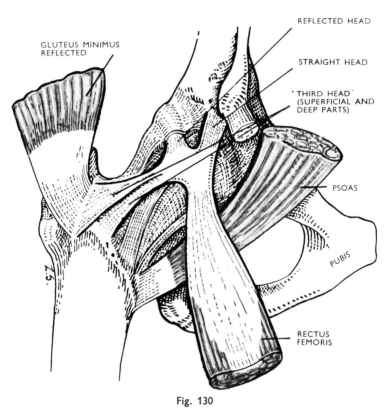

REFLECTED HEAD

GLUTEUS MINIMUS
REFLECTED

STRAIGHT HEAD

`THIRD HEAD`
(SUPERFICIAL AND
DEEP PARTS)

PSOAS

PUBIS

RECTUS
FEMORIS

Fig. 130

The 'third head' of rectus femoris (after Paturet). Its deep part joins the iliofemoral ligament and the trochanteric line ; its superficial part joins the tendon of gluteus minimus on the front of great trochanter. (The tendon of sartorius is not labelled.)

ANTERIOR APPROACH TO THE FEMUR COMBINED WITH SMITH-PETERSEN'S EXPOSURE OF THE HIP JOINT

These two are complementary procedures, a fact of special value in a fracture dislocation (Fig. 131).[1]   And so in passing from

---

[1] Referred to in a paper on that subject (*British Journal of Surgery*, 1934, **22**, 205) written with Bayumi. Mahmud Bayumi died in 1940, only a short while after the Royal College of Surgeons of England had conferred his Fellowship without examination—a good friend, a loyal follower of Sir Robert Jones, and pioneer in Egypt of common sense in orthopædic methods.

the femur to the hip continue the incision to the level of at least the highest point of the iliac crest—four fingerbreadths behind the anterior superior spine. Then you can raise the twofold gluteal bonnet and turn it back sufficiently to bring the deeply situated hip joint to the *surface.* For that you must, if you are working in the opposite direction (from joint to femur), be sure to rip the seam between the rectus femoris and vastus lateralis at least a wide span

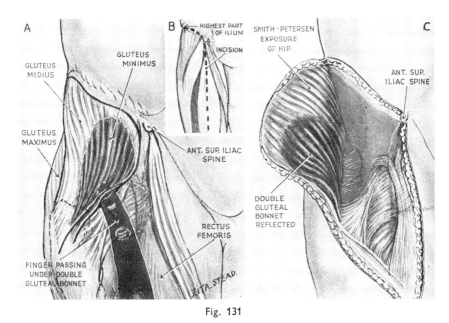

Fig. 131

The double gluteal bonnet and the combined approach to hip and femur

A. Gluteus medius fits over minimus to cover the top of hip joint. B. The incision. Note that it must reach (1) the highest point of iliac crest ; (2) at least a span, distal to the anterior superior spine. This lets you hinge back the muscles sufficiently to bring both joint and femur to the *surface.* C. Shows how the anterior approach to femoral shaft merges with the Smith-Petersen exposure of hip.

distal to the ' spine.' A skimping of the wound, in either case, will leave this deep joint cribbed about by muscle.

I have preferred to *cut* away the glutei from crest and outer face of ilium, instead of peeling off the periosteum : the knife leaves two things that are useful—a carpet on the outer face of ilium ; a fringe along its crest. The fringe will serve for reconstructive suturing ; the carpet lets us catch with ordinary forceps divided vessels in its pile of cut gluteal fibres. But if instead we peel the muscles off, we set ourselves the task of stopping bleeding from a *bone.*

Repair.—Sutures at the crest of ilium bring the great mass of muscle back in place, and pressure keeps it there. Healing is sound in young or old ; for fleshy fibres cut from bone (unlike a tendinous detachment) unite again both fast and well.

EXPOSURES OF THE POPLITEAL FACE OF FEMUR

This face can be approached and dealt with from the inner or the outer side ; or from the back. Each mode of access has its use. That from the *inner* side is not so easily continued up the shaft : the field is crossed by major vessels which must be mobilised and looped away (p. 215).

The *outer* access on the other hand can be at once prolonged far up the thigh—with due respect for perforating vessels. A medial or lateral sinus requiring excision will frequently decide our choice of route.

Fresh injury, again, may need the third or *mesial* approach, but use of it in face of fibrous matting courts danger to the nerves and vessels. Then, too, a hypertrophic scar may form behind the knee—a chance event, outweighed by ease of access and facilities obtained in tracing nerves and vessels up or down the limb ; the place in that respect is like a no-man's-land through which attack may go in two directions. (Description of this midline route comes later—with the calf, p. 251.)

THE INNER (MEDIAL) APPROACH

A plan intending to exploit the rear of any situation solely from the flank might seem a hopeless paradox. But in our surgical assault we hold this clear advantage over generals—the *place* can turn obligingly and let us in.

Try it yourself—or on a skeleton—while one (or other) lies upon the back with limbs extended. Rest the outer edge, say, of the *right* foot on the left shin, letting the right knee sag. This turns the popliteal face towards the left—round, nearly, through a right angle. Then, with a sandbag, raise the other buttock (or decorously tilt instead the pelvis of your skeleton) : the popliteal surface turns still farther round and looks not only left but up, towards the ceiling.

The vessels and the bone.—In all exposures of the popliteal face we must negotiate the popliteal *vessels*. That is made easy by a thumbwide gap which parts the vessels from the bone and owes existence to the fact that while, above, the trunks lie close against the shaft, below, the condyles (bridged, of course, by capsule) fend both artery and vein away from femur—much as a backward flexion of the fist will fend a ruler, lying lengthwise, off the dorsum of the carpus (Fig. 132).

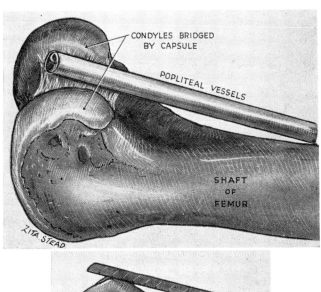

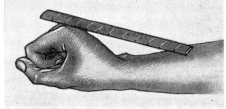

Fig. 132

Showing how the bridge of capsule between the condyles fends the vessels off the popliteal face, leaving a useful thumbwide interval.

The *guiding tendon of the adductor magnus* is overlaid by muscle ; sartorius and gracilis cover its medial side. But, when the knee is bent and fascia divided, these bellies slip right back and show the tendon ; only a loose, thin membrane just behind this whitish cord remains to part us from the popliteal space.

THE OPERATION

Position.— A sandbag underneath the buttock of the sound side tilts the recumbent patient. Place the foot of the affected limb so that its outer edge rests on the other shin as near the knee as possible [1] (Fig. 133).

Incision.—Cut *lengthwise* for an ample span, crossing adductor tubercle. The knife follows the bend of the limb and only severs

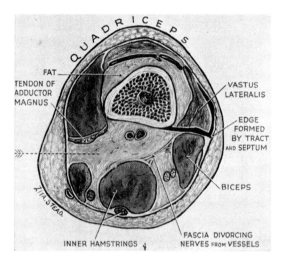

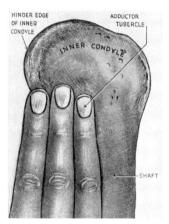

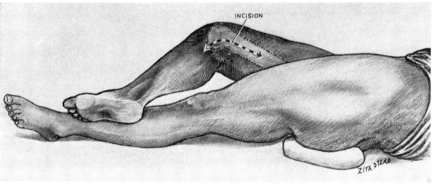

Fig. 133

Position and incision for inner popliteal approach

The knee is shown raised in order to demonstrate the incision clearly ; in practice it rests on the table. Note above a three-finger method of locating adductor tubercle. When the 'free' edge of the hinder finger is at the hinder edge of inner condyle the pulp of the anterior finger covers the tubercle. Note, too, the way in, as shown by the arrow in the cross-section.
(This has been adapted from Eycleshymer and Shoemaker, Section 88, p. 146.)

skin and surface fat. Three fingerbreadths of this incision are distal to the tubercle, the rest and major part is proximal (Fig. 133). Be careful here : a medial condyle has often been mistaken for adductor tubercle ; incisions then lie too far back. Locate the

[1] If the knee of the affected side does not flex easily, work from the *opposite* side of the table.

hindmost margin of the condyle ; the tubercle is found three fingerbreadths in front (Fig. 133).

Dissect the hinder edge of skin back for about an inch ; expose sartorius above the level of the adductor tubercle ; divide the fascia in front of it ; then (with Mayo scissors ' on the flat ') detach the deep surface of the muscle, avoiding thus a risk of injuring synovial membrane that lies between the condyle and sartorius.

The free sartorius falls back and leaves exposed the guiding tendon of adductor magnus in front of which the large saphenous nerve leaves the canal of Hunter. The nerve is sometimes carried off upon the deeper aspect of sartorius ; or else lies loosely, strung across the wound. With it is found the superficial branch of the descending genicular artery—the old anastomotic. The *deep* branch of this vessel runs along adductor tendon surrounded by some fibres of the inner vastus. Nor do we see the great saphenous vein (which lies upon the surface of the sartorius), if we have rightly placed our skin incision.

Immediately behind the adductor tendon pick up and open the loose thin fascia—the last impediment before you reach the fossa. Slide a finger in, keeping its back against the tendon, till you touch the centre of the popliteal face (Fig. 134). The *vessels* lie, we know, a thumbwidth from the bone, so bend the finger-tip to find them. Widen the entry to the space and let the finger mobilise the vessels —up to the opening in the adductor magnus, down to the condyles of the femur. As we retract them gently back, some twigs they send to bone string out across the wound and thus are easily controlled and cut. The popliteal face of the femur then lies bare (Fig. 134). (The major *nerves* do not appear in this exposure ; they run remote from bone and from the surgeon (p. 221 and footnote to p. 241).)

THE MEDIAL ROUTE EXTENDED TO FEMOROPOPLITEAL TRUNKS AND TO THE SHAFT.—Prolong the upper part of the incision *towards* the mid-point between anterior superior spine and pubic symphysis—in the direction of the femoral artery (Fig. 135). Find the anterolateral edge of the sartorius ; liberate and move the belly inwards off the membrane roofing Hunter's femoral canal. Then split the roof and find the vessels. When the knee is bent the femoropopliteal trunks will come to hand with gentle separation and be loose enough to loop aside. The *outward* twigs which moor the bundle here are few and widely spread ; one set of these, much larger and more constant than the rest, lies about seven fingerbreadths above the adductor tubercle. A little blunt dissection

made along the leash and on the outer aspect of the parent
bundle will let us raise the major vessels like a bucket-handle
and clear an access to the shaft.[1]

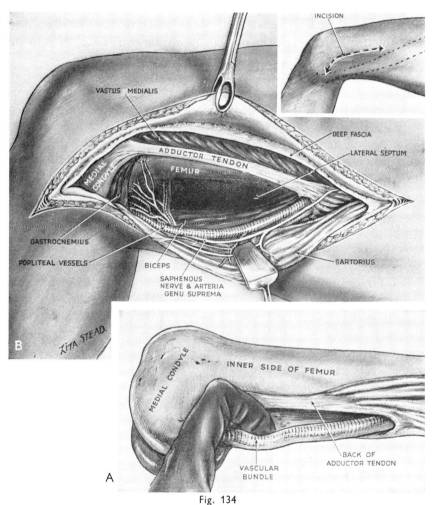

Fig. 134
Exposure of the popliteal face from the inner side
A. Open the flimsy fascia just *behind* adductor magnus tendon ; slide a finger into the fossa
keeping its back against the tendon ; touch the *centre* of the popliteal space. Hook the finger
to locate the vessels. Widen the opening and mobilise the vessels. B. The popliteal face
exposed.

[1] *Mutual relations of femoropopliteal vein and artery.*—Sartorius will help us to remember
them : down the *thigh* sartorius and vein have *opposite* relations to the artery. So,
where sartorius is lateral, near Poupart's ligament, the vein is medial ; in Hunter's canal
sartorius lies in front, the vein behind ; beside the popliteal face of femur sartorius is
medial, the vein is lateral. Still farther down, within the bottle-neck produced between
the condyles and the heads of gastrocnemius, the vein—as if perforce—lies close behind
the artery. But in the *leg* it holds once more a medial position—just as it does near
Poupart's ligament. (See legend to Fig. 157.)

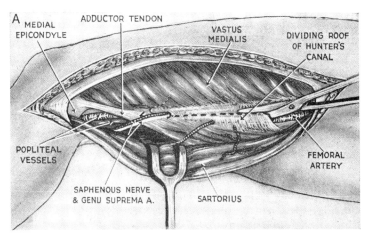

A
MEDIAL
EPICONDYLE

ADDUCTOR TENDON

VASTUS
MEDIALIS

DIVIDING ROOF
OF HUNTER'S
CANAL

POPLITEAL
VESSELS

FEMORAL
ARTERY

SAPHENOUS NERVE
& GENU SUPREMA A.

SARTORIUS

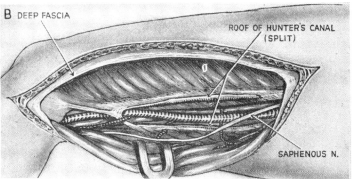

B   DEEP FASCIA

ROOF OF HUNTER'S CANAL
(SPLIT)

SAPHENOUS N.

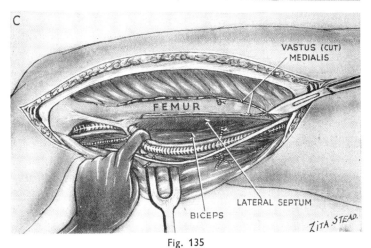

C

VASTUS (CUT)
MEDIALIS

FEMUR

LATERAL SEPTUM

BICEPS

ZITA·STEAD.

Fig. 135

**Extension of the medial approach to expose first the femoro-
popliteal trunks in continuity, then the shaft**

A. Displace sartorius from the roof of Hunter's canal which is then split.
B. Bend the knee and mobilise the femoropopliteal trunks. In doing this
the leash of very large vessels which binds the trunks to vastus medialis seven
fingerbreadths above adductor tubercle can be cut, or liberated with Mayo
scissors. (In the figure it is cut.) C. Loop the main trunks aside—like a
bucket-handle—and clear a path to femoral shaft.

Then, working at the *back* of the vastus medialis, detach the muscle from its slender hold on bone ; for there, as if to help us, the fibres spring from linea aspera and cover, but have no attachment to, the inner side of femur. So, by a mere extension of the route of Fiolle and Delmas, we expose a span or more of shaft in continuity with popliteal surface.

THE OUTER (LATERAL) APPROACH

Exposure of the popliteal surface from the outer side is simple. We take advantage of a loop-hole leading straight into the fossa, and widen it to reach the bone.

ANATOMY

The loop-hole.—Close to the outer condyle the short head of biceps lies ' free ' behind the septum, and there a touch—once fascia is opened—will separate the belly and reveal (between the biceps, the septum and the condyle) a loop-hole opening in the popliteal fossa—a crevice we shall presently enlarge (Fig. 136). But we must find it first. And what a mess if we should fail ! For cuts that blunder into quadriceps through tract or septum will sometimes cause a singular confusion, incredible till actually seen.

The iliotibial edge.—Provided that the knee can be even slightly flexed, mistakes, for once, are almost inexcusable. We can enlist the certain guidance of a hard and constant edge which marks the union (at an angle) of lateral septum with the hinder margin of the iliotibial tract (Fig. 136, A and B). The *edge* will therefore lead us in behind the septum to the loop-hole.

We have a choice of ways for finding it. The wise use both.

THE TWO-FINGER METHOD.—With the knee partly flexed run your middle and index fingers (side by side and touching) *lengthways* down the outer surface of the thigh—your left fingers for the left thigh, your right for the right. When the tip of your middle finger touches the back of the fibular head the pulp of index rests on skin that shifts across the stable hinder edge of iliotibial tract (Fig. 136, c). Behind this edge (which merges, inwards, with the septum) is a loose, soft mass of biceps—so different with anæsthesia from the cord we feel behind a wakeful knee.[1]

---

[1] The biceps 'tendon' just above the joint is *not* the cord-like structure which often seems so obvious to eye or touch. It is instead a *lamina* that coats a wider belly and goes slack with it. " *Les deux portions de ce muscle s'attachent à l'extrémité supérieure du péroné par un tendon considérable qui monte en s'élargissant derrière ces deux portions réunies.*" Little escaped the Baron Boyer.

THE TEST OF RELATIVE MOBILITY.—Grasping the soft and mobile biceps belly close above the condyle we find it moves across the stable edge (Fig. 136, D). This simple test will guide our knife and bring us opposite the loop-hole.

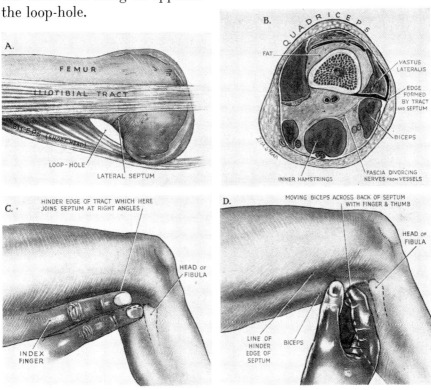

Fig. 136

The outer popliteal approach

A. The loop-hole. B. Cross-section showing how the guiding edge which lies in front of the loop-hole is formed by the junction of iliotibial tract with lateral septum. At this low level (but not higher up) tract and septum form a right angle. C. *Two-finger method of finding the edge.* Use right middle and index fingers for the right side, left for the left. Slide them lengthwise down the thigh till the tip of middle finger strikes the back of fibular head. The pulp of index feels the edge. D. *The test of relative mobility.* Find the edge by moving biceps across the back of septum. (This test is useful when the knee cannot be flexed.)

The biceps, passing to the fibula, crosses the outer head of the gastrocnemius, and, on the outer side of lateral condyle, lies for a little space against the synovial membrane of the knee—a fact to keep in mind.

THE OPERATION

Position.—Place the patient on the sound side with the sound limb straight. Lay the knee of the affected side just before its fellow knee so that the heel will rest on the ' sound ' shin and tilt the popliteal face to a convenient angle (Fig. 137).

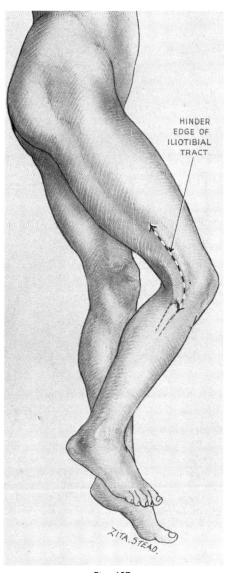

HINDER
EDGE OF
ILIOTIBIAL
TRACT

Incision.—A longitudinal cut a span in length— through skin and fat but *not* through deeper fascia—exactly maps the hinder, guiding edge of the iliotibial tract, down to the head of the fibula (Fig.137). Make *doubly* certain of this guiding edge before you seek the loop-hole. Then, close above the condyle, pinch up fascia just behind the edge ; divide it lengthwise with the edge as guide. A finger-breadth above the condyle a touch with Mayo scissors will detach the ' free ' part of the biceps belly from the septum and reveal the loop-hole. (Avoid the use of pointed scissors which might prick synovia round the condyle.)

Enlarge the loop-hole with the finger. Work gently up along behind the septum, and free the slight attachment of the biceps. As you do this you meet with two or three resistant strands—twigs which

Fig. 137

Lateral popliteal exposure

Position and incision. The *position* serves, too, for exposing fibula (p. 292 below).

biceps before they pass (through septal arches) to the quadriceps (p. 205). Divide and tie these twigs. Avoid the cramp of working down a pit by separating the biceps upwards to the *limit* of your skin incision. Then through the gap slide in a finger close above the condyle, keeping its back against the hinder surface of the septum. Touch with the nail the centre of the bony plane, and hook the finger gently to catch and mobilise the rope-like parcel of the vessels ; divide a few unpaired and variable offsets that moor it loosely to the femur. Retraction then displays the popliteal face in full (Fig. 138).

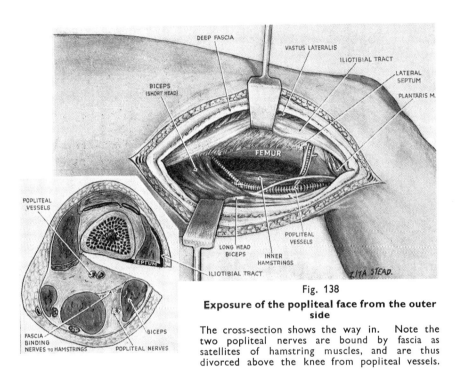

Fig. 138

Exposure of the popliteal face from the outer side

The cross-section shows the way in. Note the two popliteal nerves are bound by fascia as satellites of hamstring muscles, and are thus divorced above the knee from popliteal vessels.

The major nerves—like persons with too many aliases [1]—keep in the background : reaching the fossa from behind, they lie, as one might guess, behind the vessels (which reach it from in front). The nerves, in fact, are satellites of the hamstring bellies and have (above the knee) a mere, and easily divorced, *proximity* to vessels. That is why, when the popliteal artery and vein are hooked up by a finger, the nerves are unperceived and left behind : until they reach the leg, a sheet of intervening fascia postpones the linkage which creates a neurovascular bundle (Fig. 138, inset).

[1] For comment on these aliases see footnote, p. 244.

THE LATERAL POPLITEAL ROUTE EXTENDED TO THE OUTER FACE OF SHAFT.—Ten inches more of femur can be seen by this extension. No main trunks cross the field ; we deal instead with transverse branches of the perforating vessels (Fig. 139).

Let us continue the incision of the skin (Fig. 137) a handbreadth

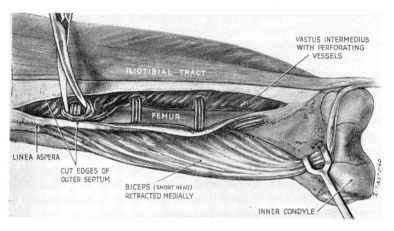

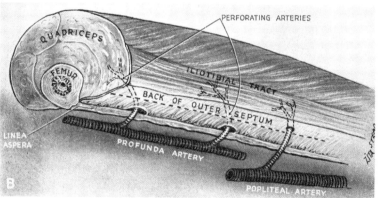

Fig. 139

Lateral popliteal exposure extended to the shaft of femur

A. Split the outer septum lengthwise from behind. Trace the ladder-like lay-out of vessels through the vasti ; then work between the ' rungs ' and bare the bone.
B. Shows the anatomy in diagram.

up beyond the length of shaft we wish to bare ; and, in the same direction, pursue the stripping of the biceps from septum and (as well) from the linea. This will expose the naked back of the septum.

The vascular bundles.—The terminals of perforating vessels from profunda cross the field to reach the outer vastus group in series with some lower twigs that spring from the popliteal trunks. But none—except this lower singleton or pair—are obvious : *it* runs a little way in view before it perforates the back of septum, contrasting thus with branches of the profunda that disappear, as soon as they have crossed the linea, through septal *arches* ranged along the shaft.

If then we split the septum lengthwise from behind, we come directly on the *back* of the quadriceps (on the vastus intermedius below, and half-way up the shaft, on the vastus lateralis, Fig. 119, D). Beginning at the linea we trace the bundles through the rather open texture of the vasti. A very little care will keep the vessels safe while a rugine strips off the flimsy hold of muscle from the outer side of shaft.[1] This leaves the bone conveniently accessible between and underneath the bundles, which now lie spaced like ladder rungs across its naked flank (Fig. 139). And, if we wish, we can divide a rung or two.

A METHOD OF EXPOSING THE FEMOROPOPLITEAL TRUNKS WIDELY FROM BEHIND

For a maximal exposure the *incision* begins in the leg behind the tendon of semitendinosus and passes up along the medial hamstrings to reach the midline *above* the popliteal fossa and continues there as high as the gluteal fold. The level of this corresponds roughly with the apex of Scarpa's femoral triangle four fingerbreadths below the midinguinal point. Open the deep fascia parallel to the several parts of the skin incision but not immediately deep to them. Above and close to the femoral condyles, slide the palmar face of the fingers inwards across the backs of the two inner hamstrings—semitendinosus and mem-branosus. Curve the fingers so that their tips go *deep* to the superficial pair of *medial* muscles—gracilis and sartorius (Fig. 140, A). Begin below at the tendon of adductor magnus and part the medial edge of magnus from the lower end of sartorius, and also from the deep face of gracilis. Draw the magnus belly out towards the femoral shaft and with it bring the longus : their full retraction opens a plane of cleavage that lets us reach and enter into Hunter's canal from behind (Fig. 140, B).

---

[1] The clearance of the *inner* face of femur from the back is troublesome ; it is most difficult in the approach to peel off tough insertions of adductors without progressive injury to major veins. For, with the patient prone, the perforating vessels are jammed between adductors and the femur. In contrast it is simple, as we have seen, to push these vessels backwards—clear of bone—when working from the front (p. 205).

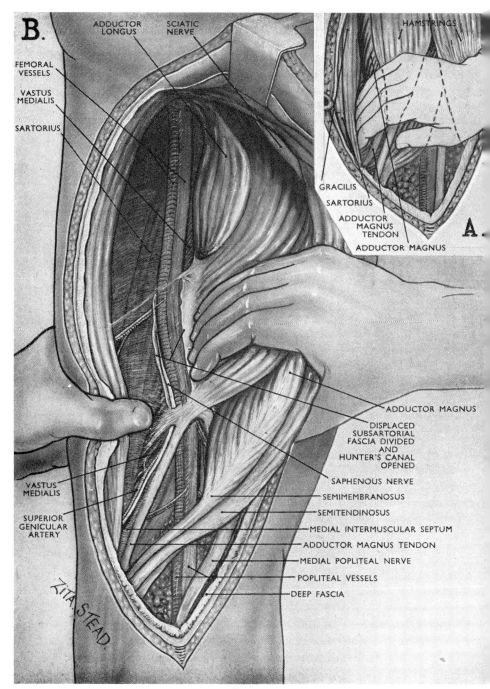

Fig. 140

Exposure of right femoropopliteal trunks from behind

Inset A shows how the palmar face of the fingers slides inwards across the back of medial hamstring. The tips of the fingers dig deep to gracilis and then to sartorius ; they thus curve round the separabl inner edge of adductor magnus. This they draw outwards together with adductor longus, and thu (as in Fig. 141, B) bring the subsartorial fascia round *behind* the femoral trunks. The trunks are disclose when the fascia is opened.

Inset B shows the *en masse* retraction of adductors, which—like café journals slung by the edge on a rod– are turned towards the femur (see p. 237).

The length of the exposure is illustrated.

Access through a displaced fascia.—The line for entering 'Hunter' follows the direction of the medial edge of the belly of adductor magnus. Incision up this line opens the canal, not as one might expect through its thin posterior fascial wall, but through the much thicker subsartorial fascia. The reason for this is that though the subsartorial fascia, while undisturbed, spreads

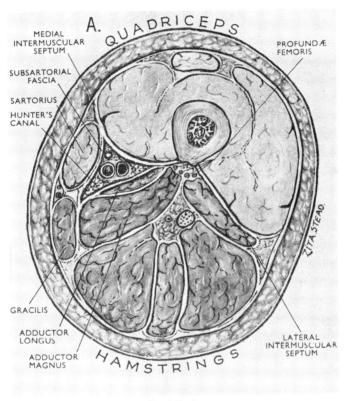

Fig. 141, A.
The subsartorial fascia undisturbed.

in a sagittal plane (Fig. 141, A) through the lower two-thirds of thigh, the strong retraction we have put on the adductor mass has drawn the fascia away from sartorius and has then dragged it round *behind* the femoral trunks (Fig. 141, B). Emergence through this fascia of the supreme genicular artery, the saphenous nerve or its accessory (Fig. 142), and sometimes, too, of a communication with a posterior obturator branch, guides us straight into Hunter's canal.

During the strong retraction of adductors the subsartorial

fascia becomes concealed in a gutter bounded and overlapped by adductor muscle and vastus medialis—a concealment that is of no consequence once the clue of emerging nerve or artery has led us to the main femoral trunks above the opening in adductor magnus :

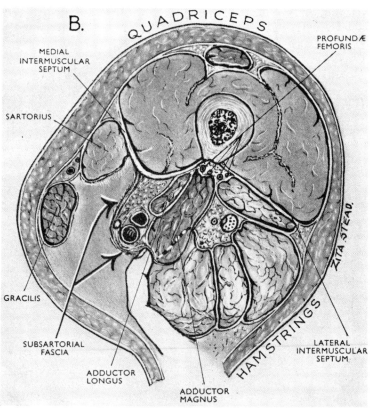

Fig. 141, B.

Cross-section showing how the strong lateral retraction of great and long adductors distorts Hunter's canal—displacing the subsartorial fascia from the deep face of sartorious and dragging it round *behind* the superficial femoral trunks so that we reach them by opening it (see Fig. 140, B).

after that we merely slit through the subsartorial fascia and follow them.

Thus, finally, these trunks themselves become our guide in extending their own exposure upwards—which finger separation achieves. The higher we go the deeper we get, but 9 in. of superficial femoral vein and artery are easily available, plus 4 in. of popliteal above the knee-joint line, and some 3 in. below. And happily the *backs* of femoral artery and vein are relatively free from offsets.

The saphenous nerve.—Our early medial thrust of fingers by displacing sartorius and gracilis will have already moved the nerve—which passes between these two muscles—away from the medial side of the superficial femoral artery so that we can easily catch the nerve by bending a finger up into this neurovascular angle. (The nerve, as we trace it *from below*, lies first in front of the magnus tendon and then approaching the artery touches its medial side for a few fingerbreadths before turning to pass up the anterior wall of the vessel.)

EXPOSURE OF DEEP FEMORAL VESSELS

Global wars multiply lesions otherwise rare. Yet, excepting in the scale of personal distress, the toll that reaches ' base ' from deep femoral trunks is slight : Homer, and others after him, record the quick deadliness of relevant wounds. Wars then, especially, or some new need, may give sporadic currency to pages that stem from a ten-year-old request by Sir James Paterson Ross in a most kindly review.

I shall deal with problems that arose, and then summarise the actual procedure.

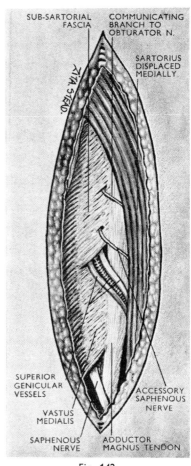

SUB-SARTORIAL FASCIA

COMMUNICATING BRANCH TO OBTURATOR N.

SARTORIUS DISPLACED MEDIALLY

LIFE STEAD.

SUPERIOR GENICULAR VESSELS

VASTUS MEDIALIS

ACCESSORY SAPHENOUS NERVE

SAPHENOUS NERVE

ADDUCTOR MAGNUS TENDON

Fig. 142

This figure shows nerves and vessels, some or all of which may pierce the distal part of the subsartorial fascia. These include superior genicular veins and artery, the saphenous nerve and its accessory, a twig communicating with the posterior branch of the obturator nerve.

The subsartorial fascia in this figure is *undisturbed* (compare Fig. 141, A and B).

BARRIERS OF MUSCLE, BONE, AND
MAIN FEMORAL TRUNK

Much of the 12 in. length of profunda vein and artery lies
" where the cluster of muscles in a man's thigh is thickest." That
is one of three facts which dominate the problem of complete
exposure. The second is that the profundæ, in their distal 5 in.
reach, are fastened near or actually stripe the medial lip of linea

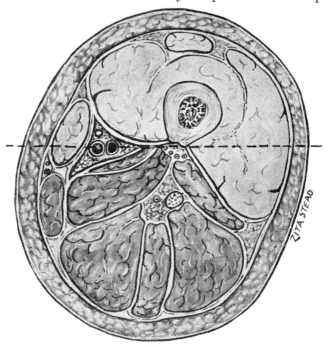

Fig. 143

Recumbent femurs are like stranded boats : the spread or *flare* of
the sides obstructs a frontal access to the keel (or linea aspera) and so
to the profunda vessels that stripe its length. (The broken line
shows the horizontal plane.)

aspera ; and linea, in the limbs of recumbent patients, is like a
keel from which the sides of femoral shaft bulge or slope up
towards the surgeon, exactly as the sides of boats are said to
flare (Fig. 143). The shaft then will overhang and mask the keel-
like linea, together with the satellite and distal 5 in. of profundæ.

Thus for *complete* exposure of the deep femorals, which course
in the front and back of thigh, a posture is required that will
relax muscles and will also turn the femur in such a way that *one*
position of the limb lets us open the thigh in front and on its
hinder face (p. 233).

The third fact—dominating proximal approach—is also exigent. Profunda artery frequently springs either from the back or from the outer side of the common femoral trunk—most often at some level between the two transverse planes that graze the upper and lower borders of the pubic symphysis. From the outer origin the vessel winds down in a loose half-spiral curve to lie behind the superficial femoral artery, parted from it by two veins, the femoral and its own deep companion. This anteroposterior arrangement of four large vessels (femoral artery, femoral vein, profunda femoris vein, profunda artery—in that order from before back, but often, too, with a slant from within out) calls for *oblique* approach to the deeper pair—a fact brought home to me by a ' slip of the knife,' not perhaps the sort that Kipling honoured as ' predestined,' but one which undeservedly was fortunate.

During a hasty cadaver demonstration of the femoral-shaft exposure (described on p. 197) I made an incision aimed, as I thought, at the lateral angle of patella. This, however, with the leg and foot, was covered by a cloth, and when deep fascia was divided I found I had reached the *wrong* side of rectus femoris— the medial instead of the lateral.[1]

I then discovered that the whole limb, owing to a fractured femoral neck, lay in the fullest possible eversion. My mistake was, of course, due—like so many at all stages of operative procedure— to losing touch with bony points. Happening, however, to move the rectus femoris outwards during a distasteful review of the field, I saw that I had obtained access to the upper 7 in. of the deep femoral vessels- an access which, because it was oblique, was excellent (Fig. 144).

The cloak of nerve branches.—Viewed, however, from the lateral side near Poupart's ligament a cloak of nerves, formed by the sudden terminal branching of the femoral trunk, screens the outer face of the great vessels, deep and superficial. But the cloak is easily displaced, for some of its constituents supply or are linked with the two mobile bellies of the front of thigh— sartorius and rectus. So when we draw these muscles outwards most of the cloak of nerves tends to move out with them and thus uncover the outer and, for us, strategic face of the main vessels in Scarpa's triangle.

[1] " Do you know," said d'Artagnan, " why master pastrycooks never work with their own hands ? "
" I wish you'd tell me," said Porthos.
" Well, the fact is they fear to scorch a tart or curdle cream in front of apprentice pupils : it might raise a laugh, and you mustn't laugh at master-cooks."

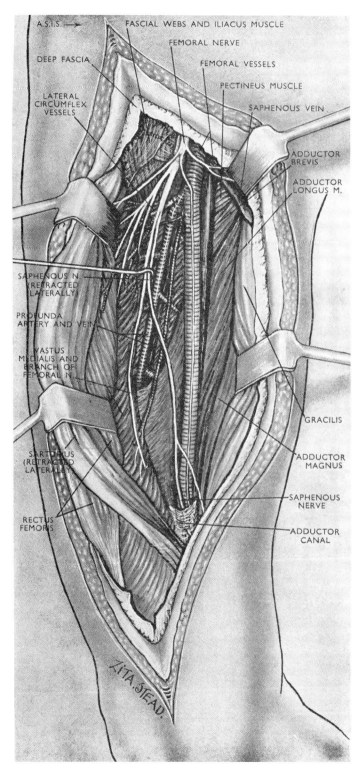

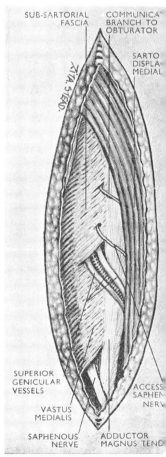

Fig. 144

The oblique lateral view of fe⋯ arteries

Because rectus femoris and sartori⋯ supplied by the femoral nerve, ou⋯ retraction of these two muscles⋯ that nerve trunk away from the a⋯ ing arteries and will thus educ⋯ pattern of the femoral nerve wh⋯ peculiar to the patient—a patterr⋯ prone to vary.

Only a scrap of the sheet of subsa⋯ fascia has been preserved. The⋯ shows *one* arrangement of the stru⋯ that may pierce the distal part ⋯ fascia. (It is this subsartorial shee⋯ is drawn round *behind* the vess⋯ retracting adductor magnus (p.⋯ Fig. 141, A and B) in a posterior fe⋯ popliteal approach.)

A check to this movement comes from one or sometimes two fine threads which slope inwards from the nerve cloak and cross or may embrace the femoral vessels. When these threads have been cut the major part of the cloak is free to move out with the two muscles : sartorius carries off the intermediate cutaneous branches and its own nerve supply ; rectus femoris also carries off its own supply and that of vastus lateralis. The branches to the other vasti muscles (intermedius and medialis) *already* lie lateral to the great vessels, while the saphenous nerve (and its accessory) make a lateral approach before actually reaching the front wall of the superficial femoral artery.

All these nerves, therefore, either (1) lie lateral to the vessels or (2) move away from the vessels when we retract the two mobile muscles, or (3) are, like saphenous, easily dissected off and drawn aside by separate retraction.

The accessory saphenous nerve.—This finds no place in standard British textbooks. It was first described by Cruveilhier (1791-1873), and is firmly established in French teaching : Poirier, Hovelacque, and Paturet treat of it in almost identical detail. The nerve would seem to share an origin from the intermediate and medial cutaneous nerves of British anatomy. An offset of the accessory saphenous may enter Hunter's canal to lie as a satellite nerve on the front of the femoral artery. This satellite may pierce the anteromedial wall of the canal at any level and reach medial skin above the knee ; it may also end at any level by fusing with the saphenous nerve.[1]

OTHER CONSIDERATIONS

After a course of about a handbreadth in ' Scarpa ' the profundæ leave the superficial femorals and pass behind adductor longus, lying between its belly and that of adductor brevis. Some 2 in. lower down the short adductor ends. Near this level, for some three fingerbreadths, the vessels lie and are bound in

---

[1] French anatomists describe the *femoral nerve* as dividing into four terminal parts : two deep parts—our own saphenous nerve and the trunk to quadriceps ; two superficial parts—the internal and external musculocutaneous nerves of the thigh, both of which supply sartorius and skin. The external of these two superficial nerves gives origin to the *accessory* saphenous. The satellite nerve to the femoral artery is sometimes equated in French illustrations—though not in the text—with the *whole* accessory saphenous (Hovelacque (1917), *Anatomie des nerfs*, Plate LXXX ; Paturet (1951), *Traité d'Anatomie*, vol. ii, Fig. 718) : it is, however, only one of the nerve's two branches ; the other branch is the satellite of the long saphenous *vein* and corresponds to part of our medial cutaneous nerve of the thigh.

satellite relation to nacreous bands of a medial aponeurosis that is part of vastus medialis. There, as they pass down the limb, the vessels veer slightly out to meet the inward slope of femoral shaft. This veering occurs about 9 in. above the upper face of the medial femoral condyle ; it is important and I shall return to it. Below this spot all three adductor attachments join to form a tough sheath that binds the last 5 in. of profundæ to or close to the back of linea aspera.

The three parts of profundæ.—For purposes, then, of surgical approach the average 12 in. length of profundæ may be divided into three parts : (1) a *proximal part* about 5 in. long, moored chiefly by its own offsets and lying first near the groove between psoas and pectineus, then in front of pectineus, then behind adductor longus, where it is briefly sandwiched by longus in front and brevis behind ; (2) a 2 in. *intermediate part* held at the ' 9 in. spot,' as though pasted on to the nacreous aponeurosis of medial vastus by a thin imperfectly translucent fascia ; (3) a 5 in. *distal* or *asperal part* surrounded and affixed to linea by dense insertions of adductor muscle.

Of this foot-long vein and artery about seven upper inches are accessible by an anterior approach passing medial to rectus femoris, while the lower 8 in. can be reached from behind. Thus it will be seen that roughly 3 in. (the fifth, sixth, and seventh, counting from above down) are found by using either route.

Discovery of the distal 5 in. of the deep vein and artery is simplified if we first find the intermediate portion of the vessels and use it as a guide to their asperal continuation.

' **The 9 in. spot.**'—The intermediate portion of profundæ lies at a spot about 9 in. (a *full* span) above the upper surface of the medial femoral condyle, and I keep the term ' 9 in. spot ' for convenience. T. P. Garry, however, has devised a manual way of marking it, more accurate by far than linear measurement. I shall describe his method with the technique of operation.

THE OPERATION

Postures.—A *supine position*, with the limb fully everted, serves for access to the proximal 7 in. of profundæ and at the same time to the whole length of the common and superficial femoral vessels, plus some 4 in. of popliteal trunks (p. 215). The *prone position* allows us to reach the distal 8 in. of profundæ together with (should need arise) the whole 7 in. of popliteal trunks, plus nine distal inches of superficial femorals, amounting thus to a length of some 16 in. of femoropopliteal vessels (p. 226).[1]

THE SPECIAL POSTURE FOR COMPLETE EXPOSURE OF PROFUNDÆ. —This posture is required for simultaneous access to the proximal and distal parts of the deep femorals ; as, for example, when a communicating aneurysm is thought to lie at the intermediate part of these 12 in. trunks, or where there is doubt as to whether superficial or deep femorals, or both, are involved. For though this doubt is most likely to arise in relation to proximal lesions, the four femoral vessels, superficial and deep, remain relatively close together for some distance below Scarpa's triangle where they neighbour the ' 9 in. spot.' Unless, then, we are completely confident of reaching a sufficient length of profundæ, either in front or from behind, the special posture for full access is indicated.

The patient lies on the *sound* side with the ' sound ' scapula flat on the table. Bend the ' sound ' hip and ' sound ' knee each to a right angle and make the lateral face of the sound limb touch the table. (This position of the sound limb gives exactly the right amount of rotation to the trunk.)

Then (*a*) *in a thin, long-limbed patient*, flex the knee and hip of the ' operation ' side each through 20 degrees, making the *medial face of the knee* lie flat on the table. No change of posture is required in the tall and thin when passing from the proximal to the distal approach.

(*b*) *In a stout or short-limbed patient*, put the *sound* limb as at first described ; but—in order to avoid the cramping of your access to ' Scarpa ' which might here result from flexion at the groin—keep the ' operation ' limb with knee and thigh extended and its foot in pure plantar flexion till you have completed the proximal exposure. *Then* flex the hip and knee of the operation side through 20 degrees, as in the thin and long-limbed, and lay the inner face of the knee on the table. (This slight move, if made gently, calls for no change of towels.)

INCISIONS

The anterior incision runs for a full span from a point two fingerbreadths medial to the anterior superior iliac spine towards the medial angle of the patella. Divide deep fascia and with it raise and displace inward the superficial inguinal glands when,

---

[1] It is, however, well, after exposing eight distal inches of the 12 in. profundæ, to check the natural urge to go still higher and reach the upper four : depth and gluteus maximus are hindrances, while the hip joint parts us from the two top inches.

as so often, they mass in front of the femoral trunks. Mobilise the medial edge of sartorius first, keeping a fingerbreadth medial to the muscle so as to avoid intermediate cutaneous nerves linked with the sheath. Then mobilise the medial edge of rectus femoris, taking care not to injure the very large lateral circumflex vessels that cross immediately deep to the muscle some three fingerbreadths below ' Poupart.'

The nerve cloak.—Look for any fine nerve threads sloping down medially across the main vessels. Divide the threads and retract sartorius and rectus laterally, thus removing the major part of the cloak of femoral-nerve branches from the outer face of the vascular trunks (pp. 229 and 231).

Find the more deeply running nerves (to vastus medialis and vastus intermedius) which lie just lateral to the superficial femoral vessels. Look for and detach the saphenous nerve or nerves that approach the artery from without before they come to lie along its anterior wall ; retract these deeper nerves laterally to expose the outer face of the superficial and deep femoral trunks. These tend to lose their sagittal arrangement in the lower part of Scarpa's triangle where the profundæ shift out towards the inward slope of the femur, so that of the four great vessels the profunda artery instead of lying farthest back is now most lateral.

The deep femoral vessels below ' Scarpa ' leave the superficial trunks and pass behind the long adductor where they can be followed for about three fingerbreadths after mobilising the upper edge of that muscle.

Some seven proximal inches of profundæ are now accessible.

The posterior incision at the level of the popliteal space should run behind the inner hamstrings and *then* pass up the midline of thigh. (The course of these long incisions must often vary on account of wound or scar resection, and provided they do not cut vertically through a flexor crease their actual line loses much importance in virtue of the access we can get by skin reflection.)

After dividing deep fascia, clear the field sufficiently to reach the back of adductor magnus : part the medial and lateral hamstrings, controlling several large isolable vessels that feed these muscles and intervene ; mobilise the sciatic nerve and displace it medially, working on its ' safe ' *outer* side, from which (as Grant points out) only one collateral branch springs—that to the short head of biceps.

Define the asperal edge of adductor magnus ; it lies beside and medial to this short head which reaches up as far as the gluteal fold. Two fingerbreadths below the fold define the spot that I have loosely termed '9 in.,' where profundæ are satellite to vastus medialis and veer obliquely out to stripe or closely link with linea aspera. This spot is marked as perfectly as vascular anatomy allows by means devised by Mr T. P. Garry, to which we can presently resort (Fig. 145).

Garry's marking.—The spot lies near the back of the inner side of femur at the intersection of two planes : (1) a sagittal plane in the midline of thigh, and (2) a transverse plane a handbreadth distal to the ridge that bounds the lower edge of great trochanter. The surgeon works from back to front along this intersection. (The *ridge* is plainly felt, through skin or towels, by moving the hand *up* the outer face of the femur. It lies three fingerbreadths below the top of great trochanter.)

The asperal edge of magnus.—While defining this edge and parting it from the short head of biceps we may note that the relaxed fleshy fibres of magnus bulge slightly in across linea and curve out again to reach their asperal insertion. In this way they overlap short, *longitudinal* segments of tendon that link them with bone. When the fleshy fibres are carefully detached and drawn outwards a translucent membrane appears, and if this is divided some three fingerbreadths above the opening in adductor magnus, the profundæ vessels in general appear, sandwiched between the membrane and the tough asperal aponeurosis of adductor longus. In some subjects no vessels are seen—a condition that may be unilateral, and this and other handicaps have led me to suggest the plan that follows :—

A. *We have explored ' Scarpa '* sufficiently far to find, isolate, and put a guiding loop round the segment of profundæ that is satellite to the nacreous vastus bands. Then we can work *down* from it by detaching the asperal edge of magnus.

B. *We have not explored ' Scarpa.'*—We shall then begin detachment of the asperal edge of magnus some three fingerbreadths above the magnus opening and look for profundæ where they lie on or close to linea, sandwiched between translucent membrane and the tough aponeurosis of longus. Then (1) we find the vessels and follow them ; or (2) we fail to find them, in which event we must expose the satellite segment from *behind*, and make it guide us downwards to the distal reach of profundæ. We therefore note the point where Garry's planes intersect, and there we separate the coarse fibres of magnus, which at this level is from one to two fingerbreadths thick. We come then *as a rule* on a thin areolar layer in which a leash of small vessels passes transversely outwards, arranged sometimes like a fan. These

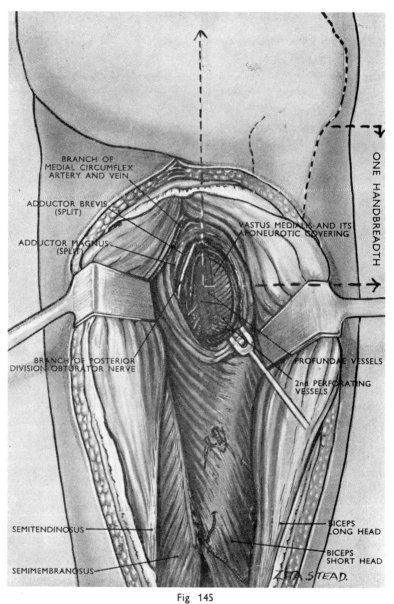

Fig 145

Garry's marking (see text) for finding the upper (satellite) reach of profunda vessels. The blue profunda vein is fastened to the nacreous aponeurosis of vastus medialis by a thin fascia through which both structures show faintly.

structures mark the plane of cleavage that parts adductor brevis from the front face of magnus. When, however, the brevis muscle has an exceptionally low (or high) attachment to linea, this station on our path may be absent. Usually the vascular leash must be cut and tied and we must split the $\frac{1}{4}$ in. thickness of the brevis belly, whose fibres at this level have exactly the same slant as those of magnus but are less coarse.

As soon as we have split completely through adductor brevis we reach a surface barred with sloping nacreous bands, through which the femur can be felt. The lustre of these bands is reduced by a thin fascial covering which fastens bands and profundæ in satellite relation at the ' 9 in. spot '—much as the visceral branches of internal iliac are pasted to the side walls of pelvis (p. 170). A careful division of the fascia covering the bands will therefore liberate this portion of profundæ and let the vein show blue against the nacreous background. The bands together form the aponeurotic covering of vastus medialis as it clothes the femur ; they have accordingly the slope of medial vastus fibres, contrasting sharply with adductor slope.[1]

It is a comfort to know that we can at any moment compress the distal portion of profunda vein and artery against bone ; but the hinder field is rich in anastomoses of muscle branches that link the perforating vessels.

COMPLETE COMBINED EXPOSURE OF MAIN THIGH VESSELS

The synthesis needs no elaboration. The reader will perceive that the posture described on page 233 for full access, back and front, to profundæ femoris (from Scarpa's triangle down, p. 235), when joined with the method of reaching the femoropopliteal vessels from behind (p. 223), allows—with *one* position of the patient—complete exposure of the whole 12 in. length of profundæ together with the twenty-odd inches of femoropopliteal trunks.

The ' journals-on-a-rod ' procedure.—For we can treat the two

---

[1] These nacreous bands arising from linea are an essential feature of the vastus medialis, their deep surface gives a needed extra hold to fleshy fibres that clothe—but do not spring from—the medial face of femoral shaft. Lower down the thigh the bands unite with adductor fibres and thus produce the medial intermuscular septum. (If the profundæ are drawn inwards at the ' 9 in. spot,' they reveal the beginning of this union in the shape of a slip of fibres from adductor longus coming down in *front* of the vessels and crossing the slope of the nacreous bands.)

Poirier gives the *medial intermuscular septum* a more robust constitution than it receives from most anatomists. He describes it (1) as formed essentially from the aponeurosis of origin of vastus medialis ; (2) as taking part in forming the lateral wall of Hunter's canal ; (3) as accompanying the tendon of adductor magnus to the medial (epi)condyle after joining with the aponeurotic insertions of adductor muscles.

Poirier's view appears just : the aponeurosis of the medial vastus sends a strong contribution to the investing fascia of the thigh.

adductor muscles, magnus and longus, like two journals that one sees in clubs and continental cafés, slung for convenience by an edge on the same rod or shaft. Through the posterior approach we reach them from behind. Then, if we curve a hand round the free edge of these linked adductor ' journals ' (Fig. 140), we can draw them both towards the shaft of femur and thereby gain posterior access to Hunter's canal (p. 225). Thus we can extend exposure from popliteal vessels to superficial femorals as far as ' Scarpa ' ; while, if we leave the back of magnus *flat* beside the femur, we can set free its fixed or asperal edge—working, of course, down the shaft into the stripping angle. When that is done gently and piecemeal, a little patience will reveal intact the 5 in. distal reach of the profunda vein and artery. For the rest, the exploitation of Garry's marking (Fig. 145) and of an *oblique* access to Scarpa's triangle (Fig. 144) completes both femoral exposures, the deep and superficial.

ACCESS TO PROFUNDÆ OFFSETS

Proximal portions of these offsets are seen when the main trunks are exposed. Remoter parts may require separate approach. (To simplify descriptions of direction I shall deal only with arteries, leaving the reader to supply companion but counterflowing veins.)

The medial circumflex artery.—This springs from the back of profunda some two or three fingerbreadths below ' Poupart ' and has a backward course of about a thumbwidth before leaving Scarpa's triangle, where it is often visible if we draw the femoral trunks *laterally* so as to uncover the deep groove between psoas and pectineus. This thumbwidth of artery enters the groove in a sagittal direction ; it cannot be traced beyond ' Scarpa ' without detaching or at least mobilising pectineus.

Leaving Scarpa's triangle the vessel lies beneath the femoral neck and there is stated to divide into (1) an *ascending* offset which goes behind the neck to meet the great trochanter, and (2) a so-called ' transverse ' portion which, in fact, *prolongs* the circumflex and feeds the hamstrings. (See Cunningham's clear diagram, Fig. 146.)

In my day Dublin students, ignoring the distinction between ' transverse branch ' and parent artery, employed six handy words to memorise the course of medial circumflex through intervals between three *pair* of muscles : " Parish-Priest Of-Bray

Queer-Man " stood helpfully for Psoas-Pectineus, Obturator-Brevis, Quadratus-Magnus—' Obturator ' being externus, ' Brevis ' and ' Magnus,' adductors. That six-word ' open sesame ' will guide us through these barriers. For first, in Scarpa's floor, lie ' Psoas-Pectineus ' ; and while psoas must remain inviolate, we can mobilise and if need be dislodge pectineus. Beginning therefore at the pubic tubercle, which marks the upper and medial end of the oblique cleavage line between pectineus and

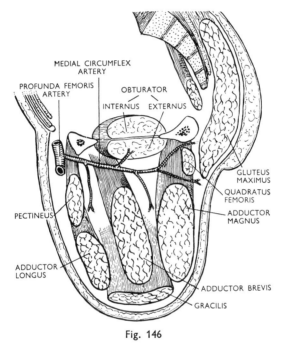

Fig. 146

The sagittal course of the medial circumflex artery
(after Cunningham).

adductor longus, part the two muscles cleanly for about four fingerbreadths. Mobilise the belly of pectineus, working from within out on its deep surface. It is then often possible to reach the artery after it has passed the upper and outer edge of the muscle. If the access is cramped, detach pectineus from its linear and J-shaped origin on pubic ramus. The muscle lifted and gently drawn out, serves both as buffer and retractor for the femorals (see also p. 174). A thumb along the ramus should continually guard the femoral veins when we detach the muscle. In front of pectineus lie minor vessels, which we shall cut and then retract along with it—the deep and superficial external pudendals whose veins discharge into the arch of great saphenous, which also lies in front of pectineus and slightly shares its outward shift.

Remoter lesions of medial circumflex—behind the ' Obturator-Brevis ' barrier—require a division of adductor brevis, the sectionable lower member of the pair. Lesions deeper still, such as those affecting the hindmost part of medial circumflex itself or ascending branches that pass from it (with no mnemonic) between quadratus femoris and obturator, such lesions will lie *behind* the ' Quadratus-Magnus ' plane and so be *subgluteal*. They are reached by hinging back the lid-like maximus (p. 180).

Incision for the medial circumflex vessels will as a rule prolong upwards the one already made to explore ' Scarpa ' ; it will thus cross in front of ' Poupart ' and extend a handbreadth up the belly. Deepen this abdominal handbreadth to reach (and leave intact) external oblique aponeurosis. This permits reflection inwards of the skin and lets us clear the field sufficiently to loop spermatic cord or round ligament from pubic tubercle and either mobilise pectineus or detach its origin.

The lateral circumflex artery (Fig. 198), which often springs from femorals instead of from profunda, goes laterally out of ' Scarpa ' sandwiched first between the sartorius and iliacus, then, farther out, between rectus femoris and vastus intermedius. The main need, therefore, with lesions close to ' Scarpa,' is to relax sartorius and rectus fully. If that is not achieved sufficiently for rectus by the posture used in the *complete* exposure of profundæ (p. 233), turn the patient on his back, straighten the knee, and prop the heel well off the table.

Lesions of lateral circumflex that lie some distance *out* from the profundæ will need the upper span of an incision used to reach the front of femur—the one beginning at the accurate bisection of the notch immediately beneath anterior superior iliac spine and aimed towards the outer angle of patella (p. 200). (The patient lies recumbent with the heel raised.) Tensor fasciæ is parted from sartorius, then rectus femoris from outer vastus. Most of the fan of lateral circumflex—the transverse and descending part—is then displayed. The third, ascending, portion of the fan lies covered by the distal free edge of a fascial web that shows, with others, just below the ' spine ' on parting rectus femoris from tensor (p. 209).

The perforating arteries—1, 2, 3, 4 (but they may number two or six).—No single route will fully expose their circuitous courses (Fig. 139). Short lengths of 1, and often 2, are visible by the anterior access to profundæ (Fig. 144), while proximal extremes (and nothing more) of 2 and 3 are seen from *behind* on separating great adductor heads—when that is feasible—and reaching parent trunks. But this route bares the whole of 4, except the outer terminals.

The outer terminals of 2, 3, 4.—During the exposure of the femur from in front we can see a proximal fingerbreadth of each terminal, where each lies framed within its arch of lateral septum against the keel of linea (Fig. 125). We get this view by looking level with the wound when we have split and liberated vastus intermedius and drawn *back* its outer half from bone. Beyond these single naked fingerbreadths the vessels vanish in the substance of the outer parts of vasti and form therein a set of ' ladder-rungs,' curved forward round the shaft of femur.

This ladder-rung *quartet* of terminals (if we include a common supplement from popliteal trunks) is reached by widening upwards the outer route to popliteal surface (p. 222). The hinder face of lateral intermuscular septum, already partly cleared from biceps, is further bared. If, then, the septum be bisected lengthwise, retraction of each severed edge displays the backs (though often fused) of outer portions of *two* vasti—below (as Poirier makes clear), the back of vastus *intermedius* ; above, of lateralis (Fig. 119). McBurney cleavage of the slanting grain reveals the ' rungs ' (Fig. 139).

REFLECTIONS ON RELATED POSTERIOR EXPOSURES IN THIGH AND LEG AND ON THE LEG IN GENERAL

An old approach of Guthrie's through the calf—a method which of late received new life and grace—gives origin to several exposures. In these we separate the heads of the gastroc-nemius, proceeding proximally for the thigh, distally for the leg. Attack on either part where it adjoins the other will of necessity involve the fellow segment ; for nerves and vessels hold so fast in each that if we limit our approach to leg or thigh we cannot mobilise the neurovascular ' bundle.' [1]

[1] '*Bundle*.'—We have already noted (p. 221) as a point of practical importance that popliteal nerves and vessels are divorced above the knee ; they therefore fail (above the knee) to constitute a veritable neurovascular bundle. The fact is obvious when we approach these structures from the *side* : the finger hooks up vessels only, for fascia segregates the nerves and binds their trunks as satellites to hamstrings (see the cross-sections, Figs. 136 and 138). That, we saw, is why the nerves elude our search in medial or lateral approach. But if we enter from the back and reach as deep as popliteal vessels, we must in doing so destroy the crucial sheet of thin, divorcing fascia ; and then—when that is gone—the mere proximity of nerve and vessels will let us hook them up collectively in what *appears* to be a bundle. (This note explains why ' bundle ' has inverted commas here, and on pp. 251 and 253.)

The 'bundle' dominates the popliteal space; control of it is vital, whether we wish to deal with its constituents or draw it sideways from our path.

The gastrocnemial heads.—First we must separate these heads which are surprisingly disposed; for though the widest part of

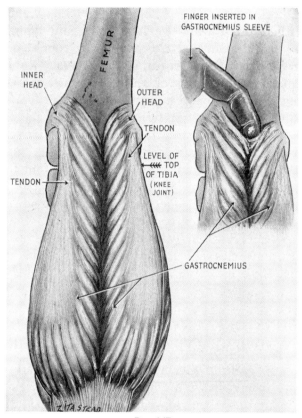

Fig. 147

Showing how the gastrocnemius V is formed *above* the level of the knee joint. A finger can define the V which marks the entrance to the half-sleeve covering the back of leg.

femur lies between their origins, they do not form, as that might lead one to expect, a long V pointing down the limb. Instead they meet before they leave the thigh and make a shallow midline V above the joint; and there, if other guides default, a finger may be hooked between the heads (Fig. 147).

The mesial guides.—The early union of the heads gives value to guides that help in parting them below; for swollen calves are soon deformed by posture, and midline structures shift. Two guides—a vein and nerve—will almost always set us right : they mark the groove between the bellies of the gastrocnemius—the seam to rip, Fig. 148. The vein (the blue guide) is the short saphenous ; it rests on fascia covering the groove. (A deep elastic layer of superficial fascia—the kind used recently in plastic work—invests

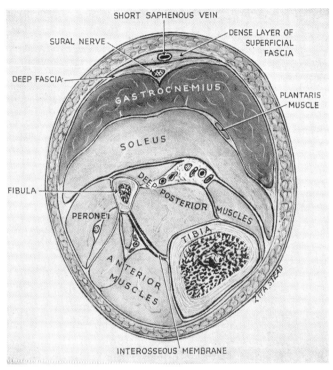

Fig. 148

Guides to the gastrocnemius seam

Note how the blue guide (short saphenous vein) is bridged by deep fibres of *superficial* fascia which bind it to the surface of deep fascia. (Sometimes the vein is deep to deep fascia.) The white guide (sural nerve) is regularly deep to deep fascia and *occupies* the groove between the gastrocnemial heads.

the upper reach of short saphenous vein. Preserving fluids rich in phenol sometimes make this layer simulate deep fascia ; the vein then seems to occupy a level deeper than they say it should—a thing it *really* does quite frequently. My thanks are due to the Dominions officers who put me wise to this.)

Another guide (the white) lies in the groove itself, and thus within the envelope of fascia. It is the sural or calf nerve which springs from the trunk, now called the medial popliteal ; more distally, near tendo Achillis it gets a strong communicating branch from common peroneal (now called lateral popliteal).[1]

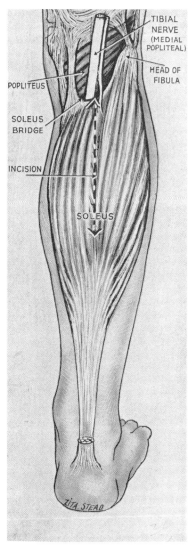

Fig. 149

The soleus bridge

The main vessels pass deep to it—between calf muscle and deep muscular group. Note where the large muscular nerve enters the edge of the bridge.

The half-sleeve and the striped seam.—The gastrocnemial heads unite to clothe the calf with a half-sleeve which we can lift with ease from underlying structure. The seam, we know, is doubly striped —in blue and white. Ripping the seam we find the popliteal bundle which goes from view beneath the slanting archway of a bridge formed between tibia and fibula by soleus belly (Fig. 149). The grain of soleus is chiefly longitudinal; so we can split the bridge and find the bundle deep to it. Nothing could be easier; the shade of Guthrie (with whom Larrey walked arm in arm through Cairo wards) might well rejoice. His method has survived the interlude when men, perhaps like Hunter's pupil, earned it the title "bloody," ranking the muscles "beefsteak number one"—and two and three.

The riddle of the bolster leg.—Indeed, this wide approach should have displaced by now the medial and cramped exposure in the calf, so indirect, so cherished by examiners,

[1] Rehearsal of these aliases is due to recent efforts aimed at making us *un*learn. We are to scrap, it seems, the painfully acquired (but excellent) "tibial" and "common peroneal" of the B.N.A.; so that, once more, internal (or medial) popliteal must change —invisibly—within a single segment of the limb and call itself posterior tibial, merely to suit the very questionable naming of an artery (see p. 246). "Tibial" plays no such tricks, and "peroneal" marks the striking early difference in course between its own deep branch and vessels *afterwards* related. Calling the other peroneal branch "the superficial," in place of musculocutaneous, prevents (I know) uncertainty regarding site—in arm, or leg—when looking through the journals.

Alice, again, in *this* peculiar nightmare, might compromise with popli-tibial, and popli-fibular.

so blind and therefore dangerous. For who knows what may lurk in swollen limbs from raid or accident? " A lucky-bag " was Ryall's word for the abdomen;[1] and, in respect of chance variety, the bloated calf becomes a kind of belly. The whole traumatic list of ' closed ' conditions must be long for I have seen the following myself : a fissured fracture causing bleeding from the arch of anterior tibial vessels, which formed a clot that blocked the crural circulation (see p. 272) ; a bruised arterial trunk with distal vasoconstriction ; aneurysm of the peroneal artery due to a broken shaft of fibula that wrenched away a *distant* branch ; the bursting of some forty varices (with no arterial injury) caused by the pressure of a wheel ; a gross œdema of each separate muscle (this in the upper limb) associated with constriction of main arteries to twine-like thinness. (The size and pulse of these diminished vessels were suddenly restored after a major slitting of fascial wrap and sheaths of muscle.)

A medley such as that in bolster limbs may wear a common mask of swelling and defective circulation, but any wholesale swaddling of these injuries in plaster—without the benefit of open exploration—will hold as grim an outlook as it would for sets of dubious ' acute ' abdomens.

Tracing the bundle down the calf, we saw, was simple ; to trace it midway up the back of thigh is simpler still. For hamstrings part behind the knee, and we prolong their separation. We shall exploit this facile cleavage in amputating through the thigh with aid of local block, reducing hæmorrhage as though we used a tourniquet ; which we shall not (p. 255).

A GLIMPSE OF LEG

Leaving the no-man's-land behind the knee let us revive a general acquaintance with the leg, not troubling greatly over detail.

The calf we have already seen ; the two great muscles, gastrocnemius and soleus, sandwich plantaris. We saw the neurovascular bundle pass beneath the bridge of soleus; there it assists in marking off the bunched mass of the calf from the flat length of *deep* posterior muscles. Let us observe the vessels first.

The main vascular bundle and its distal fork.—Once more we

---

[1] Sir Charles Ryall (1869-1922), remembered for his work on the danger of implanting cancer cells during operative interference, and better still for the affection in which he was held by his colleagues.

are the dupes of terminology. "There is," we learn, "a main popliteal trunk that ends at the distal edge of popliteus; there it divides into posterior and anterior tibial arteries." "Posterior tibial," we are told, "goes on a small way down and then gives off the peroneal branch"—a mere collateral, one might assume. We get no picture of the facts as seen by surgical approach.

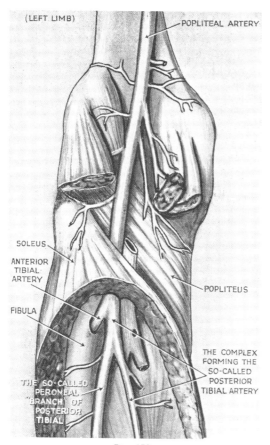

Fig. 150

The popliteal artery as currently depicted

(This is the only left-*limb* figure I have used. The drawing is after the relevant portion of Fig. 761, p. 794, Gray's *Anatomy*, 27th Edition, 1938; the indications have been modified.) A picture typical of many books, which rightly contradicts their texts: it shows conditions seen alike by artist and by surgeon—a main stem going down *beyond* its forward branch to end below by forking. (The texts end popliteal artery at anterior tibial and lump the rest of stem plus half the fork as 'posterior tibial,' having as 'branch' a vessel often larger than itself—the peroneal.) But artists, too, are fallible. The picture we have copied makes, like many others, anterior tibial come from the *side* of popliteal; in my experience (and Boyer's), it springs from the front—a point of surgical importance (pp. 272 and 273).

Looking afresh with those whose drawings contradict our texts (Fig. 150) we, too, shall see a stem—which is a 'main'—descending through the popliteal fossa, passing the popliteus muscle and going on some fingerbreadths to end by forking sharply *like a catapult*—with larger emphasis at times on one or other side. That forked arrangement must be frequent: apart from absence of posterior tibial vessels in a single leg there has been no exception in the last thirty cadavers I have seen. That, too, is what a master of anatomy, the Baron Boyer, saw and described in 1815 (Fig. 151).

"And what," you will ask, "has become of the *anterior* tibial artery?" Well, it is just a branch from the front of a main stem—a stem which Boyer calls the popliteal down to its tibioperoneal fork.[1]

We shall show presently how we can draw the proximal part of this anterior tibial branch right back into the calf and see exactly how it juts and curves (pp. 272 and 276).

But we are thinking too arterially ; the *veins* are large and thin-walled, sometimes varicose, outnumbering the branches of the

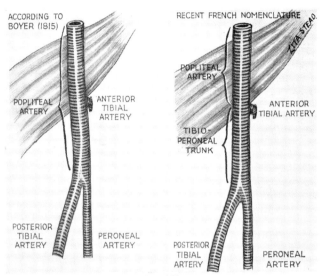

Fig. 151

Nomenclature which fits the distal forking of a main stem. (Note the term *tibioperoneal trunk*).

arteries by two to one. So veins bedevil intervention and complicate our much too simple picture of a place where vessels fork and arch—in triplicate.

The *distal portion of the bundle*, about the level where gastrocnemius and soleus join with tendo Achillis,[2] edges inwards from between the deep and superficial muscle layers, and is covered there by skin and fascia only (Fig. 152). Thence we can trace it up the leg, detaching as we go the slender mooring of soleus to the tibia, which may reach down within a handbreadth of the medial malleolus (p. 264 and p. 268).

[1] Since Boyer's day his countrymen, less simply though with clarity, make the popliteal end (as we do) at the anterior tibial branch, and then impose the name of *tibioperoneal trunk* on the last fingerbreadths of stem above the fork. We can, with those accounts, believe our eyes ; for each describes (as we do not) a major stem that goes *beyond* a forward branch and ends below by forking (Fig. 151).

[2] *Tendo Achillis*, changed in B.N.A. to *tendo calcaneus*.—This kind of make-believe at growing up is charmingly discouraged in pages cardinal to scientific outlook. " *La gentillesse des fables*," wrote Descartes, " *réveille l'esprit* " : their pleasant touch, he found, could stir the mind. (*Discours de la Méthode*, Part I.)

Leaving aside for later study the lateral peronei and the popliteus, turn for a moment to the tibial shaft.

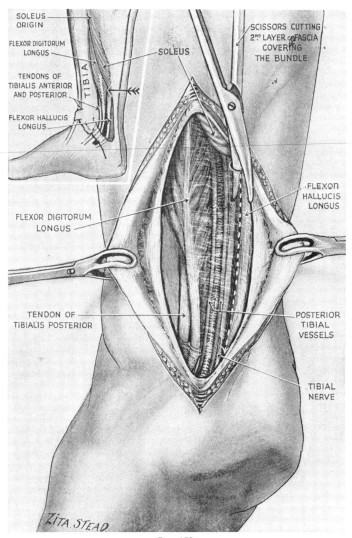

SOLEUS ORIGIN

FLEXOR DIGITORUM LONGUS

TENDONS OF TIBIALIS ANTERIOR AND POSTERIOR

FLEXOR HALLUCIS LONGUS

SOLEUS

TIBIA

SCISSORS CUTTING 2ND LAYER of FASCIA COVERING THE BUNDLE

FLEXOR DIGITORUM LONGUS

FLEXOR HALLUCIS LONGUS

TENDON OF TIBIALIS POSTERIOR

POSTERIOR TIBIAL VESSELS

TIBIAL NERVE

ZITA STEAD

Fig. 152

The distal part of the posterior bundle in the leg

It is covered here by skin and by *two* layers of deep fascia. The inset shows how tibial fibres of soleus cross and interrupt the plane of cleavage between calf and deep muscles—the plane in which the bundle lies. The deeper fascial layer and these soleus fibres serve to moor tendo Achillis more firmly on the *tibial* side (pp. 268 and 269). The arrow of the inset points to where the bundle leaves the shelter of the calf.

Anterior and deep posterior leg muscles (Figs. 153 and 154).— The subcutaneous surface of the tibial shaft separates a belly of

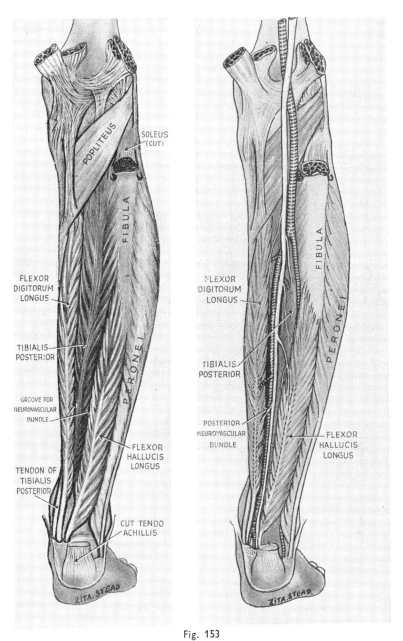

Fig. 153

The deep posterior leg muscles

Note how they form a groove for the posterior neurovascular bundle.

the deep posterior group behind from a belly in front; of these the anterior only is called tibialis; the belly behind is the long flexor of the toes.

The tibialis posterior springs from both bones of the leg; it is the deepest belly in the posterior compartment. Its *tendon*, however, comes to the surface by passing inwards, deep to the tendon of the long flexor—a relation of crossed fingers. In the distal third,

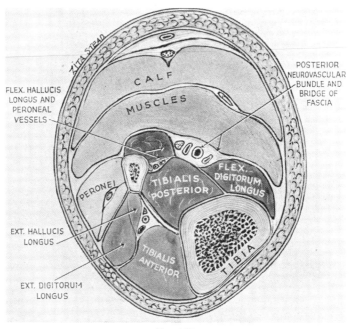

Fig. 154

The relations of deep posterior leg muscles with the anterior group

Note here, too, the groove for the posterior neurovascular bundle. A bridge of fascia makes the bundle a satellite of the deep group. Note how the subcutaneous face of tibial shaft separates the *belly* of tibialis anterior from the *belly* of flexor digitorum longus. (The inset to Fig. 152 shows how the face of tibial malleolus separates *tendons* of tibialis anterior and posterior.) Extensor hallucis longus is the only *deep* muscle of the anterior compartment.

therefore, the superficial face of tibia does actually separate two structures known as tibial—the tendons, *not* the bellies, of tibialis anterior and posterior (Fig. 152, inset).

The other muscle of the deep posterior group, flexor hallucis longus, springs (like extensor hallucis in front) from the middle two-fourths of the fibula—the 'middle half,' if you reduce the fraction. The bellies of this flexor and the flexor of the toes encroach sufficiently upon the hinder face of tibialis posterior to form a gutter for the neurovascular bundle—a gutter bridged by thin, translucent fascia which grows thick distally where it escapes the shelter of the calf (Figs. 154 and 152).

Turning now to the *anterior compartment* we find two main superficial muscles, and later we shall look between them for the neurovascular bundle (p. 276). These muscles are (1) the tibialis anterior (whose belly *and* whose tendon flank the subcutaneous face of tibia), and (2) extensor digitorum longus (coming mainly from the fibula). The off-shoot muscle, peroneus tertius—a badge (not always present) which marks us from the apes—springs with extensor longus. The one deep muscle of the anterior compartment, extensor hallucis, arises from the ' middle half ' of fibula. Going obliquely (as it must to reach the inner toe), its belly overlaps the neurovascular bundle and sets a trap (p. 278).

This general and bare account (by furnishing a sort of common back-cloth) will stage in turn exposures in the limb and let us focus on the detail.

THE MIDLINE POPLITEAL APPROACH

For this we need add little to the general reflections on p. 241. Here, too, as in exposure from the outer or inner side, we have to mobilise and then displace the intervening ' bundle.' But working this time from the back there is (in contrast with a side approach) no " open sesame " ; the place itself will not revolve and let us in. So we must take it squarely, by direct assault (cf. p. 212).

Incision.—Find first the level of the joint—a fingerbreadth above the head of fibula (Fig. 155). Incise in what you *think* the middle line—a guess which (owing to swelling and decubitus) is often wrong. Cut through skin and fat a handbreadth distal to the joint. Bring the knife sideways just below the crease behind the knee ; then upwards for a span, as shown in the inset.

The seam.—Look for the short saphenous vein (the blue guide to the middle line). It lies, remember, deep to fat, along the groove between the heads of gastrocnemius, most often on the surface of deep fascia (but sometimes underneath). If it does not appear at once, reflect a little skin at either edge. The final proof of mesiality, the sural nerve, is constantly subfascial : it occupies the groove (Fig. 156). Open deep fascia behind the calf to look for it, and not

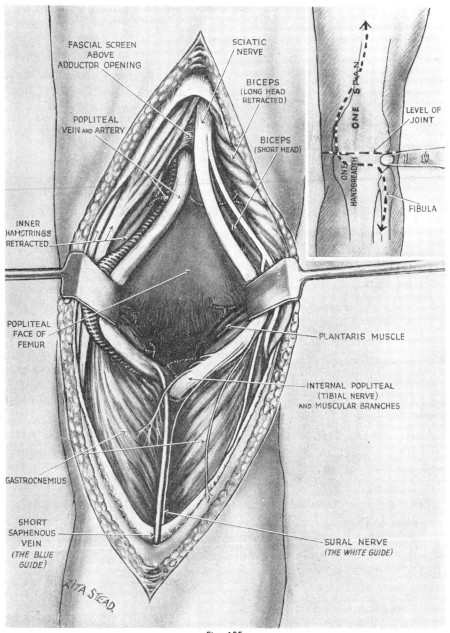

Fig. 155

Midline popliteal approach. (The figure gives a cramped and strained impression. It has been used designedly to show that freedom of the bundle and consequent exposure of the bone will only be secured when we have ripped the gastrocnemius seam.)

The long incision lets us mobilise the nerve and vessels : we either draw them bodily aside or part them (as above), moving the vessels towards the point of their fixation in adductor opening.

behind the knee joint, for there a greater trunk (medial popliteal nerve, or tibial of **B.N.A.**) lies close beneath investing fascia, and may be ripped in face of extra tension—like cortex under dura. When we have split the seam in gastrocnemius this popliteal trunk becomes a guide to separate the inner from the outer hamstrings ;

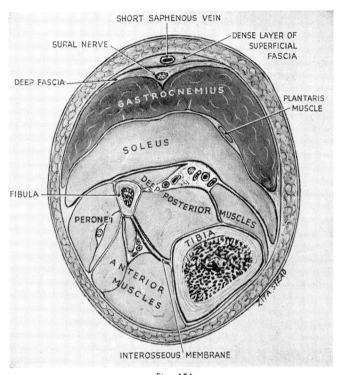

Fig. 156

Guides to the gastrocnemius seam

Note how the blue guide (short saphenous vein) is bridged by deep fibres of *superficial* fascia which bind it to the surface of deep fascia. (Sometimes the vein is deep to deep fascia.) The white guide (sural nerve) is regularly deep to deep fascia and *occupies* the groove between the gastrocnemial heads.

a finger helped a little with the knife dissolves their slight cohesion.

The ' bundle.'—Retraction of these sundered bellies in the calf and thigh reveals, beneath the inner popliteal (tibial) nerve, the close-knit popliteal vein and artery—the last impediment before we reach the bone. Then—if the finger finds it easy to displace—the ' bundle ' goes *en masse* to either side ; but, if it loosens grudgingly, we humour its constituents and pass between, moving the nerve towards its outer popliteal fellow, the vessels inwards—to the side where they are fixed in the adductor opening. The popliteal plane at once becomes accessible (Fig. 155, noting the *legend*).

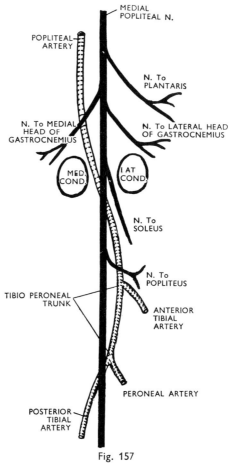

Fig. 157

The 'safe' inner side of the medial popliteal nerve (after Grant)

The popliteal artery curves away briefly towards fibula—as if drawn there by major branches. The *vein* (not shown here) parts nerve from artery throughout the fossa.

Bending the knee will loosen everything behind the joint and let the bone approach the surface. But relaxation sets peculiar traps, and semitendinosus may drift limply to the middle of the wound and there be claimed as great sciatic.[1]

---

[1] I saw this seemingly absurd mistake made twice, by reasonable men—a sign perhaps of decent equilibrium ; for those who let us know they are infallible in any field are either lunatics, "economists of truth," or in the even larger class one thinks of as 'unfortunate,' which lacks both virtue and the chance to fall.

EXTENSION OF THE MIDLINE ROUTE.—The distal part of this exposure lets us move the nerve and vessels far enough aside to cut through popliteus and expose the hinder, 'popliteal' face of tibia *without* dividing the soleus bridge (cf. p. 261 and footnote).

The next few pages show that we can use the mesial approach (combined with simple lateral posture) in the most frequent amputation of the thigh—that through the distal half.

A POSTURE FOR THIGH AMPUTATION WITH NO TOURNIQUET USING PROCAINE [1]

Custom has reconciled us to the supine posture for those who need this amputation. With that disposal limbs are slung from raised supports; or else a nurse must bear their weight. In either case we work at levels awkward for injecting nerves if

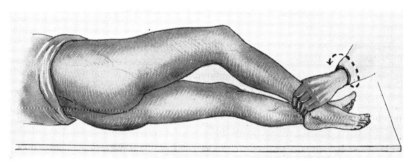

Fig. 158

The flexed limb pivots on the heel, which rests on the table. The nurse holds the leg and rotates it to present the front and sides of the patient's thigh to the surgeon without lifting the limb.

spinal block is inadvisable.[2] These troubles vanish when we place the patient on his healthy side; then, if the damaged limb will flex, the nurse need never lift the foot, but only grasp the leg and keep the heel—as *pivot*—on the table (Fig. 158). She thus presents

---

[1] *The Lancet*, 1940, **1**, 736.

[2] Procaine nerve-block, used alone or in company with gas-oxygen or minimal amounts of ether, was strikingly employed by Lotfy Abdelsamie, F.R.C.S., in my surgical unit at Kasr el Aini Hospital, Cairo, during work that much reduced mortality from crush. Abdelsamie's valuable paper should have new currency in time of war. (*The Lancet*, 1936, **1**, 187.)

each aspect of the patient's thigh : the sides in turn are brought to face the surgeon ; while to expose the back she lets the knee fall gently down across its fellow (Fig. 159). So, after infiltrating areas of flap or cuff, and *all* the operative field—most thoroughly—with procaine ($\frac{1}{2}$ per cent.), we can in comfort see and block the great sciatic trunk. While that is growing numb we shall ligate main vessels and thus avoid the use of tourniquets.

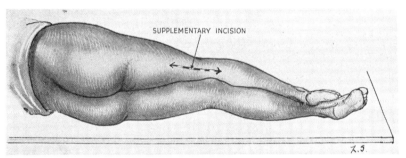

Fig. 159

The knee falling across its sound fellow gives access to the back of thigh. A long midline incision exposes the sciatic nerve for high injection and the main vessels for ligature.

The supplementary incision.—For this twin purpose make a *mesial* cut—first outlined by a weal—through popliteal skin one handbreadth distal to the joint and going upward to a spot three fingerbreadths above the site proposed for bone division (Fig. 159). We find the mesial guides (p. 242) and separate the boundaries of the popliteal space ; then we can trace the tibial or inner popliteal nerve up to sciatic trunk, which we inject with 15 c.cm. of a 2 per cent. solution of procaine—first in the sheath, then in the total thickness of the trunk.

Ligation from behind of femoral vein and artery.—The blocking of the nerve affords an interval in which to tie the two main vessels. These run, of course, at deeper levels—near the bone. And though the artery and vein do not officially become the popliteal till they have passed the opening in adductor magnus, yet, as they near the opening, only a trifling web of tissue screens them from the posterior compartment. So, if we trace the vessels *from below* (where we can hook them blindly off the femur),[1] it is extremely simple to disrupt the web and tie them well above the level for dividing bone (Fig. 159). We then proceed according to our training or experience : incisions, joining with the mesial cut

[1] A stress on " from below " is justified : the *fevered* searches that one sees begin high up where vein and artery are hard to find.

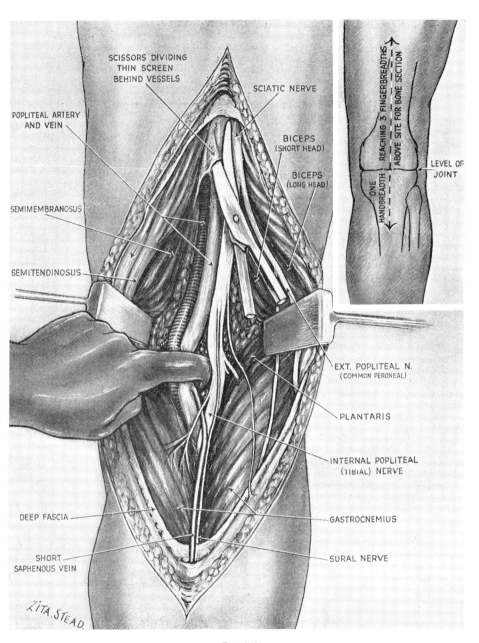

Fig. 160

The long midline incision and its use in thigh amputation under procaine

A finger introduced at the medial edge of the tibial (internal popliteal) nerve *behind the knee* hooks the main vessels up from the femur. Trace them proximally and tie them *above* adductor opening after dividing the thin fascia which screens them from behind. (The midline incision here is permissible since the knee joint will be removed.)

behind, run distally and forwards ; the flaps are made and muscles severed.

During these activities, however, the great sciatic trunk will rest in peace—until the time comes to remove the limb. With procaine infiltration not less than twenty minutes must elapse between injecting and dividing this capacious conduit of shock impulse. And that, indeed, is little time enough. Let us recall and profit by two clear and striking facts : our own distress when dentists shorten by a jot the dozen minutes *they* allow for nerves far smaller than the huge sciatic ; the sudden fading of the patient's pulse when stimuli get through a partial procaine block, unsupplemented by another anæsthetic.

The method used in the attempt to burke the later growth of axones will have prescribed already the length of nerve we first injected. I do not dare to say which method is the best, for no one knows ; but each will place the procaine to suit his own belief. It is at least important, once the limb is off, not to pull out the severed nerve and cut it short at levels unprotected by the procaine ; though I have seen this done.

We have to deal as well with the *saphenous nerve*. The guide to it—a whitish raphe on the medial side of thigh, found on displacing the sartorius—denotes the tendon of adductor magnus ; a nick with Mayo scissors made immediately in front of this will open the canal which holds the nerve. Then trace it up the thigh, inject it at the same level as sciatic, and divide it when the same long interval has lapsed.

I can confirm Abdelsamie's finding : " Amputation under *full* novocaine analgesia is a benign measure that does not shock the patient."

STUMP SEPSIS AFTER AMPUTATION FOR DISTAL INFECTION

I have seen many thigh amputations performed for this reason with careful technique after scrupulous preparation, but I have also seen, and had myself, too many septic results—perhaps because bacteria from distal foci were travelling up lymphatics during the operation, out of range of chemicals applied only to skin. In my experience sepsis came whether rubber drains were left a long or short time : if long left they seemed to determine infection ; but dangerous pooling of exudate ensued upon early removal. This pooling is prevented by placing ribbon gauze, heavily coated with dilute bipp, as a slender pack under each layer at the time of suture—for example, between bone and fascia (or muscle), and between fascia and skin. The bipped ends of the ribbons protrude as drains, and the pack is so well lubricated that it can be removed painlessly after forty-eight hours. A dry wound is left which will at once be covered with a *thickly* bipped dressing. These drains do not carry in sepsis from without, as rubber may; and certainly, too, the bipp can check bacterial growth.[1]

A relevant example of its use in another field interested some of my co-workers in this country. The large cavity left by removing a mandibular osteoclastoma was packed with bipped ribbon after thorough treatment of the wall with the high-frequency current. The cavity (lined now with dead tissue) communicated not only with the surface of the neck but also with the mouth, and the patient ate and drank as usual from the day following operation. When we removed the pack for the first time at the end of a fortnight we found a lining of clean red granulations. The pack—except on its oral surface, where saliva had washed out some of the bipp—was unaltered and fresh like the cavity.

I have no experience of the original bipp, which might be toxic in this quantity, having never used any but the dilute variety, whose value I learnt from Stoney during World War I; nor have I met with any other preparation which could so triumph in the test just described.

---

[1] The ingredients of dilute bipp are :—

Bismuth carbonate	. . 1 part	Hard paraffin .	. . .	2 parts
Iodoform powder .	. . 2 parts	Soft paraffin .	. . .	12 parts

Its preparation requires careful attention to details, of which R. Atkinson Stoney, of Dublin, has sent me the following note :—

Put the iodoform and bismuth in a large mortar and mix well. Melt the hard and soft paraffin together on a water bath ; stir well and cool slowly, stirring all the time. Take a little of the mixture of hard and soft paraffin and rub it up with the mixture of iodoform and bismuth till a smooth paste forms. Add the rest of the paraffin little by little to make a uniform ointment. The bipp should have the consistence of firm butter and should *not* be greasy. In very hot weather increase the quantity of hard paraffin and reduce the soft. (In wards the bipp is best kept in separate containers for individual patients.)

With this, I must confess, one does not quite recapture the lipstick qualities conferred on dilute bipp by pharmacists in France. But I have left the note—like that of p. 12 concerning compound fracture. For recent drugs are not the first, by many years, to start a habit of obtaining excellent results from wounds, however grossly soiled—which still, I see, claim victims.

EXPOSURE OF VESSELS AND NERVE IN THE BACK OF CALF

Incision.—Find first the level of the knee joint, a fingerbreadth

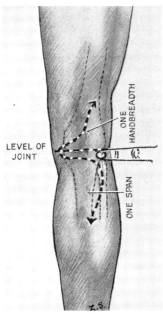

Fig. 161
Incision for midline calf exposure
Note the level of knee joint viewed from behind : it lies one fingerbreadth above fibula.

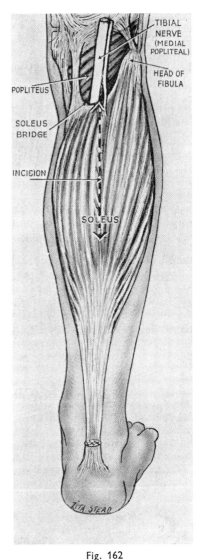

Fig. 162
The soleus bridge
The main vessels pass deep to it—between calf muscle and deep muscular group. Note where the large muscular nerve enters the edge of the bridge.

above the top of fibula. A *mesial* incision measured from this plane, runs for a hand-breadth up the thigh, a span along the calf (Fig. 161). The rest we know : the half-sleeve of the gastrocnemius, striped on its seam in blue and white, and surgically ripped to show the soleus bridge ; the lengthwise splitting of the bridge ; the underlying venous and arterial ' catapult ' (pp. 246 and 247).

The bridge-mouth of soleus.—The tibial nerve which runs behind this catapult of vessels ' bisects ' their tibioperoneal fork, but first supplies the bridge-mouth of soleus with a sturdy twig—most easily divided (Fig. 162). And so—before you split the bridge—define this entrance gently with a finger beside the disappearing vessels. (See that the foot is plantar flexed, and bend the knee to make the wound both lax and shallow.)

EXPOSURE OF THE 'POPLITEAL' FACE OF TIBIA.—This follows the exposure of the nerve and vessels whose bundles we can now displace to reach our first objective—the fan-shaped popliteus.[1]

A useful vertical extrinsic band.—The sheath that cloaks the popliteus is strengthened at its widest, medial, part by constant fibres which belong to semimembranosus (Fig. 163); these cross and stick upon the fanlike grain—a grain that yields when split a glimpse of concave bone through thick and grudging muscle. So for a better view, transect the popliteus. The knife should reach the tibia by cutting lengthwise down the band. A liberating cut is also made, respectively, along the upper and the lower margin of the popliteus. Both liberating cuts should finish *medial* to the middle line; they thus avoid the nerve to popliteus, which lies behind the muscle and ends by curving round its lower border. The upper cut should also miss the

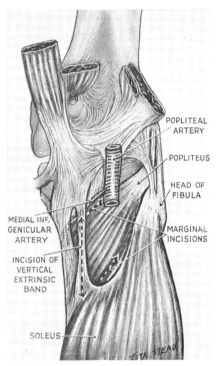

Fig. 163

The vertical extrinsic band

The knife transects the grain of popliteus by cutting lengthwise down the band. Liberating cuts are made along the margins of the muscle, sparing genicular vessels above. Retraction of the muscle towards fibula will expose the concave face of tibia. Repair by suturing *across* the band whose fibres stop the creep of sutures.

vessels (inferior medial genicular) which slope along the upper edge and are attached to it by the extrinsic band of fibres (Boyer). So, with its nerve intact, we mobilise the popliteus, raising it from bone towards the *fibula*. Then there is room to deal with our objective.

---

[1] The distal portion of the midline popliteal route (p. 251), which lets us mobilise the barrier of nerve and vessels, will also let us reach this hinder part of tibia—*without* dividing the soleus.

We make a sound repair by suturing the popliteus at right angles to the length of the extrinsic fibres ; for since they cross the fan they stop the sutures creeping through its grain.

EXPOSURE OF THE POSTERIOR NEUROVASCULAR BUNDLE IN THE LOWER PART OF THE CALF AND BELOW

Lesion of nerve and vessels half-way down the leg (or farther) is dealt with through a medial and *long* incision. The distal mark

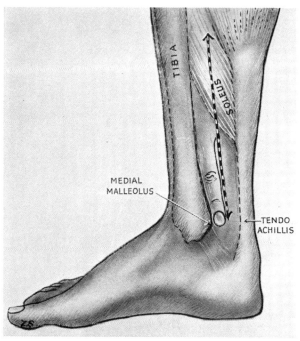

Fig. 164

Incision for the posterior neurovascular bundle of leg (distal half)

The finger with one edge pressed against the back of tibial malleolus marks with its other edge the distal end of the *artery*. Above, the knife avoids saphenous nerve and vein by cutting two fingerbreadths behind tibia. Note how fibres of soleus spring from tibia and cross the plane of cleavage that lies between calf muscles and the deep group.

for this should overlie the bundle. But where—exactly—is the mark ? Many books to-day agree in placing it " midway between the medial malleolus and the tendo calcaneus " :—a reasonable site, unfortunately countered on a previous page of one respected work, which makes the posterior tibial artery end " midway between the tip of the medial malleolus and the most prominent

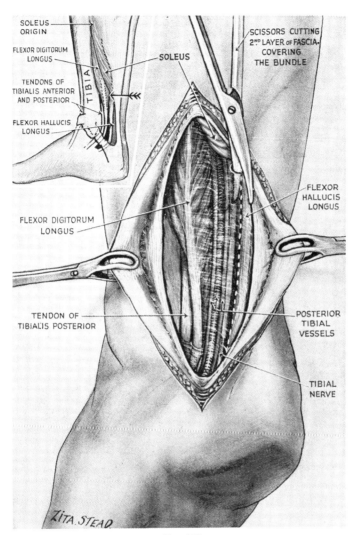

SOLEUS ORIGIN

FLEXOR DIGITORUM LONGUS

TENDONS OF TIBIALIS ANTERIOR AND POSTERIOR

TIBIA

FLEXOR HALLUCIS LONGUS

SOLEUS

SCISSORS CUTTING 2ND LAYER OF FASCIA COVERING THE BUNDLE

FLEXOR HALLUCIS LONGUS

FLEXOR DIGITORUM LONGUS

TENDON OF TIBIALIS POSTERIOR

POSTERIOR TIBIAL VESSELS

TIBIAL NERVE

ZITA STEAD

Fig. 165

The distal part of the posterior tibial bundle

Note the thick *second* layer of deep fascia covering the bundle. Above, it thins out to part deep muscles from calf. Divide it *beside* the bundle. To follow the bundle *up*, detach the tibial origin of soleus (inset). The arrow points to where the bundle leaves the shelter of the calf. If you must also reach the level of the 'catapult' extend the exposure by the wide medial access (p. 265). (For plantar continuation see p. 300.)

part of the heel." This ancient piece of imprecision (by contrast with its clear-cut fellow) haunts, I find, the memory of surgeons, and echoes widely in alternatives : " the medial tubercle of the calcaneus "; " the centre of the convexity of the heel "—uncertain places, deep to thickened skin, that serve to misdirect incisions and guide them too far back.

Let us forget this careless talk. The vessels lie a fingerbreadth behind the medial malleolus. Try on yourself. Press one edge of a finger down along the *back* of malleolus ; the other edge controls the tibial pulse. The finger therefore marks the *end* of an incision whose purpose is to amplify a plane of cleavage and thus is long enough to show the vessels without exactly following their course (Fig. 164).

Incision.— This will divide skin only. Measure a span extending from a fingerbreadth behind the medial malleolus to reach a point above, two fingerbreadths posterior to tibia—avoiding thus the long saphenous vein and the companion nerve which lies just deep to it (Hovelacque). Open the surface sleeve of fascia and then a *deeper* sheet which binds the bundle to the deeper group of muscles. This second fascial layer while it lies beside Achilles tendon is strong, opaque and tense, but passing under shelter of the calf it there becomes a thin translucent pellicle. Begin dividing it above, for down below the vessels may be slit as they approach the line of skin incision (Fig. 165). To trace it farther upwards use the plane of Fiolle and Delmas in front of the Achilles tendon—a solid strap that lets us lift the calf away from deeper muscles which hold the bundle in a satellite relation (pp. 250 and 251).

Nothing is perfect : the facile cleavage plane (which, in itself, might symbolise an influence of France on surgical technique) is crossed above by fibres of soleus. Detachment of these lower fleshy fibres allows, as I had previously described, a further view of nerve and vessels ; but with such limited detachment a second means of access—through the middle line—was needed to expose the region of the ' catapult ' (pp. 241-247). Complete detachment of soleus from the tibia extends and simplifies exposure.

WIDE MEDIAL EXPOSURE BY THE COMPLETE
DETACHMENT OF SOLEUS FROM TIBIA

Wounds of the calf must frequently claim use for midline access ; but while the twofold character of gastrocnemius favours surgical approach, *veins* [1] in the belly of soleus may prove troublesome at operation.

Thus half a dozen large veins are likely to be cut in any central splitting of soleus belly ; and, aside from special indications, this induces a return to medial approach—one, however, widely different from the old and often futile exercise of groping through a medial slit, compared with which the midline route, however bloody, gives what Binnie called a " soul-satisfying view."

The present method rests on the two piers of the arch by which soleus bridges the main neurovascular bundle. Each pier of the arch has a linear attachment, one to tibia, one to fibula. The longer tibial attachment has two *continuous* parts : the upper, oblique part rises from short stiff fibres that help to fashion the rough soleal line ; the lower, longitudinal part of the attachment descends immediately behind the inner edge of tibia, but, being *fleshy* and not fibrous, fails to mark the back of the bone (Fig. 166).

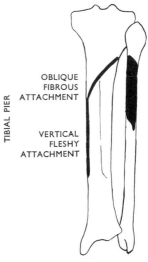

Fig. 166

The attachment of the piers of the soleal arch, tibial and peroneal

The tibial pier arises in two continuous segments—an upper oblique and fibrous, attached to the rough soleal line ; a lower and vertical fleshy segment which does not mark the back of tibia.

If we detach both these continuous linear origins from tibia (Figs. 167 and 168), then, by virtue of the plane of cleavage that parts soleus from the deeper muscles, we can rotate soleus (and

---

[1] These veins are apt to thrombose early in a long decubitus and form potential launching sites for emboli. Later, if the blocked veins should become recanalised and thenceforth valveless, the pumping action of soleus will drive blood *down* towards their union with the triple set of veins—so often rediscovered and forgotten—that normally should drain the favourite site of varicose ulcer into the deep, posterior tibial veins. The soleus pump, disposing now of an excessive downflow, will force the valves belonging to this triple set of veins, making the venous blood reach skin instead of draining from it. So, with the stress of venous irrigation, and by seepage, the healthy but predestined site for ulcer becomes an ill-drained, ill-fed, pigmented swamp. (See F. B. Cockett and Elgan Jones, *Lancet*, 1953, **1**, 17.)

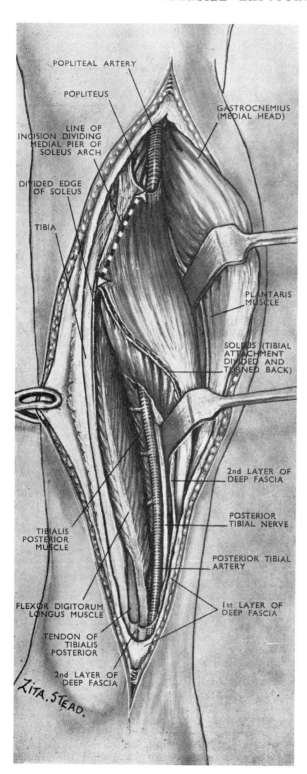

POPLITEAL ARTERY

POPLITEUS

GASTROCNEMIUS
(MEDIAL HEAD)

LINE OF
INCISION DIVIDING
MEDIAL PIER OF
SOLEUS ARCH

DIVIDED EDGE
OF SOLEUS

TIBIA

PLANTARIS
MUSCLE

SOLEUS (TIBIAL
ATTACHMENT
DIVIDED AND
TURNED BACK)

2nd LAYER OF
DEEP FASCIA

POSTERIOR
TIBIAL NERVE

TIBIALIS
POSTERIOR
MUSCLE

POSTERIOR TIBIAL
ARTERY

FLEXOR DIGITORUM
LONGUS MUSCLE

1st LAYER OF
DEEP FASCIA

TENDON OF
TIBIALIS
POSTERIOR

2nd LAYER OF
DEEP FASCIA

ZITA. STEAD.

Fig. 167

The posterior tibial neuro-vascular bundle ; a medial extension of its distal exposure

Stage I.—After separating the thin, longitudinal attachment of soleus from the medial edge of tibia, continue to detach the muscle from the soleal line. This *oblique* attachment forms the medial pier of the soleus arch in front of which the popliteal vessels and medial popliteal vessels and medial popliteal nerve change their names and pass down the leg.

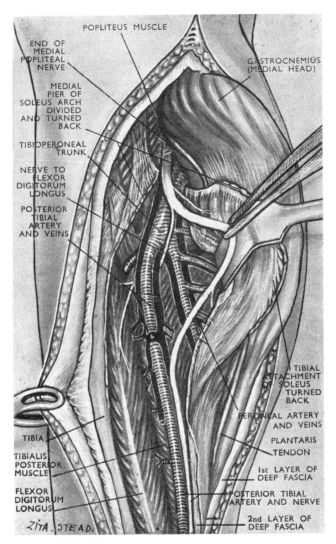

POPLITEUS MUSCLE

END OF
MEDIAL
POPLITEAL
NERVE

GASTROCNEMIUS
(MEDIAL HEAD)

MEDIAL
PIER OF
SOLEUS ARCH
DIVIDED
AND TURNED
BACK

TIBIOPERONEAL
TRUNK

NERVE TO
FLEXOR
DIGITORUM
LONGUS

POSTERIOR
TIBIAL
ARTERY
AND VEINS

TIBIAL
ATTACHMENT
OF SOLEUS
TURNED
BACK

PERONEAL ARTERY
AND VEINS

PLANTARIS
TENDON

TIBIA

1st LAYER OF
DEEP FASCIA

TIBIALIS
POSTERIOR
MUSCLE

FLEXOR
DIGITORUM
LONGUS

POSTERIOR TIBIAL
ARTERY AND NERVE

2nd LAYER OF
DEEP FASCIA

ZITA. STEAD.

Fig. 168

**The posterior tibial neurovascular bundle ; a medial
extension of its distal exposure**

Stage II.—Now—with its tibial attachment cut—we can turn soleus
back and out through two right angles. This will expose all the main
neurovascular structures of the leg: the distal end of the medial
popliteal nerve and its posterior tibial continuation, the tibioperoneal
trunk (p. 247), the posterior tibial and peroneal vessels together with
portions of all the deep muscles of the posterior compartment.

the whole calf) outwards through two right angles on the hinge formed by the short fibular pier.

The incision, made when the foot is plantar flexed and the knee bent, runs longitudinally. It starts from a handbreadth above the tip of the malleolus and ends three fingerbreadths below the line of the knee joint; its upper end should lie two fingerbreadths behind the inner edge of tibia; the rest, a fingerbreadth behind. The long saphenous vein and the saphenous nerve both run in surface fascia in front of the incision and are carried forward with the side-curtain.

Detachment of the tibial pier is almost bloodless. A finger will protect the neurovascular bundle where it is bridged by the soleus arch.

The access to the bundle is as complete as that got by the midline approach, but the ' catapult ' division of the tibioperoneal trunk (pp. 246 and 247), accompanied by veins, is now seen bunched in profile instead of full face. The posterior tibial nerve, continuing the medial popliteal, goes down immediately behind the trunk.

(Note that the distal portion of the tibial nerve has kept its relative position in the bundle : it still lies just behind and lateral to tibial vessels—exactly as it does when it ' bisects ' the catapult.)

Exposure of this hinder bundle is easily continued to the sole, if we should need to trace the plantar distribution of nerve and vessels (p. 300, and *legend* to Fig. 196, below).

EXPOSING THE BACK OF THE DISTAL END OF TIBIA

Mention of the tibia suggests the thought of an exposure from the inner side. But, if we try a simple test, we find we shall do better to employ a *fibular* approach. Kneel for a moment with the foot relaxed in plantar flexion. Then grasp and move the flaccid tendon of Achilles ; it travels farther to the inner side—away from fibula—and so uncovers more of an objective which spreads across the middle line. One reason is that while its outer edge is ' free,' soleus fibres reaching down the shaft (it may be almost to a handbreadth from the medial malleolus) tie the Achilles tendon to the tibia. So, like a dog, it moves most easily towards its leash. Another—dominating—factor is that on the medial side Achilles tendon is more firmly fixed, than on the lateral, against the *denser* portion of the sheet of fascia covering the deeper muscles of the leg (*legend* to Fig. 152, p. 248).

Displacement of Achillis is not the sole advantage of an outer access, for that will let us liberate as well the belly of the flexor hallucis—a muscle which arises from the fibula and spreads at once to hide the tibial surface. This belly (by the aid of a strategic interval) is readily displaced towards the *in*accessible and medial fixation of its tendon down the foot. Fig. 169 shows *one* occasion for this approach.

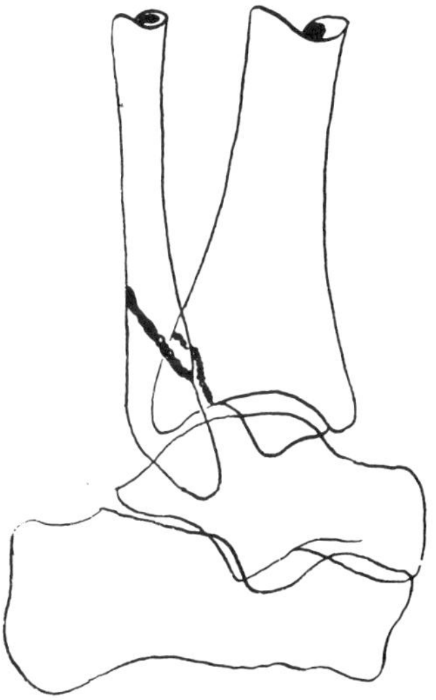

Position and incision.—A sand-bag laid beneath the instep of the 'face-down' patient bends his knee and keeps the foot in plantar flexion. The skin incision curves from a point a full thumbwidth below the fibular malleolus and goes a largish handbreadth up the leg, close to the outer edge of the Achilles tendon—a line that will avoid the sural nerve which otherwise is likely to be cut above and also distally (Fig. 170, A).

After incising fascia the knife once more will enter fat, crossed as a rule two fingerbreadths above os calcis by an artery, which must be severed; its parent stem, the peroneal, accompanied by veins that may be very large, lies here on bone and stripes the shaft of fibula just medial to the hinder edge.

A further opening of the fat will show a spot where we can reach the back of tibia, between hallucis and the fibula—an angular strategic interval (Fig. 171, A, inset).

Fig. 169

The 'third malleolus' of Destot (from an X-ray tracing by M. Levine)

This is an inconstant local exaggeration of the normal excess in length of the *hinder* lip that bounds the distal face of tibia. Its function is to check such backward trends of the foot as threaten a downward step or landing from a jump.

When Destot's malleolus is prominent a relatively small force that stretches ligaments will break and thrust it backwards. (A car in one case stopping short, slid its passenger off seat to bump her sitting on her ankle.) More violent occasions make wider sweeps and shear through two or even three malleoli—Destot's plus the medial and lateral—each displaced backwards. The X-ray was taken after reduction of the displaced third malleolus which, like the broken fibula, was then fixed by a screw.

But first be sure you *have* identified hallucis. The common, disconcerting slip is to mistake for it the peroneus brevis whose belly has a way of bulging in towards the tibia. To test the matter embrace the doubtful muscle from behind with thumb and finger; and if in front of it you pinch the narrow fibula, your grasp includes not hallucis but *both* the peronei. The hallucis lies farther medially and deeper (Fig. 170, c).

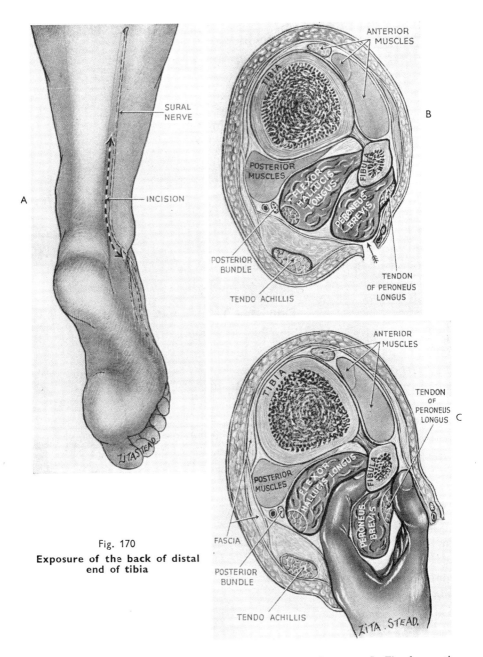

Fig. 170
Exposure of the back of distal end of tibia

A. The incision close and *lateral* to Achillis, avoiding sural nerve. B. The frequently deceptive bulging of peroneus brevis that simulates hallucis. C. Recognition of peroneus by closing on the narrow fibula in front with an embracing thumb and finger.

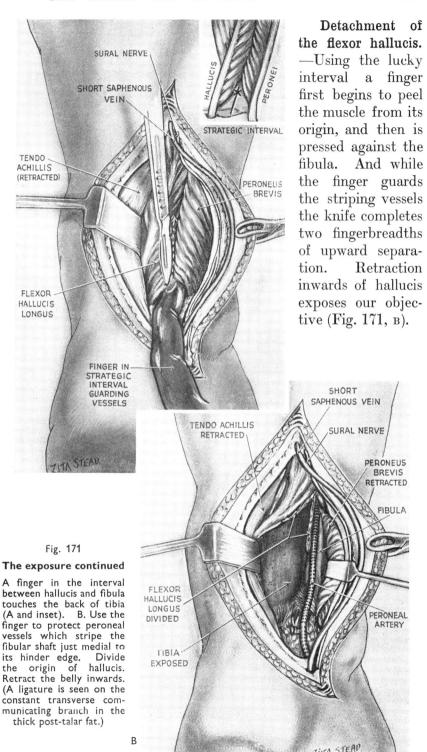

SURAL NERVE

SHORT SAPHENOUS VEIN

HALLUCIS

PERONEI

STRATEGIC INTERVAL

TENDO ACHILLIS (RETRACTED)

PERONEUS BREVIS

FLEXOR HALLUCIS LONGUS

FINGER IN STRATEGIC INTERVAL GUARDING VESSELS

ZITA STEAD.

SHORT SAPHENOUS VEIN

TENDO ACHILLIS RETRACTED

SURAL NERVE

PERONEUS BREVIS RETRACTED

FIBULA

FLEXOR HALLUCIS LONGUS DIVIDED

PERONEAL ARTERY

TIBIA EXPOSED

ZITA STEAD.

B

Detachment of the flexor hallucis. —Using the lucky interval a finger first begins to peel the muscle from its origin, and then is pressed against the fibula. And while the finger guards the striping vessels the knife completes two fingerbreadths of upward separation. Retraction inwards of hallucis exposes our objective (Fig. 171, B).

Fig. 171

The exposure continued

A finger in the interval between hallucis and fibula touches the back of tibia (A and inset). B. Use the finger to protect peroneal vessels which stripe the fibular shaft just medial to its hinder edge. Divide the origin of hallucis. Retract the belly inwards. (A ligature is seen on the constant transverse communicating branch in the thick post-talar fat.)

EXPOSURE OF THE ARCHED SEGMENT AND UPPER THIRD OF ANTERIOR TIBIAL VESSELS [1]

Our study of the *leg* began behind—the master site and starting place of crural trunks; the answer, thus, to Dupuytren's perplexity when faced with local bleeding: " But *which* is cut? Is it anterior or posterior tibial? The peroneal or the popliteal? One or else several at once? "

Transition from the back comes easily; the arching forward of anterior tibial vessels leads straight into the front compartment. Distal to the knee this deep, sequestered segment juts from the popliteal stem, and passing through or above the interosseous membrane turns down—like a tap.

Records of bleeding from the arch are rare enough to leave at least some surgeons unprepared to stop it by direct exposure. Yet this hæmorrhage is dangerous: the mass of blood (or clot) is placed exactly where it shuts both tap and main as well.

Fiolle and Delmas (1921, *Surgical Exposure of the Deep Seated Blood Vessels*, London, p. 21) describe how Pierre Duval (to reach an aneurysm of the arch) cut through and drew aside the upper third of fibula. For that he bared the bone, dividing peroneus longus, the outer head of gastrocnemius, and part of soleus—liberating first the common peroneal nerve and looping it aside.

The poor condition of my only patient with bleeding from the arching segment led me to try a quick alternative. I therefore used a tiny ' Mikulicz '—a tampon placed exactly where a finger-tip controlled the unseen vessel. But that might sometimes fail to stop the hæmorrhage, or might (like clot itself) impede the circulation.

Looking for other means I found a simple one.

THE OPERATION

With Dupuytren, no doubt, we wondered what was bleeding and have (I trust) begun to reconnoitre from the back. So— through a mesial incision of at least a span—we shall by now have ripped the sleeve of gastrocnemius and traced the popliteal vessels downwards to the bridge-mouth of soleus; and, if the mouth has overhung and masked the branching of the major trunks, we have already cleared a prospect by splitting lengthwise through the bridge.

But still there is no sight of our objective: the arch juts

[1] *The Lancet*, 1943, **1**, 141.

forward and away. Nor can we yet persuade it backwards into view for it is fastened out of reach—in front. So, turning to the front, we *there* release the arch and draw it out behind.

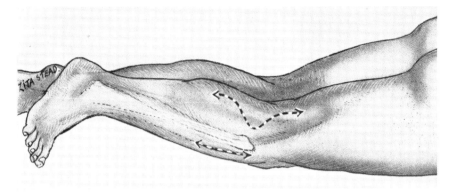

Fig. 172

Exposure of arched anterior tibial segment

With the patient face-down cant the foot across the sound ankle. You then have easy *simultaneous* access to front and back compartments of the leg.

Position.—Till now a sand-bag lifts the instep of the 'face-down' patient, bending his knee to slack the calf. Now (without altering the posture of his trunk) take the foot from the bag and lay its medial edge across his other ankle (Fig. 172). The trivial change gives access to the front compartment and leaves the hinder wound in sight and in control.

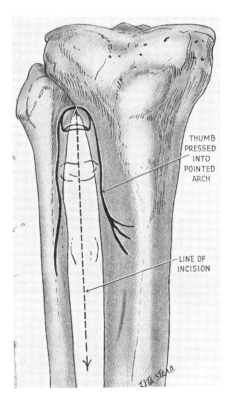

THUMB PRESSED INTO POINTED ARCH

LINE OF INCISION

Fig. 173

Finding the intermuscular plane for opening the upper reach of the anterior compartment

The thumb, pressed up from below, fits lengthwise into the pointed arch between tibia and fibula. Open skin and fascia along a line bisecting the thumb from nail to wrist. The line marks where the curved plane of cleavage comes to the surface (see text); it does *not* mark the course of the anterior tibial bundle which here lies deep to the lateral muscle.

A rule of thumb for the anterior incision.—First we must separate the pair of muscles that cover the front of the vascular arch and its continuation down the leg. Between the two the

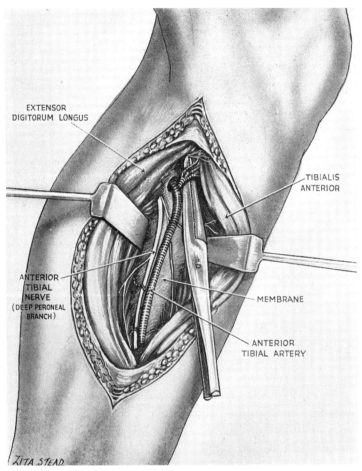

Fig. 174

Cutting the leash of anterior recurrent tibial vessels to free the arch

A pair of forceps slides up the interosseous membrane medial to the main neurovascular bundle and lifts the leash for section. A few small nerve twigs may run with it and can be spared: they do not moor the arch. If they are cut, tibialis anterior remains well supplied.

cleavage plane is *curved* : the belly of extensor longus digitorum bulges into that of tibialis. This curving plane comes to the fascial surface along a line which can be found with ease. Approaching from below press and fit the pulp of your thumb into the pointed, gothic archway formed above by tibia and fibula (Fig. 173). Divide the patient's skin as if you were bisecting the guiding thumb from nail to wrist—a method of location more robust than ghostly pointers to the plane of cleavage (the academic groove or petty artery or whitish line) which soon fade out with trauma. Using this guide again, we open fascia along the same line, *not* tearing muscle. A finger separates the interlock of bellies and shows the bundle of anterior tibial vessels. These are deep to long

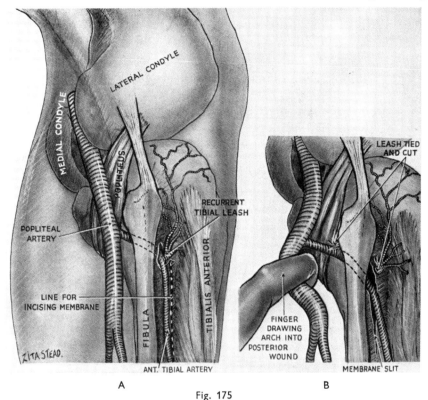

A   B

Fig. 175

A. The arch set free in front, and B, drawn back and brought to view in the posterior wound. A narrow opening through interosseous membrane has been widened medial to the vessels.

extensor and so lie lateral to our incision (see the *legend* to Fig. 173). When we have made them visible throughout the wound against the background of interosseous membrane we can proceed to mobilise their arch.

Impediments of leash, membrane, and muscle.—The arch is moored in front by its recurrent branch and venous tributaries— a wide-flung leash whose narrow end we cut (Figs. 174 and 175).[1]

---

[1] John Bell—brother to Charles, the physiologist—says of the anterior recurrent tibial:
"It is a branch which comes off the fore part of the tibial artery instantly after it has pierced the interosseous membrane; it turns immediately upwards under the flesh of the tibialis anticus; it gives many muscular branches, some to the head of the tibialis,

Variable, small, peroneal recurrent vessels—the posterior which curls up in front of fibula, the anterior which *rises* in front of it—may also require section, or be torn through unnoticed.

Then, if the opening in the membrane is large enough already, we are at liberty to draw the arch back into the calf. But, if the hole itself is small—or narrowed by encroachment of the hinder tibialis—we must enlarge the passage, slitting the membrane downwards medial to the bundle (to avoid the nerve); and then, if need be, stretching with a finger a pathway through or over tibialis. That will remove the last impediment and let us bring the arch from front to back for safe and unrestricted access (Fig. 175).

EXPOSURE OF THE DISTAL TWO-THIRDS OF THE ANTERIOR TIBIAL NEUROVASCULAR BUNDLE

The long incision of Fiolle and Delmas so greatly simplifies the operation that those who read of it incline to over-confidence. Its virtue dwells in length : it reaches down to where the *tendons* have replaced a close-packed interlock of bellies ; and using tendons we can cleanly split extensor digitorum from the tibialis. So all we have to do is choose correctly. And that is just where many fail : they take a near-by tendon for the tibialis and lose their way at once.

A little care avoids discomfiture. We know (pp. 248 and 250) that in the leg tibialis anterior borders its namesake shaft throughout : *that* is its certain countersign. The tendon lateral to tibialis (except immediately above the ankle—where hallucis comes forward to replace it) must, during anæsthetic relaxation, be a tendon of extensor digitorum longus ; the interval between is the required interval.[1] But first let us divide the skin.

---

others to the upper part of the extensor digitorum, and branches go round the head of the fibula to the origin of the long peronæus muscle. One branch goes directly upwards and spreads all over the front of the knee-joint mixing its branches in the common muscular net-work." (John and Charles Bell, 1816, *Anatomy and Physiology of the Human Body*, London, vol. ii, p. 28.)

[1] The text-books here are rather careless ; or do they merely illustrate once more the striking difference in outlook of surgeon and anatomist ? Their pictures show the tendon of extensor hallucis already flush with tendons of digitorum and tibialis, as high as midway up the leg. But, coming from the *depth* of the anterior compartment and springing from the ' middle half ' of fibula, hallucis (when relaxed) *can* only reach the level of its superficial fellows a very little way above the ankle. The tendons, too, of longus digitorum are often drawn as though they formed a single strap within the leg—another point that might seem trivial were it not misleading. In fact, their segmentation as a rule goes about half-way up towards the knee ; and, even where it fails to be complete, the *signs* of it (as Boyer wrote) are visible—" almost throughout the tendon's length." It would be only fair to mention that Baron Boyer practised as a surgeon and had the chance to guess what surgeons want.

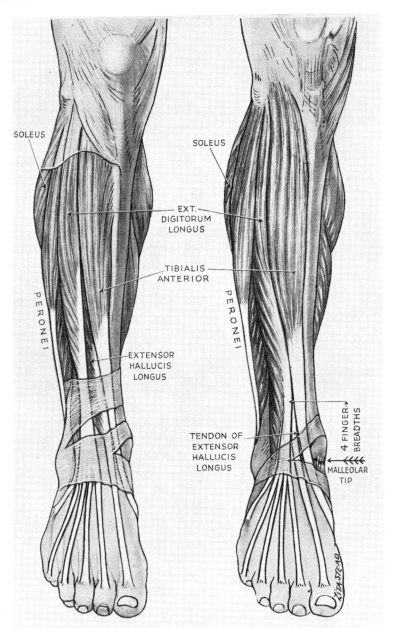

Fig. 176

The surfacing of extensor hallucis longus

A is the almost universal picture which affects to show an undisturbed relation, thus inducing surgeons to believe that hallucis reaches the surface midway up the leg and *there* begins to part tibialis anterior from extensor digitorum longus. Anatomists, perhaps, may cock a toe and say (like Galileo) : "But it does ! "— unmindful that our patients, properly anæsthetised, do not cock toes. B. Hallucis, when relaxed, comes to the surface three fingerbreadths above the ankle joint. When fully active, tightness of the fascial sleeve combined with structural cohesion will merely let hallucis raise a ridge that carries up a covering of laxer muscles but does not sunder them.

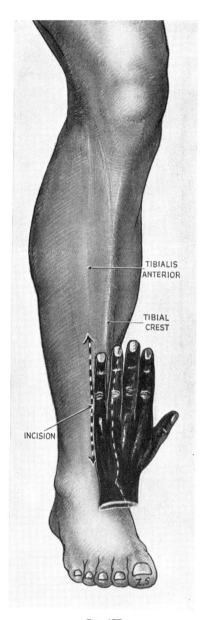

Fig. 177

**Incision for anterior tibial bundle
(distal two-thirds)**

'Rule' this a little-fingerbreadth to the fibular side of tibial crest. As it goes up the leg, incline the cut towards the bisected-thumb mark of Fig. 173, above. Below, a small medial reflection of skin finds the tibial crest; next to it is tibialis tendon.

Incision.—Press—in the distal half of the leg—your *little* finger against the outer (fibular) side of tibial crest (or shin). Then ' rule ' a cut along the outer edge of where your finger lay—*not* opening through deep fascia. Cut for about a span (Fig. 177).

The bone and the tendon.— Now for the small precaution. Reflect a little skin at just one distal spot—enough to give a quite indubitable glimpse of tibia. Open the fascial sleeve in line with the incision. The tendon that is flattened close against the bone (and looking rather like it) is tibialis tendon; the interval we want lies at the tendon's outer edge, and *there* begins our separation.

The last pitfall.—But we can still contrive to go astray. Extensor hallucis, the only deep anterior muscle of the leg, slopes from the fibula to screen the neurovascular bundle. So, if we wander *lateral* to hallucis, we find, perhaps, another artery—or none at all.

You will avoid this terminal collapse by keeping touch with tibialis: work on its outer face, and find the bundle backed above by interosseous membrane, and distally by tibia (Fig. 178). The nerve (deep branch of peroneal, or anterior tibial), which starts upon the neck of fibula, curves gently in to lie in front of the companion vessels, and then, below, recedes a little out again towards the fibula.

That, at least, is what we learn. Nor can I give at first hand figures to dispute it; but Hovelacque in his *Anatomie des Nerfs*,

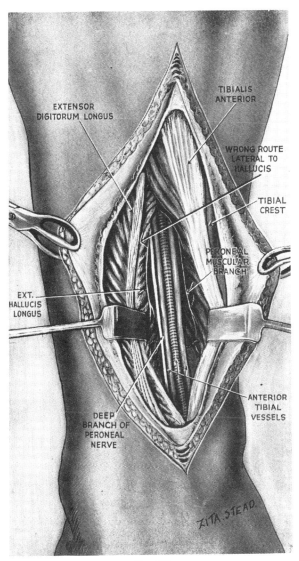

Fig. 178

Showing how the deeply placed extensor hallucis longus overlaps the bundle. The arrow shows the *wrong* route that may be taken—lateral to hallucis. (In this figure the nerve lies lateral to vessels.)

Paris, 1927, p. 609, describes the normal path of the anterior tibial as crossing to the *inner* side of its companion vessels, and shows this transit at the middle of the leg (Plate LXXXIX). He also cites Marcellin-Duval who notes that in 450 legs the nerve had crossed the vessels in all but one per cent. For Boyer, too (in 1815), this transit was the common disposition.

One might from these divergences suspect a strange, cross-channel difference in gross anatomy; or even that (as Pascal said of truth) *meridians* decide the course of nerves—a thing I rather doubt.[1]

The distal reach of this approach to the anterior compartments of the leg merges directly with the late Willis Campbell's 'all-purpose' incision down the instep. I had omitted this extension from the previous edition, leaving a gap to which I returned with renewed distaste as a tongue will to a sore tooth.

This repugnance centred chiefly on my recollection of the gross ankles that go with mere removal of the talus, a rare necessity

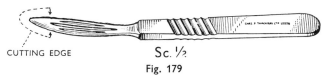

CUTTING EDGE　　　　　Sc. ½

Fig. 179

Knife for dividing moorings of talus from within the ankle joint.
(It is a Kocher's dissector toughened and sharpened.)

required only after certain comminuted fractures or more rarely still by local bone disease.

Of late, however, a new description of an old use for talectomy had partly countered my dislike. In 1911 Lorthioir, to arthrodese a palsied foot, resected and decorticated the talus; then, after due removal of adjacent cartilage, he placed the bone back in its original position, as a *graft*.[2]

I owe a final liquidation of a 'talectomy complex' to the quick understanding and skill of a fourth-year student, my demonstrator, Mr M. Stranc, who in a brilliant academic career had not till then performed an operation of any kind whatever. For that reason I asked him to test the clarity of notes on talectomy which I had long shelved. I suggested, too, that he should try on the cadaver the efficacy of the knife made at my

[1] The more so since the artist in a recent 'Gray' refutes the text and shows the nerve as lying *tibial* to the artery within the lower segment of a leg. (Gray's *Anatomy*, 27th Edn., 1938. Compare Fig. 655, p. 649, with the statement in the first two lines on p. 1127.)

[2] W. S. Hunt and H. A. Thompson, *Journal of Bone and Joint Surgery*, 1954, 349. It was from an illustration in this paper that I first learnt of Hatt's spoons and their connection with talectomy. I imagine (for it is suggested but not described by these authors) that their use resembles that of the knife in Fig. 179, which, however, does not derive from them; Messrs Thackray of Leeds had it on order two years before the paper came into my hands.

request by Messrs Thackray to simplify the operation. This he did quite independently, demonstrating the knife (Fig. 179) and the foot (together with its talus resected and unblemished) before an audience that chanced to number professors of surgery from four universities.

The **'all-purpose' incision** devised by Campbell begins a handbreadth above the malleoli and goes in superficial fat midway between them to the web that joins the two outer toes. It is only rarely that the lateral division of the musculocutaneous nerve can be spared (Fig. 180).

The sling-like extensor retinaculum. — This is our next objective. It may be shaped like a prostrate X or a prostrate Y.

1. *If like a* Y, detach the *double* stem of the Y from the upper face of the front of calcaneum and with it the included bony origin of extensor digitorum brevis.

2. *If like an* X—by reason of a surplus fastening to the fibular malleolus—divided this fastening too.

Once free of lateral attachments the whole sling of retinaculum can be turned over towards the medial side

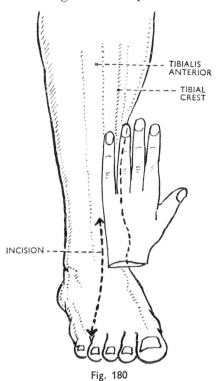

TIBIALIS ANTERIOR

TIBIAL CREST

INCISION

Fig. 180

This incision (which is Willis Campbell's) continues that on the front of the leg shown in Fig. 177

of the foot carrying off within its several compartments the long tendons of the instep (peroneus tertius and extensor digitorum longus, extensor hallucis longus, tibialis anterior) *with* their synovial sheaths. The anterior tibial neurovascular bundle remains to hug the deeper plane of bone and ligament.

Draw the retinaculum and tendons forcibly inwards, exposing the front of the ankle joint and the upper face of the mid-tarsal joint. Peroneus tertius provides a good buffer for this strong retraction. Then if talectomy is purposed, a transverse incision opens the front of the ankle joint after the anterior neurovascular bundle has been moved laterally.

The dorsal line of the mid-tarsal joint.—Viewed from above the line begins to cross the instep directly behind the navicular tubercle, a thumbwidth in front of the medial malleolus. (Both these points stand out with slight inversion of the foot and comfortably lodge the thumb between their two projections.) The line has two opposite curves : the rounded head of talus forms a medial and forward convexity ; the recessive face of calcaneum, a lateral and forward concavity. The curves are crossed at their junction by the two parts of the bifurcate ligament which binds calcaneum to the cuboid and navicular bones. In addition there is the thin dorsal calcaneocuboid and talonavicular ligaments together with navicular fibres that come forward from the deltoid ligament. To open the mid-tarsal joint for the purpose of erasing cartilage follow the curves, cut these ligaments, and ' break ' the foot downwards like the breech of a shotgun.

TALECTOMY FROM IN FRONT

Counting *all* the ligaments and bands that have been described as fixed to talus, ten (apart from the thin capsule of the ankle joint) must be cut to free the bone. Two are fascial derivatives not mentioned in British textbooks : one of these, the peroneo-talocalcanean, comes away (at least in part) when deeper-lying ligaments—posterior talofibular and posterior talocalcanean—are detached ; the other, spreading from the flexor retinaculum, helps (with posterior talocalcanean) to bridge the talar groove for the long flexor tendon of the big toe. The occurrence of another ligament, the medial talocalcanean, seems to be inconstant, or is absorbed into the back of the deltoid expansion.

There are thus some nine (or ten) moorings that require section. All these, except two, can be severed from talus by working from *within* the synovial cavity of the ankle, using the knife shown in Fig. 179. This was modelled on the stout shape of a Kocher's dissector whose curve, I found, would fit the upper face of talus. The thick ' blade ' is sharpened only at the end and at *adjacent* parts of either edge, the sharpened portions having thus the same extent as the end and edges of a small finger-nail. It thus forms a strong 6 in. tool, which—were it magnified by 8— could trim the margins of a lawn.

The rota of ligament division.—*From outside the ankle joint* cut the two ligaments already exposed : (1) the anterior talofibular ligament on the outer side of the neck of talus ; (2) the dorsal talonavicular ligament (unless the mid-tarsal joint has already been opened).

From inside the ankle joint, after twisting the plantar-flexed foot *out* to tense the medial ligament, keep the knife against the medial face of talus and cut the *deep* part of the deltoid ligament attached to it. Then twist the foot *in* and cut the stretched lateral talocalcanean ligament. (The lateral fibulocalcaneal ligament which overlaps it will probably be divided at the same time.)

Next divide the two layers of the interosseous talocalcanean ligament, beginning with the thick and often separate pivotal piece of the anterior layer ; drive the sharp knife tip along the oblique course of the tarsal tunnel, from without, inwards and backwards. (The interosseous ligament should till now be left undivided so that talus and calcaneum will move together when we twist the foot to tighten medial and lateral ligaments for section.)

The *posterior*, remoter moorings are brought to the knife by catching the neck of the talus with bone forceps and drawing it forward.

The role of the ' trigonal ' (lateral) tubercle.—Find first the prominent tubercle at the back of talus which sometimes remains separate as an os trigonum ; it forms the *lateral* lip of the deep groove that lodges the tendon of flexor hallucis longus. Engage the groove with the knife tip, keeping the slightly concave surface of the blade against the bone. Turn the tip so that its sharp adjoining *edge* moves heelwards on the *lateral* wall of the groove to meet and cut the fibres that bridge the tendon posteriorly. As you turn the knife the blunt *back* of the tip thrusts the tendon aside. The liberated tendon, thus displaced, remains behind when forceps draw the talus forward.

Apart from the uncertain hope of its action after tarsal fixation, the long hallucis tendon is worth preserving, *if only as a buffer*. It lies between the blunt back of the knife's end and the posterior tibial neurovascular bundle, which it neighbours (as horse or harlot) in mnemonics as widely known as Grimm's fairy tales.

The lower end of the posterior tibial bundle—the only part of a main neurovascular structure that comes at all near the knife during this talectomy—lies about $\frac{1}{8}$ in. behind the medial talar tubercle of Stieda and is there separated from the bone by hallucis tendon [1] and the fibres that bridge it ; and then, from the inner

---

[1] Division of hallucis tendon was the solitary flaw in Strane's first talectomy—a fortunate accident that taught us to avoid its repetition in the way described.

side of the same tubercle, by deep posterior fibres of the deltoid ligament (Figs. 183, D, and 184).

Still hugging the trigonal tubercle the knife proceeds first to free its hinder end, then its outer face from the long reach of the posterior talofibular ligament, which—at the end of the tubercle— lies behind and blends with the posterior talocalcanean so that *there* both structures are detached together.

Once the safety of the long hallucis tendon (and therefore of

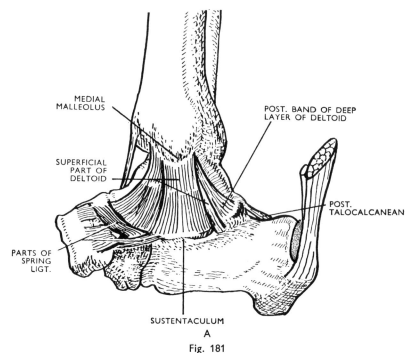

Fig. 181

Medial view of moorings of talus

A. The *superficial* fibres of the deltoid ligament cover all the deep (talar) fibres anteriorly. The deep fibres are seen posteriorly, and are fully exposed when the superficial fibres are reflected (Fig. 182).

posterior tibial bundle) is assured, any bands that still check the delivery of talus can be cut at the bone's surface. (One such check might be a widespread form of the peroneo-talocalcanean ligament, the *fascial* derivative of Rouvière and Canela and therefore lying heelward of the ordinary ligaments ; so that, at least in part, it shares their separation.)

Perhaps the table on pages 286-287 may serve to chart a sequence for dividing talar moorings.

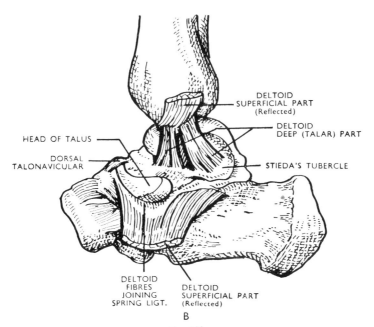

DELTOID
SUPERFICIAL PART
(Reflected)

DELTOID
DEEP (TALAR) PART

HEAD OF TALUS

DORSAL
TALONAVICULAR

STIEDA'S TUBERCLE

DELTOID
FIBRES
JOINING
SPRING LIGT.

DELTOID
SUPERFICIAL PART
(Reflected)

B

Fig. 182

Medial view of moorings of talus

B. The *deep* fibres of deltoid seen after reflection of superficial layer.

Note the strong posterior band sloping to Stieda's tubercle. Fibres of this band may escape early section and are then cut when talus is drawn forward in the last stage of liberating the talus. (The medial talocalcanean ligament was absent here.)

TALAR LIGAMENTS ARE DIVIDED FROM OUTSIDE

AND

FROM INSIDE THE ANKLE JOINT

BY

ANTERIOR ACCESS

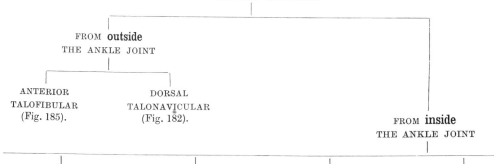

FROM **outside**
THE ANKLE JOINT

ANTERIOR TALOFIBULAR (Fig. 185).

DORSAL TALONAVICULAR (Fig. 182).

FROM **inside**
THE ANKLE JOINT

Lateral Talocalcanean
(The fibulocalcanean over-lies this and may become detached too, Fig. 185.)

Deep part of the Medial (Deltoid) Ligament of Ankle (Fig. 182).

Medial Talocalcanean
May be absent or blended with the posterior deep band of the deltoid liga-ment which crosses and covers it. Its fibres join the medial talar tubercle of Stieda to the back of sustentaculum.

Interosseous Talocalcanean
plus its pivotal core (Fig. 183, A).

Cut after twisting the foot medially.

Cut after twisting the foot laterally.

Cut by inserting the k. tip at the outer end sinus tarsi and working and heelwards through tunnel.

res bridging the ar Sulcus for allucis Tendon		Posterior Talocalcanean	Posterior Talofibular	Peroneo-talocalcanean
ey are derived a two inter-linous septa that e from the deep of flexor retina-m. The posterior calcanean liga-t also contri-s.) To cut these es, keep the con-face of the blade t the proximal of talus. Engage end of the blade the posterior us. Then, turn end to hug the r wall of the us. Cut heel-ds with the short adjoining edge (Fig. 183, D).	With hallucis tendon free draw the talus forward and thus bring the next three moorings to the knife.	is overlain by the next and, like it, is attached to the tip of the 'trigonal' tubercle.	Its end reaches the tip of the 'trigonal' tubercle; it also has a long attachment to the outer side of the tubercle (Fig. 183, B and D).	ligament of Rouvière and Canela derived from deep fascia, it thus lies heelward of posterior talofibular and so is detached with it (Figs. 183, D, and 184)

Of these three ligaments the first is deepest; the second intermediate; the third superficial. They may thus be detached *en masse* from the **end** of the trigonal tubercle when forceps draw the talus forward. Part of a *widespread* peroneo-talocalcanean sheet may escape and require separate division.

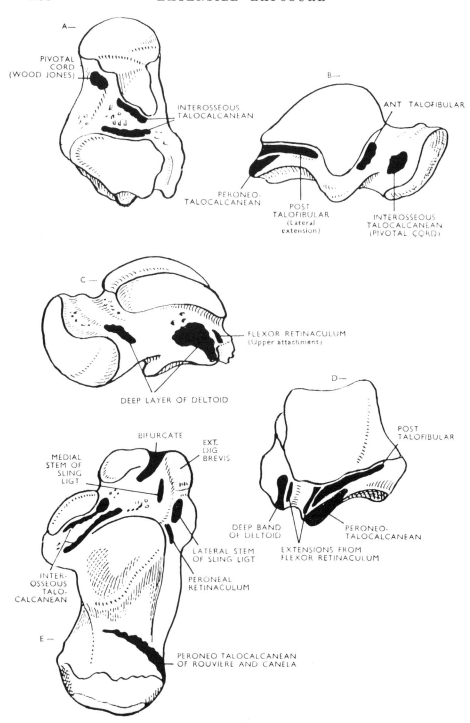

A—

PIVOTAL
CORD
(WOOD JONES)

INTEROSSEOUS
TALOCALCANEAN

B—

ANT TALOFIBULAR

PERONEO-
TALOCALCANEAN

POST
TALOFIBULAR
(Lateral
extension)

INTEROSSEOUS
TALOCALCANEAN
(PIVOTAL CORD)

C—

FLEXOR RETINACULUM
(Upper attachment)

DEEP LAYER OF DELTOID

D—

POST
TALOFIBULAR

BIFURCATE

EXT.
DIG
BREVIS

MEDIAL
STEM OF
SLING
LIGT

DEEP BAND
OF DELTOID

PERONEO-
TALOCALCANEAN

EXTENSIONS FROM
FLEXOR RETINACULUM

LATERAL STEM
OF SLING LIGT

PERONEAL
RETINACULUM

INTER-
OSSEOUS
TALO-
CALCANEAN

E—

PERONEO TALOCALCANEAN
OF ROUVIERE AND CANELA

Fig. 183

These tali and the calcaneum are all of the **right** side. Ligamentous attachments are marked in black, muscular attachments in colour.

A. **Inferior aspect.**—The strong pivotal cord was not described by Wood Jones, but he has emphasised its function in relation to Inkster's work on talocalcaneo-navicular movements.

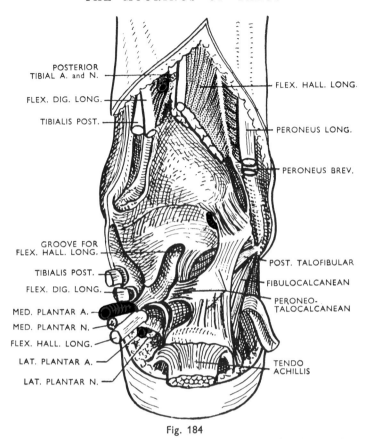

POSTERIOR
TIBIAL A. and N.

FLEX. DIG. LONG.

TIBIALIS POST.

FLEX. HALL. LONG.

PERONEUS LONG.

PERONEUS BREV.

GROOVE FOR
FLEX. HALL. LONG.

TIBIALIS POST.

FLEX. DIG. LONG.

MED. PLANTAR A.

MED. PLANTAR N.

FLEX. HALL. LONG.

LAT. PLANTAR A.

LAT. PLANTAR N.

POST. TALOFIBULAR

FIBULOCALCANEAN

PERONEO-
TALOCALCANEAN

TENDO
ACHILLIS

Fig. 184

The extrinsic peroneo-talocalcanean ligament (after Paturet)

This fascial derivative is fixed above to the lateral malleolus and to the postero-inferior tibiofibular ligament. Descending, it gives a process to the trigonal tubercle of talus and then goes on to join calcaneum. Only part of the sequence of ligaments from surface to depth is seen—peroneo-talocalcanean overlies posterior talofibular; the deepest ligament—posterior talocalcanean is concealed.

Fig. 183 (*continued*)

B. **Lateral aspect.**—Note the long lateral attachment of the posterior talofibular ligament and also the site of the pivotal cord which is lodged here in a bony pit.
The peroneo-talocalcanean ligament of Rouvière and Canela is seen in full in Fig. 184. Paturet describes it as an *extrinsic* ligament, derived from fascia, and belonging to two joints —tibio-tarsal and posterior talocalcanean.

C. **Medial aspect.**—This shows the attachments of the *deep* layer of deltoid ligament which is fixed *solely* to talus. The posterior attachment is particularly strong; it clothes the medial face of Stieda's tubercle—the inner boundary of the groove for the tendon of flexor hallucis longus. Fibres of this ligament may escape section till the talus is drawn forward.

D. **Posterior aspect.**—The long attachment of the posterior talofibular ligament runs out and forward from the trigonal tubercle—the outer boundary of the groove for flexor hallucis longus tendon. The bundle lies behind and medial to the tendon, p. 283.

E. **Right calcaneum, upper face.**—The bifurcate ligament forks in front to reach navicular and cuboid. The two stems of the sling ligament—the frondiform of Retzius and the inferior part of our extensor retinaculum—sandwich the origin of flexor digitorum brevis. The pivotal ligament has no separate attachment to calcaneum in this specimen, for it has sloped down and merged with the anterior sheet of the interosseous talocalcanean, a sheet described in Gray's *Anatomy* as the " posterior ligament of the talcalcaneo-navicular joint."

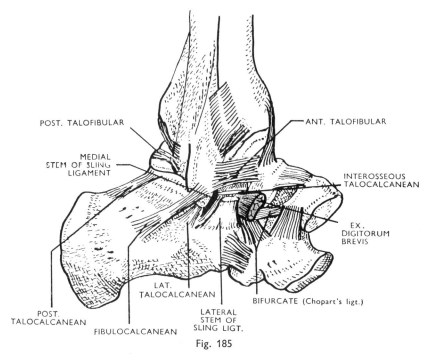

POST. TALOFIBULAR

ANT. TALOFIBULAR

MEDIAL
STEM OF SLING
LIGAMENT

INTEROSSEOUS
TALOCALCANEAN

EX.
DIGITORUM
BREVIS

LAT.
TALOCALCANEAN

BIFURCATE (Chopart's ligt.)

POST.
TALOCALCANEAN

LATERAL
STEM OF
SLING LIGT.

FIBULOCALCANEAN

Fig. 185

Lateral view of moorings of talus

One of the two ligaments divided from *outside* the ankle joint is visible—anterior talofibular. The fibulocalcanean is often cut in company with a true talar mooring that lies
on a plane deep to it. (The double stem of the sling ligament has been divided along
with the origin of extensor digitorum brevis at an early stage in the operation—of course
outside the ankle joint.)

Note that the pointer to *interosseous talocalcanean* lies just too low and touches instead
the medial stem of the sling ligament.

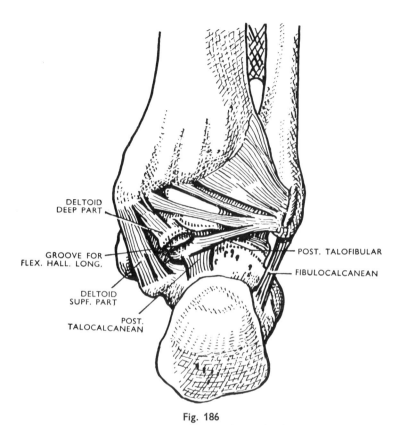

DELTOID
DEEP PART

GROOVE FOR
FLEX. HALL. LONG.

DELTOID
SUPF. PART

POST.
TALOCALCANEAN

POST. TALOFIBULAR

FIBULOCALCANEAN

Fig. 186

Posterior view of moorings of talus

The hindmost band of the deep deltoid layer is seen attached to Stieda's
tubercle. Fibres of this band may escape section until the talus can be drawn
forward in the last stage of liberation. The fibulocalcanean ligament is sometimes cut in company with the lateral talocalcanean.

EXPOSURE OF THE FIBULA AND NERVES
RELATED TO IT [1]

ANATOMY

The neck and upper third of the fibula are in direct contact with nerves. Muscles surround three-fourths of the shaft.

The relations of the nerves to the upper part of the bone are insufficiently described in many text-books, which give the impression that only the *neck* of the fibula is in contact with the branches of the external popliteal nerve (common peroneal B.N.A.). A glance at Fig. 187 modified from that which accompanies Poirier's excellent account of the peroneus longus, shows in diagram the true extent of this contact (*Anatomie Humaine*, 2ème Edn., vol. ii, fasc. 1, p. 251, Paris, 1901).

It is, of course, at the fibular neck (where the nerves are thinly covered by the origin of the long peroneus) that they are most often exposed to violence ; but the surgeon whose intervention is not to come within this category should be familiar with the true anatomy of the region.

The lateral popliteal (common peroneal, B.N.A.) gives off its last three branches as it lies upon the fibular neck : first, the recurrent tibial nerve, which is often double ; then, anteriorly, its deep (or anterior tibial) branch ; and, posteriorly, its superficial (or musculocutaneous) branch. This last nerve descends almost vertically along the shaft, separating the diaphyseal origin of the long peroneus into anterior and posterior moieties, and keeping contact with the upper third of the shaft. Distal to this the peroneus brevis separates the nerve from the bone.

Exposure of the upper half of the fibula requires a full mobilisation of these nerves. This can be safely done by defining the trunk of the common peroneal as it descends behind the head of the bone (Fig. 189). When the nerve is raised, it leaves a shallow groove which separates the muscles of the calf from the fibular head. This groove is a strategic point, and gives the surgeon entry to a plane of cleavage which allows him to separate the peronei from the soleus muscle, and thus expose the bone with least damage. In exposing the distal half of the fibula a plane of

---

[1] Except for the addition of a final paragraph (and the correction of a slip) the text of these pages on the fibula is copied from *Exposures of Long Bones and other Surgical Methods*, Wright and Sons, Bristol, 1927.

cleavage between the peroneus brevis and the extensor muscles can easily be found at the apex of the triangular subcutaneous area, but an exposure along this line should be limited to the distal half of the bone.

The following is a description of a complete exposure of the fibula.

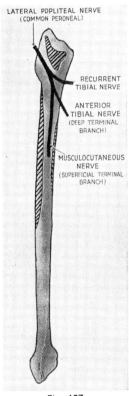

Fig. 187

Diagram of right fibula (modified from Poirier) showing extent of bone in direct contact with nerves. The shaded areas are the three fibular origins of the peroneus longus. (No other muscle is represented.)

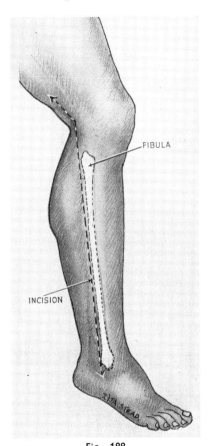

Fig. 188

Divide skin and superficial fascia from the back of external malleolus to the back of fibular head. Continue the incision one handbreadth along the biceps tendon.

THE OPERATION

Position.—The patient lies on the sound side with the sound limb extended. Place the knee of the affected side just in front of the other knee so that the heel of the affected side rests upon the other shin (as in Fig. 137).

Incision.—(Fig. 188). Divide the skin and superficial fascia from the back of the external malleolus to the back of the fibular head; continue the incision along the biceps tendon for one handbreadth beyond this. Open the deep fascia proximally, at the medial edge of the biceps tendon; continue its division with blunt-nosed scissors down behind the fibular head. Find the

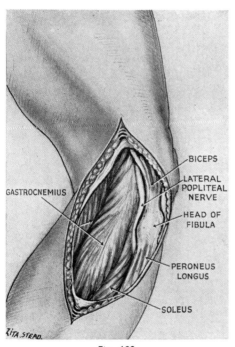

common peroneal (lateral popliteal) nerve where it lies flush with the tendon at the inner side of the biceps insertion. The tendon overlaps the nerve in the proximal part of the wound (Fig. 189). Mobilise the nerve proximally till a loose loop of it can be drawn out across the tendon and the fibular head. Slip one blade of the scissors down along the groove which the nerve has left. Divide the deep fascia in the direction of the groove, and thus open the plane of cleavage between the soleus and the peroneal muscles.

Fig. 189

Open deep fascia over the biceps tendon. Expose the distal end of the outer popliteal nerve (common peroneal); it lies in a groove which separates soleus from the fibular head. **This groove is the key to the plane of cleavage between the peronei and calf muscles.**

Next, draw the nerve-loop distally (towards the foot); turn the knife's edge away from the nerve against the lower border of the fibular head, and divide the thin slip of peroneus longus which bridges the nerve as it branches upon the fibular neck (Figs. 189 and 190). The nerve-loop can thus be drawn still farther out and away from the bone, while the peronei are raised after it and turned forward.

Stripping the rest of the shaft.—When we have safely bared the upper third of fibula the major task is done, but we should finish well and leave no scarecrow, distal spectacle of ragged bone and tattered tissues. Two sets of things demand and rarely get attention: the different stripping angle for muscles and interosseous membrane; the close adhesion of the peroneal vessels

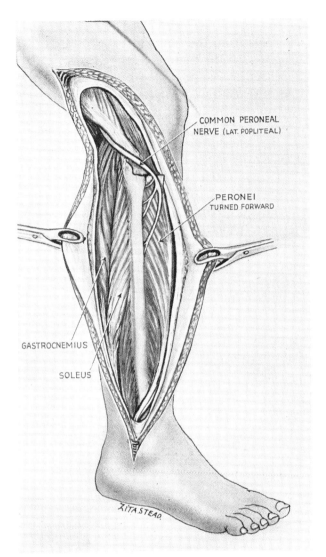

COMMON PERONEAL
NERVE (LAT. POPLITEAL)

PERONEI
TURNED FORWARD

GASTROCNEMIUS

SOLEUS

XITASTEAD

Fig. 190

Mobilise the nerve and lift it from the groove behind the head
of fibula. Slip one blade of blunt-nosed scissors into the groove
and divide the deep fascia throughout the wound. Separate
soleus from peroneus longus. Draw the nerve-loop forwards.
Turn the knife edge away from the nerve, and cut through the
thin slip of peroneus which bridges it. Detach the peronei and
turn them forward, keeping the nerve-loop taut.

to periosteum—a contact that begins about a handbreadth distal to the knee.

The *muscle fibres* from the fibula stream towards the foot ; the edge of the rugine should therefore travel kneewards, into their narrow angle with the shaft. At the fibular malleolus, pass the rugine deep to the tendons of peroneus longus and brevis *from behind*. Used from in front and working up the limb the handle of the instrument might strain emerging branches of the musculo-cutaneous (much better called the superficial branch of peroneal), just where the nerve is liable to form neuralgic trigger-spots.[1]

The *peroneal artery and veins* are seen to hug the lateral malleolus just medial to its hinder edge. A lengthwise cut through periosteum lets the rugine displace them safely from the shaft in company with flexor hallucis. Clean the whole shaft of muscle, working towards the knee. Till that is done do nothing to the *interosseous membrane*; its fibres slope in the reverse direction ; so you can strip the membrane *down*, towards the foot.

THE ELKIN-DUVAL METHOD OF EXPOSING THE ANTERIOR TIBIAL ARCH BY FIBULAR RESECTION

Elkin and his colleagues have made new and admirable use of a means that was first but only once employed by Pierre Duval (p. 272)—a means by which the awkward lodgment of the arch becomes an open field. But while Duval's objective was the arch itself, Elkin bares it incidentally in course of dealing with com-municating aneurysms at any part of the upper two-thirds of the leg.

Where such communications flourish, anastomoses open, neighbouring vessels dilate, and even small twigs that pierce the interosseous membrane enlarge and grow dangerous. For should they break under traction, they may withdraw through the membrane and bleed on its farther side—remote perhaps from an approach which enters only *one* of the leg's three osteofascial compartments.

---

[1] *Mononeuralgia in the superficial peroneal nerve.*—In 1941 I saw three patients thus afflicted whose *only* pains were in that distribution. These were made worse by turning in the foot with plantar flexion—an act which stretched the nerve ; and, during lulls, pains could be sharply reproduced by pressing on it near but distal to its exit from deep fascia. The nerve just there is clothed in fat, and this—in all three patients—was full of hard and tiny nodules, each very sensitive to needle-prick.

These patients all attributed their pains to sudden twists of foot or ankle. Two were sufficiently improved by procaine ; the third for whom injectional relief had shrunk from weeks to hours, was cured by nerve resection at the trigger-spot.

Elkin and Kelly (*Annals of Surgery*, 1945, **122,** 529) stress the need for " direct visualisation of these transmembranous branches." They therefore open all three compartments ' at a stroke,' widely and together. This they do by resecting the upper two-thirds of the fibula.

These authors have generously acknowledged the assistance gained in fibular resection by looping the lateral popliteal (common peroneal) nerve forward off the fibular neck in the way described above.

THE OPERATION

This procedure—which comes so simply from the practised hand of Elkin—for me was full of pitfalls, and could, I know, humiliate when first attempted. I have accordingly endeavoured to provide myself and other tyros with aids, such as the following.

When the nerve is mobilised and looped the muscles and inter-osseous membrane can be safely stripped from the fibula. Avoid injuring the anterior tibial arch and the peroneal vessels by keeping really close against the bone. Move the rugine upwards to strip the fleshy fibres of the muscles. Work round successively from front to back *without* detaching the interosseous membrane ; otherwise the membrane, whose stripping angle (p. 4) is *opposite* to that of the muscles, will tear and strip raggedly and thrust the rugine off from the bone, endangering the vessels. Detach the membrane last, moving the rugine *down* along the bone. (A leaf likewise strips best if you direct force into the *sharper* of the two angles it makes with the stem.)

Turn the stripped peronei forwards. Turn the soleus attachment back and with it the weak fibular prong of the cleft at the top of tibialis posterior muscle—the cleft which transmits the arch of anterior tibial vessels. Cut the biceps tendon close to the fibular head, leaving it in fascial continuity with peroneus longus (Fig. 191).

Divide the bare shaft a span below the upper tibiofibular joint. Then, with the biceps tendon cut, we have a mobile bony rod that we can twist on its long axis so that each ligament comes in turn for section, and so sets free the upper part of fibula.

A landmark and a clue.—The articular facet now seen upon the lateral condyle of tibia is a good landmark ; the arch of anterior tibial vessels lies two fingerbreadths below it. The clue—which is the anterior tibial nerve—comes (before displacement) obliquely down and inwards from the neck of fibula ; it joins its fellow vessels three fingerbreadths below the facet (Figs. 191 and 192).

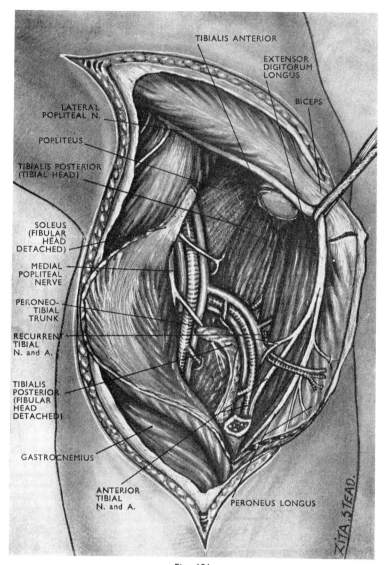

Fig. 191

**Exposure of the arched segment of anterior tibial vessels
by fibular resection**

The lateral popliteal trunk and (in this subject) its *bisection* into anterior tibial
and musculocutaneous branches have been freed and turned forward as in
Fig. 190 after dividing the fibrous arcade with which peroneus longus covers
these nerves as they lie against the neck of the fibula. Traction on the clue
provided by the anterior tibial nerve has at once retrieved its fellow artery
from the flat unfeatured field left by fibular resection, and so has led to the
detection of the arched segment of anterior tibial vessels.

In the figure the anatomical elements have been separated and labelled "for
information," but not "for necessary action." Still, if it's anatomy you're
after, be careful to mark the interosseous membrane with recognisable forceps
before you part it from the fibula ; otherwise you may lose the distinction
between front and back compartments of the leg.

(The pointer to peroneus longus also indicates musculocutaneous nerve.)

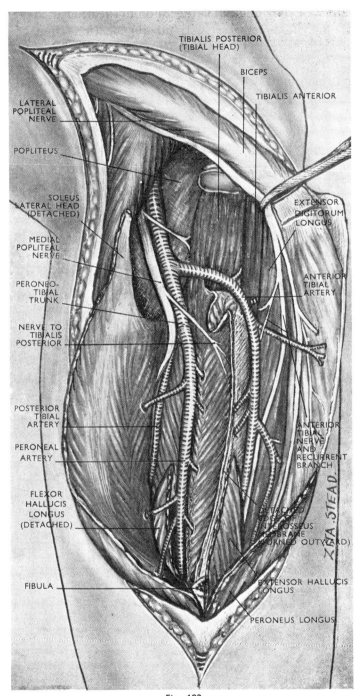

TIBIALIS POSTERIOR
(TIBIAL HEAD)

BICEPS

TIBIALIS ANTERIOR

LATERAL
POPLITEAL
NERVE

POPLITEUS

SOLEUS
LATERAL HEAD
(DETACHED)

EXTENSOR
DIGITORUM
LONGUS

MEDIAL
POPLITEAL
NERVE

PERONEO-
TIBIAL
TRUNK

ANTERIOR
TIBIAL
ARTERY

NERVE TO
TIBIALIS
POSTERIOR

POSTERIOR
TIBIAL
ARTERY

PERONEAL
ARTERY

ANTERIOR
TIBIAL
NERVE
AND
RECURRENT
BRANCH

FLEXOR
HALLUCIS
LONGUS
(DETACHED)

DETACHED
EDGE OF
INTEROSSEOUS
MEMBRANE
(TURNED OUTWARD)

ZITA STEAD.

FIBULA

EXTENSOR HALLUCIS
LONGUS

PERONEUS LONGUS

Fig. 192

A greater length of fibula has been removed than in Fig. 191 so that the
long extensor and the long flexor of the big toe are detached.

This neurovascular junction is the guide to the otherwise precarious exposure of these vessels : without its location they are easily missed or cut in the flat unfeatured surface left by fibular resection (*legend* to Fig. 191)—a surface thoroughly delusive ' in the raw.'

The safe course is to neglect the arch until our clue has led us to the neurovascular junction. This it will do if we pull gently upwards on the freed loop of lateral popliteal trunk : the trunk pulls on our clue (its own anterior tibial branch) ; the clue pulls on and reveals its junction with anterior tibial vessels. The junction lies a fingerbreadth below the arch, and thus locates it.

INDICATIONS FOR USE OF THE TWO METHODS OF EXPOSING THE ARCH

The paper by Elkin and Kelly implicitly assigns respective roles to either means of exposing the anterior tibial arch—the fore-and-aft method (p. 272) and their own. In presence of a communicating aneurysm even the light pull that draws the arch back into the hinder wound might tear enlarged transmembranous twigs.

The Elkin method, therefore, is the one for aneurysm ; and we may link the fore-and-aft exposure with *recent* local bleeding when routine search incriminates the arch.

EXPOSURE OF PLANTAR STRUCTURES

Except for pointing abscess, incisions through the sole are best avoided ; they give no comprehensive view, and cicatrise at times with deeply creviced, cornifying scars. Convenient and benign approach is made from the inner side of the foot, or is continued there from the leg (p. 268, and *legend* to Fig. 196).

ANATOMY

The muscle.—Seldom do we find so many grouped as if to aid the memory ; and here, yet once again, *muscles* (and their tendons) are the key to surgical exposure. They lie in layers— 1, 2, 3, 4, counting from skin to bone. Layers 1 and 3 (the odd numbers) are both triads : each consists of three muscles—a central belly flanked by two companions. Layers 2 and 4 (the

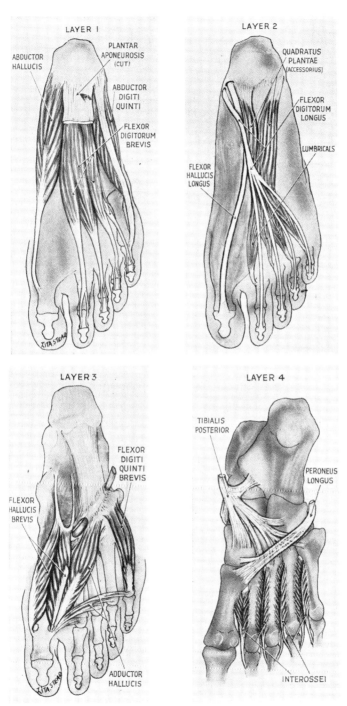

Fig. 193

The four plantar layers

The odd numbers, 1 and 3, are symmetrical with central and flanking bellies; the even numbers, 2 and 4, have each two long tendons and short muscles. Layers 3 and 4 lie to the *front*—except for slips from tibialis posterior. The transverse adductor springs from ligament, not from bone (Wood Jones). (To fit the plan on p. 302 the two adductors are counted as one.)

even numbers) differ from 1 and 3 but are themselves akin:
each consists of two long tendons plus short muscles (Fig. 193).
The layers alternate as follows :—

Layer 1 (a triad)

ABDUCTOR	FLEXOR DIGITORUM	ABDUCTOR
OF	BREVIS	OF
GREAT TOE		LITTLE TOE

Layer 2 (Two long tendons   +   Short muscles)
            Flexor hallucis longus   *Lumbricals*
            Flexor digitorum longus   *Quadratus plantae*
                                                                  (=*accessorius*)

Layer 3 (a triad)

SHORT FLEXOR	ADDUCTOR HALLUCIS	SHORT FLEXOR
OF		OF
GREAT TOE		LITTLE TOE

Layer 4 (Two long tendons   +   Short muscles)
            Peroneus longus   *Interossei*
            Tibialis posterior

It must be noted that (with one exception) the various components of layers 3 and 4 are placed towards the *front*, and are
related thus to metatarsal bones and to the distal row of tarsus.
So, in the hinder portion of the foot (where 3 and 4 are absent),
constituents of layer 2 must lie next ligament and bone, with here
and there an intervening slip of tendon from tibialis posterior
(Fig. 193)—the one exception just referred to.

The door of a cage.—The foot when standing on a level surface
forms with its skeleton a vaulted cage that opens widely at the
inner side. The door which keeps it closed is the abductor hallucis
of layer 1 (Fig. 194) ; and if we free the upper fastenings of abductor
and hinge the belly solewards, then we can reach the contents of
the cage ; though, for the moment, these may be screened by
fascia ; and even when we open it the muscles are so packed and
linked that, till we part them cleanly, the view is worthless.

The long tendons of layer 2 and hallucis brevis.—These are
the bonds which hold the plantar layers close against the tarsal
vault and bind them to each other. The master knot controlling
this assemblage is found about a thumbwidth lateral to the navicular tubercle. Here, where the tendons cross (with hallucis above
the digitorum), they both are tied against the summit of the vault.
Here, too, and just outside the crossing of the tendons, the origin
of flexor hallucis brevis (Figs. 195, 197 and 198) suspends its
fellow structures ; for this intrinsically trifling belly procures

through its relations a veritable nexus of the first three layers—the three which chiefly count in this approach.

It happens thus. The tendon of flexor hallucis longus lies in a lengthwise groove on brevis' belly and straps it to the plantar face of first metatarsal. Next to, and sometimes joining with, the inner side of brevis is abductor hallucis of layer 1—an intimate relationship which often leads to tearing of the brevis belly during the opening of the cage. Then, on the outer side, abductor hallucis

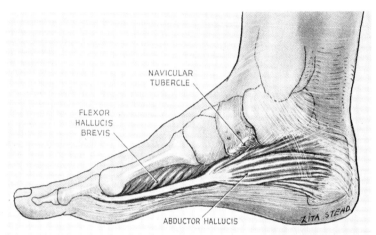

NAVICULAR
TUBERCLE

FLEXOR
HALLUCIS
BREVIS

ABDUCTOR HALLUCIS

ZITA STEAD.

Fig. 194
The cage door
The cage is opened by hinging abductor hallucis down through a right angle on a plantar hinge. Note the relation of abductor with flexor brevis. Deep to abductor is a sheet, more aponeurotic than fascial, which sometimes comes away with the belly but often stays behind and partly screens the cage.

is sometimes linked with flexor brevis—a chance event that turns to our advantage and lets us move both muscles solewards as a *sheet* which bears off on its plantar face (besides the tendon of hallucis longus) the lumbricals arising from the fan of longus digitorum tendons.

If therefore, working on the master knot, we first set free the two long tendons of the second layer, and then the origin of flexor hallucis brevis, we can at once retract a major bulk of muscle from the tarsus and leave the plantar ligaments exposed.

THE OPERATION

Position.—The foot lies on its outer edge; the knee is partly flexed.

Incision.—Divide the skin and superficial fascia at the inner side of the foot, from the ball of the great toe to the heel, by an

incision curving up to cross the tuberosity of navicular (Fig. 196).
Identify and catch the veins.

The guide to the cage door.—Find the tendon of abductor
hallucis at the inner side
of first metatarsal. Mobilise
the tendon, taking care
to leave intact adjoining
fleshy fibres of flexor hallucis
brevis. Use the tendon as a
guide for separation of the
less distinctive margins of
abductor belly. Detach this
belly, first from its fascial
bond with the navicular
tuberosity, then from the
indefinite anterior part of
the vague annular 'ligament'
(laciniate of B.N.A.).[1]
Continue the detachment
down to the inner tuberosity
of calcaneus. *Then* you can
hinge the muscle solewards
through a full right angle
(Fig. 197), taking care to save
the pair of twigs it gets from
the medial plantar nerve.
Both twigs lie fortunately
close to the hinge, two and
three fingerbreadths respectively behind the tuberosity
of navicular.

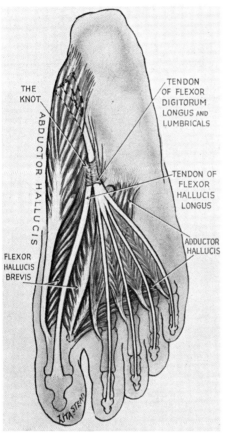

Fig. 195

Flexor hallucis brevis

A vital link of layers 1, 2 and 3. Note the
relations of the belly. Its tarsal *origin*—by
means of tails, or by a fusion with the fibrous
screen *deep* to abductor hallucis—shares in the
master knot that fastens long hallucis and
digitorum tendons to tarsus.

**The screen, the 'knot' and
the neurovascular bundles.**—
When that is done we see the
partial screen of fascia, rough
perhaps with broken fibres of abductor. The fascia is defective
fore and aft, and aft of it we can locate the plantar nerves and
vessels. These form two bundles, medial and lateral. Find where

---

[1] " Its proximal border . . . is very imperfectly defined. Its distal margin but little more
distinct, being continuous more or less with the tendinous origin of the abductor hallucis
which arises from it." (T. H. Bryce in Quain's *Elements of Anatomy*, 1923, 11th edn.,
p. 248.) This band is now appropriately termed *flexor retinaculum.*

they first diverge, three fingerbreadths behind the tuberosity of navicular; then they are covered by the screen, and this we must divide.

Next we cut loose the master knot, a thumbwidth lateral to the tuberosity of navicular, dividing first the fibres which attach the two long second-layer tendons to the vault, and after that (a trifle farther out and forward) the strap-like origin of flexor hallucis

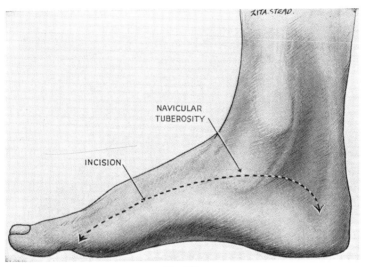

Fig. 196

Divide skin and superficial fascia from the ball of the great toe to the heel. The highest part of the incision crosses the scaphoid tuberosity. Reflect the skin flap downwards and find the tendon of abductor hallucis at the inner side of first metatarsal.
Should there be need to trace nerves or vessels from leg to sole, turn the incision *up the leg*, instead of down the heel. This will leave ample room for skin reflection—sufficient even to ' decorticate ' calcaneus.

brevis. Then we can draw the muscles solewards and trace the nerves and vessels on the dorsal side of layer 1.

The *medial bundle* skirts the inner aspect of the long hallucis tendon, and after that runs forward in a gutter thinly roofed by fascia. This gutter lies upon the *dorsal* face of layer 1—between abductor hallucis and flexor digitorum brevis. The *lateral bundle*, slanting out towards the base of fifth metatarsal, skirts the inner surface of quadratus, then lies within a fellow gutter bounded here by flexor digitorum brevis and abductor digiti quinti. Reaching the outer metacarpal base, part of the bundle curves once more, but this time inwards. A portion of the outer bundle, therefore, passes *twice* across the sole : first out, between layers 1 and 2 ; then in, between layers 3 and 4. The fact, perhaps, of chief

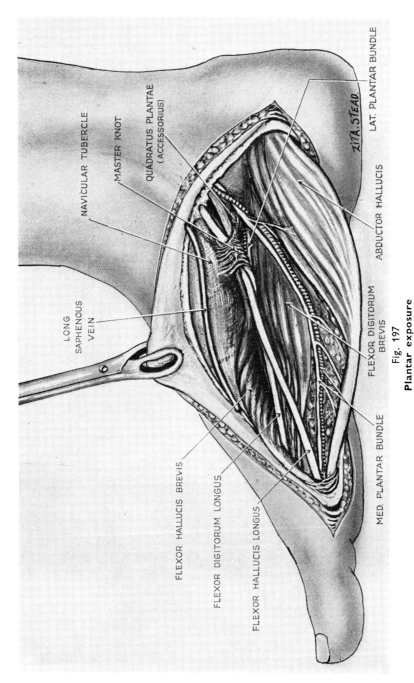

NAVICULAR TUBERCLE

MASTER KNOT

QUADRATUS PLANTAE
(ACCESSORIUS)

LONG
SAPHENOUS
VEIN

FLEXOR HALLUCIS BREVIS

FLEXOR DIGITORUM LONGUS

FLEXOR HALLUCIS LONGUS

MED. PLANTAR BUNDLE

FLEXOR DIGITORUM
BREVIS

ABDUCTOR HALLUCIS

LAT. PLANTAR BUNDLE

ZITA STEAD

Fig. 197

Plantar exposure

Abductor hallucis has been hinged down through a right angle ; with it has come the fibrous screen. When that occurs you see at once the crossing of the two long tendons (flexor hallucis and digitorum), a thumbwidth lateral to navicular tubercle. Take care not to injure the medial plantar bundle near the hinge. The parting of the bundles lies three fingerbreadths behind the tubercle.

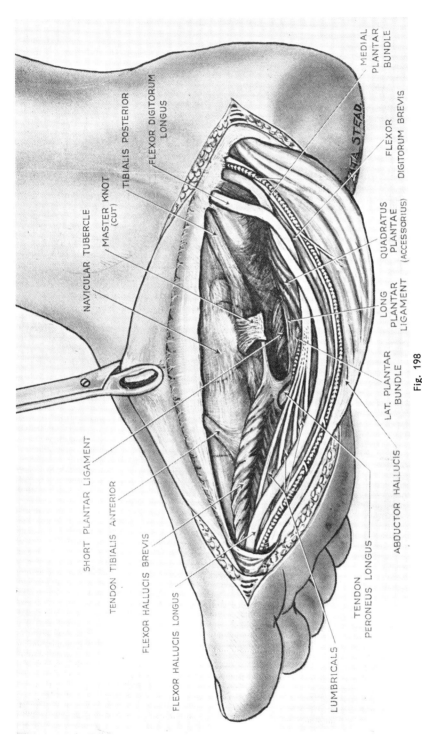

MEDIAL PLANTAR BUNDLE

FLEXOR DIGITORUM LONGUS

TIBIALIS POSTERIOR

MASTER KNOT (CUT)

NAVICULAR TUBERCLE

ITA STEAD

FLEXOR DIGITORUM BREVIS

QUADRATUS PLANTAE (ACCESSORIUS)

LONG PLANTAR LIGAMENT

LAT. PLANTAR BUNDLE

ABDUCTOR HALLUCIS

SHORT PLANTAR LIGAMENT

TENDON TIBIALIS ANTERIOR

FLEXOR HALLUCIS BREVIS

FLEXOR HALLUCIS LONGUS

TENDON PERONEUS LONGUS

LUMBRICALS

Fig. 198

The exposure continued

The master knot consisting of fibrous derivatives (from screen or from flexor hallucis brevis) has been detached from tarsus letting us retract layers 1, 2 and 3 sufficiently to show ligaments. Most obvious of these is the short plantar. Only the hinder end of hallucis brevis has been disturbed.

importance is that both the plantar bundles (in the especial segment of their course which can be mobilised most easily) are linked *as satellites* with layer 1. So, when we part this layer from the tarsal vault the bundles too will move away.

Ligaments.—The first to come in view is the *short plantar*; its fibres slant towards the great toe between the *long plantar ligament* laterally and the ' *spring* ' *ligament* medially (Fig. 198). This last (the inferior calcaneonavicular), by fusing at its inner edge along the base or distal margin of the deltoid ligament, forms a resilient hanging shelf suspended from the medial malleolus. The strap-like tendon of tibialis posterior loops round beneath the shelf, and thus combines to bear the weighted head of talus.

The structures of the sole are now at our disposal and further steps will vary with the object of procedure. Whatever that may be take care to leave the field as dry as though it were the site of toxic goitre : the sponge of venules which infests the foot tends, if it can, to seep in aftermath. And so where circumstance allows, and if you have the right to treat the individual and not the mass, drain, when you close the wound, as you would drain deceitful dryness in a thyroid bed, and raise the fixed and firmly bandaged foot. Then, in a day or two, when drains are out—but not till then, unless you tolerate or disregard *occasional* calamity—then only will you seal the limb in plaster.

It is the fate of detailed ' practical ' descriptions to wear the desultory look of curves mapped out with points : each is a series of related but disjoined minutiæ—the " static snapshots " which the mind demands before it can proceed to the direction of a complex, uninstinctive act. So, it is both a consolation and a stimulus to be aware that in the due performance of the act itself (as in the swift, unhurried hands of surgeons like de Martel) " there is no detail." And closing thus these pages have acquired merit ; they chance to link the memory of two great gentlemen— de Martel and Roy Dobbin.

INDEX

F